MEDICAL
INTELLIGENCE
UNIT

CHALLENGES IN PEDIATRIC SURGERY

Thomas C. Moore, M.D., Ph.D. (Cantab.)

Harbor-UCLA Medical Center
Torrance, California

R.G. LANDES COMPANY
AUSTIN

Medical Intelligence Unit

CHALLENGES IN PEDIATRIC SURGERY

R.G. LANDES COMPANY
Austin

CRC Press is the exclusive worldwide distributor of publications of the Medical Intelligence Unit.
CRC Press, 2000 Corporate Blvd., NW, Boca Raton, FL 33431. Phone: 407/994-0555.

Submitted: May 1994
Published: August 1994

Please address all inquiries to the Publisher:
R.G. Landes Company, 909 Pine Street, Georgetown, TX 78626
or
P.O. Box 4858, Austin, TX 78765
Phone: 512/ 863 7762; FAX: 512/ 863 0081

ISBN 1-57059-048-6
CATALOG # LN9048

Library of Congress Cataloging-in-Publication Data
Moore, Thomas C. (Thomas Carleton), 1921-
    Challenges in pediatric surgery / Thomas C. Moore.
      p. cm. — (Medical intellignece unit)
    Includes bibliographical references and index.
    ISBN 1-57059-048-6 (hardcover)
    1. Gastrointestinal system—Surgery. 2. Children—Surgery.
  3. Abdomen—Surgery. I. Title. II. Series
    [DNLM: 1. Surgery, Operative—in infancy & childhood.
  2. Gastrointestinal Diseases—in infancy & childhood.
  3. Gastrointestinal Diseases—surgery. WO 925 M824c 1994]
  RD540.M843 1994
  617.4'3'0083—dc20
  DNLM/DLC   94-27363
  for Library of Congress   CIP

Dedicated to Beth

CONTENTS

PREFACE

The new *Oxford English Dictionary*[1] describes a preface to a literary work as an introduction containing some explanation of its subject, purpose and scope and of the method of treatment.

The author elects to begin this preface by a narrative detailing his initial exposure to, acquaintance with and fascination by pediatric surgery. At the time of this writing (1994), the author is quietly celebrating the 50th anniversary of his first contact with the clinical surgical discipline of pediatric surgery and in the most hallowed and stimulating of environments—Harvard and the Children's Hospital of Boston in the heady days of the mid and late 1940s.

In 1944, the author, as a senior medical student at the Harvard Medical School, elected to take one of the then most popular senior medical student elective clinical rotations which was in pediatric surgery at the nearby (next door) Children's Hospital of Boston. The chief resident in pediatric surgery at that time was H. William Scott, Jr. and the Surgeon-in-Chief was Professor William E. Ladd. Professor Ladd's faculty backup was a brilliant young surgeon named Robert E. Gross. What a Camelot! Bill Scott was the consummate chief resident, excelling and superlative in every possible and significant way—and he hasn't changed.

After a straight surgical internship at the Peter Bent Brigham Hospital under Professor Elliott Carr Cutler and a two year active duty stint in the U.S. Navy, the author returned to Boston and a year of residency in pediatric surgery under the new Surgeon-in-Chief, Professor Robert E. Gross who had succeeded Professor William E. Ladd in the interval. The chief resident's first name was still Bill. However, the last name had changed from Scott to Clatworthy. After a truly fabulous and unforgettable year, the author returned to his home and native state of Indiana to complete his residency including the Chief's year at the Indiana University Medical Center in Indianapolis under Professor Harris B. Shumacker Jr., one of the truly great Department of Surgery Chairmen of this country and this century. This experience was quite fortuitous in a number of ways, particularly in the area of pediatric surgery as approximately one half of the clinical experience at this Medical Center was in pediatric surgery as the James Whitcomb Riley Hospital for Children was not only the only children's hospital in the state of Indiana with a then population of 5,000,000 but also was located in the center of both the state and the Medical Center campus and an integral part of it in every way. As the sole chief resident, the author was able personally to do a very large volume of complex and interesting pediatric surgery of all sorts and to initiate a variety of then current and retrospective studies of a number of important and interesting congenital disorders of the newborn. These studies accelerated in a following year of full-time research as a new full-time junior faculty member (see Appendix A for publications during this period).

After this research year, the author returned to his home town of Muncie, Indiana to join his father, Dr. Will C. Moore (one of the state's busiest and most talented and skilled surgeons) in the private practice of surgery at the Ball Memorial Hospital which was located on the campus of the Ball State University. Thanks to the truly remarkable support of Professor Harry Shumacker, the author was able to continue as a "de facto" full time faculty member with an active research laboratory and teaching responsibilities. One full day a week (Wednesday) was spent in the surgical research laboratory and this was topped off with a concluding weekly one hour lecture to the junior (3rd year) medical students in Pediatric Surgery. The author during the ensuing 14 year period was responsible for the medical student lectures in pediatric surgery with the exception of one year (1962-1963) when the author took a one year "sabbatical" from private practice to move to Lexington, Kentucky to join Professor Ben Eiseman's new and founding faculty in surgery at the brand-new University of Kentucky Medical Center as a full time full Professor and as Chief of the Division of Pediatric Surgery. Also with Professor Eiseman, the author's laboratory research metamorphosed from macro- and micro-vascular surgical research to the molecular, with study of vasoactive neurotransmitter (and modulator) molecules such as histamine and serotonin in isolated-perfused canine and porcine livers and lungs.

On returning to private practice in Muncie and research and teaching at the Indiana University Medical Center in Indianapolis, the author initiated a new line of research investigating the role of histamine and related molecules in cellular immunity (a new concept as histamine then was thought to be involved only in immediate hypersensitivity and anaphylaxis and allergy and with no involvement whatsoever in delayed hypersensitivity and cellular immunity). The initial vehicle for these studies was the urinary excretion of histamine following skin allografting in rats. These studies were quite exciting and did establish for the first time a role of importance for histamine in cellular immunity and allograft rejection.

In mid-1966, the author elected to return to full-time academic surgery and research in association with Professor David M. Hume at the Medical College of Virginia in Richmond and in his pioneering transplantation program which then involved skin, kidney, liver and heart. Thanks to the kindness of Professor Arnold Salzberg, a continuing involvement in pediatric surgery was an additional bonus. This was an excellent research environment in which to continue histamine involvement in transplant rejection. The first publication from this new line of research appeared in the August 19, 1967 issue of the prestigious journal *Nature*[2] and was concerned with the prolongation of rat skin allograft survival by inhibition of the histamine formine enzyme, histidine decarboxylase. A solid role for histamine formation in cellular immunity and allograft rejection was further identified in this period by collaborative studies with Richard W. Schayer employing a new isotopic method of histidine decarboxylase activity assay developed by him. Elevated levels of histamine formation from elevated levels of histidine decarboxylase enzyme activity were identified in both rejecting skin allografts[3] and in the spleens[4] of host/allografted animals/rats. Pediatric Surgery was not totally neglected during this Richmond period as the author coauthored with Professor Arnold Salzberg an article involving Pediatric Surgery in the February 1970 issue of *Surgery*.[5]

In 1968, the author accepted an offer to come to UCLA as a full-time full Professor with clinical responsibilities as Chief of Pediatric Surgery and Chief of Clinical Renal Transplantation at the Harbor-UCLA Medical Center. In 1978, the author gave up clinical renal transplantation responsibility for clinical concentration and teaching in Pediatric Surgery. He has exercised senior responsibility in Pediatric Surgery for the past 26 years at Harbor-UCLA with the exception of a five year period of a sabbatical from UCLA in clinical (liver) and research transplantation at the University of Cambridge (England) with Professor Sir Roy Calne, followed shortly by a basic science Ph.D. at the University of Cambridge (Trinity College) in Molecular Immunology. The Ph.D. research was carried out in the MITI (Mechanisms In Tumor Immunity) Unit of the Laboratory of Molecular Biology (MRC Centre, Cambridge, UK). This comparatively small research laboratory complex was nestled in the center of the Medical School of the University of Cambridge and in a period of 20 consecutive years (including the five years of the author's residence in Cambridge) had generated an awesome average of one Nobel prize every other year—a rather impressive and formidable "track record".

Last year, 1993, the author published a book relating to his long-time research interest in neurovascular immunology, an area to which he had contributed some 195 personal journal publications. This book *Neurovascular Immunology: Vasoactive Neurotransmitter and Modulators in Cellular Immunity and Memory*[6] and published by CRC Press, Inc. (Boca Raton, Ann Arbor, London, Tokyo) started out as an "updating" of the author's Ph.D. thesis[7] but rather rapidly became something much more as the author discovered that for just one of the chapters ("Serotonin") 10,000 new publications had been listed in the *Cummulated Index Medicus* in the eight years since the completion of his Ph.D. thesis. This single author book ultimately came to 464 printed pages and involved a mega effort of literature searching and writing.

The writing and completion of this 1993 book triggered a determination to do something similar with respect to the author's equally long interest in Pediatric Surgery, an area in which his first paper was published in 1950 and in coauthorship with Robert E. Gross.[8]

The author elected a somewhat novel and hopefully innovative approach as there were already plenty of good text-books in Pediatric Surgery and furthermore he had *zero* interest in writing a traditional "text book".

Over the years, the author has made a practice of selecting a title for an article before writing anything. For the Pediatric Surgery book he selected the title *Challenges in Pediatric Surgery*. He purposely and scrupulously avoided the word "controversies" as this word implies confrontation, hostility, etc., when the author's real goal and most fundamental intent and desire was to achieve and foster innovative and creative ideas and approaches.

As with the 1993 book, the first undertaking was a massive literature search of some 40 years, photocopying of articles deemed significant and of importance, arranging these photocopied articles chronologically and numbered and securing them in pressboard binders by topic. Before a word was written, all articles were read with care, including the author's own publications, and the main points and observations were written down and in major categories. Only then did the actual writing start.

Each chapter was devoted to a major clinical problem or occasionally to related or adjacent (anatomically) problems (Duplications and Mesenteric Cysts). Each Chapter was divided into three parts: 1) Introduction, 2) Challenges and 3) Conclusion. Early on the author, decided to solicit "Invited Commentary" for each major challenges chapter from world leaders and particularly from world leaders who had made important contributions to the topic of the chapter. It was intended that these "commentaries" should be addressed to the topic and not necessarily the author of this book's treatment of it in his writing of the chapter. The author was seeking to elicit additional thoughts and ideas of an innovative and constructive nature which might further enhance the readability and creative worth of this book. Commentaries are placed at the end of each chapter and in the order in which they were received.

Before closing this preface, the author has had both the occasion and the stimulus to reflect on important career and life-long unique experiences which may have influenced his approach to pediatric surgery over the years. An early career 14 year heavy clinical surgical experience (some 1,000 major operations per year and almost all in very major adult vascular, thoracic and cancer surgery) with only some five percent in clinical major Pediatric Surgery had both a broadening and confidence building effect especially with respect to blind faith in or thoughtless adherence to and acceptance of "traditional" dogma in any area. A career total of nine years in four year or longer episodes of exposure to full-time laboratory research (much of it basic science) has further fostered some hopefully healthy irreverence of established and "establishment" dogma. The thought keeps resurfacing (perhaps germinating from the above experiences) that innovative approaches and creative productivity are more often achieved by challenging rather than the blindly and thoughtlessly accepting of established and "establishment" dogma—what one *may* do, not what one *must* do! If some of the thoughts and approaches suggested in this book by the author may seem a bit "unorthodox" to the reader, please have patience, bear with the author—*and think about it!*

"We must always guard the liberties of the mind and remember that some degree of heresy is often a sign of health in spiritual life."

U.S. von Euler,[9] M.D. (1905-1983)
Professor of Physiology
Karolinska Institute
Stockholm, Sweden
Nobel Laureate 1970
Discoverer of substance P, prostaglandins, and noradrenaline
President, Nobel Foundation 1965-1975

The author has elected to omit chapters on cancer and on transplantation in this book as the major challenges in both of these areas involve biological scientists other than pediatric surgeons, such as molecular biologists, immunologists, geneticists, experimental pharmacologists, etc. In his 1993 book[6], the author has considered in some depth key molecules involved in the cellular immune responses to both cancer and to transplanted/allografted tissues and organs and their evolutionary roles in biological defense.

To return to the new *Oxford English Dictionary*[1] definitions of preface, this may be an appropriate spot and occasion to make use of one of its illustrative quotes and from Isaak Walton's *The Compleat Angler* i, 12, 1653, "I will preface no longer, *but proceed.*" (italics added)

1. *Oxford English Dictionary, 2nd Ed. vol XII, "preface" 1989; 342-343.*
2. *Moore TC. Histidine decarboxylase inhibitors and the survival of skin homografts. Nature 1967; 215:871-872.*
3. *Moore TC, Schayer RW. Histidine decarboxylase activity of autografted and allografted rat skin. Transplantation 1969; 7:99-104.*
4. *Moore TC, Schayer RW. Histidine decarboxylase activity of rat spleen following skin allografting. Ann Surg 1970; 171: 609-614.*
5. *Moore TC, Salzberg AM, Talman EA. Jejunoileocolic intubation and plication for intestinal obstruction caused by massive adhesions in infancy. Surgery 1970; 67: 364-368.*
6. *Moore TC. Neurovascular Immunology: Vasoactive Neurotransmitters and Modulators in Cellular Immunity and Memory. (464 pages). Boca Raton: CRC Press Inc., 1993.*
7. *Moore TC. The Effects of Inflammatory Mediators and Anaesthetic Agents upon Lymphocyte Traffic of Sheep in vivo. Ph.D. Thesis, University of Cambridge (Trinity College), 1982.*
8. *Gross RE, Moore TC. Duplication of the urethra: Report of two cases and summary of the literature. Arch Surg 1950; 60: 749-761.*
9. *von Euler US. Editorial. Circulation 1962; 26: 1233-1234.*

The Author

Thomas C. Moore, M.D., Ph.D. (Cantab.) is Professor of Pediatric Surgery in the UCLA School of Medicine. He has been based clinically at the Harbor-UCLA Medical Center in Torrance, California, since 1968 where he is also Director of Surgical Research in Molecular Immunology. From 1968 to 1978 he was also Chief of Clinical Kidney Transplantation at Harbor-UCLA as well as Chief of Pediatric Surgery.

Professor Moore received his undergraduate education at Dartmouth College. He was elected to the Phi Beta Kappa scholastic honor society during his junior year at Dartmouth and was awarded his B.A. *summa cum laude*, with distinction in his major subject (English Classics). He received his M.D. in 1945 from the Harvard Medical School where he served a special elective rotation in pediatric surgery at the Children's Hospital in his senior year. In 1982, he received a Ph.D. in Molecular Immunology from the University of Cambridge (Trinity College) in England.

Professor Moore received his surgical training at the Peter Bent Brigham Hospital in Boston (Harvard), the Children's Hospital in Boston (Harvard) and the Indiana University Medical Center/James Whitcomb Riley Hospital for Children in Indianapolis. He has served on surgical faculties at the professorial level at Indiana University, the University of Kentucky and the Medical College of Virginia prior to coming to UCLA in 1968 as a full-time full Professor of Surgery.

While on the faculty at Indiana University Medical Center (Indianapolis) and also in private practice (Muncie) from 1952 to 1966, he was responsible for third year medical student teaching in pediatric surgery (a weekly lecture) and was involved in one full day a week laboratory research in vascular, cardiovascular and esophageal surgery. During this period, Professor Moore took a one year (1962-1963) "sabbatical" from private practice to serve on the full-time faculty at the new University of Kentucky Medical School in Lexington as a Full Professor and Chief of Pediatric Surgery. Two years (1966 to 1968) at the Medical College of Virginia involved clinical and experimental transplantation surgery with the late Professor David M. Hume and Pediatric Surgery with Professor Arnold Salzberg. One year (1977-1978, on sabbatical from UCLA) was spent at the Transplantation Unit of Professor Sir Roy Calne at the University of Cambridge in England.

Professor Moore has achieved board certification in general surgery, thoracic surgery and pediatric surgery and he has specialty credentials in vascular surgery (member of the Society for Vascular Surgery since 1957) and transplantation surgery (member of the founding and organizing Committee of Four for the American Society of Transplant Surgeons and first Chairman of its Committee for Scientific Studies). Professor Moore served for four years on National Institutes of Health Surgery Study Sections. He was previously an officer (Treasurer, 1956-1959) of the Society of University Surgeons and has been a member of the American Surgical Association since 1960. His past and present society memberships, in addition to the above, include the American Pediatric Surgical Association, the Surgical Section of the American Academy of Pediatrics, the British Association of Paediatric Surgeons, the Pacific Association of Pediatric Surgeons, the American Association for Thoracic Surgery, the British Society for Immunology, the American Association of Immunologists and the Society for Neuroscience. Of Professor Moore's 312 scientific publications, 114 have been devoted to clinical and experimental pediatric surgery (largely clinical). These are listed in Appendix A.

Acknowledgment

The author is immensely indebted to Torin J. Cunningham (Pomona College BA cum laude, 1993) who has spent the 1993-1994 academic year as a Clinical Research Associate in pediatric surgery of the author here at the Harbor-UCLA Medical Center prior to starting medical school at the University of California, San Diego in the autumn of 1994. During this year, Torin has participated full-time in the clinical pediatric surgery activities (rounds, clinic, operating room, teaching sessions, etc.) In addition, he has performed brilliantly and with high efficiency and accuracy the massive task of transposing/transplanting the text, tables, legends and references for this book from the author's virtually illegible hand-written script into a beautifully organized and presented computer word-procesed manuscript ready for publication. He also, from these experiences and personal literature searching, has written all of the pediatric surgery chapters for the new *Harbor-UCLA Textbook of Surgery* which is to be published soon and which is designed to be clinical symptom-oriented and for beginning third year medical students who have had no prior clinical ward experience in surgery. Torin also has completed this with high competence, understanding and readability, as well as major involvement (and shared authorship) in at least three clinical papers submitted or to be submitted shortly for publication. This has been a thoroughly delightful and highly productive association for the most grateful author of this book.

The author also thanks Emma Alegre and her most helpful associates at the Parlow Library of the Harbor-UCLA Medical Center for their continuing superb, cheerful and invaluable assistance in the collection, transport and photocopying of large volumes of scientific articles and related material over many, many months.

═══ CHAPTER 1 ═══

IMPERFORATE ANUS

INTRODUCTION

One of the oldest historical challenges in pediatric surgery is that of imperforate anus. As the diagnosis involves only inspection of the anal area, its history is a very long one indeed. From ancient to Byzantine times, it was considered to be an incurable monstrosity and no attempt was made to cure it. The first mention of attempts at "surgical" correction is to be found in the writings of the Byzantine physician, Paul of Aegina[1] (625-690 A.D.). He recommended the blind plunge of a knife into the perineum in the hope of entering the blind-ending rectal pouch. This rather primitive and intelligent approach, followed by repeated post-"incisional" dilatations, remained the accepted treatment for centuries. The only variations in this approach involved the length, depth, and angle of the perineal "incision".

The long, fascinating and challenging history of imperforate anus has stimulated a number of excellent historical reviews includes those of Bodenhamer,[2] Matas,[3] Webster,[4] and deVries.[5] Of particular interest is the beautifully written, scholarly and superbly illustrated historical review of imperforate anus published in 1978 by Professor Alois Schärli[6] of Lucerne, Switzerland. Professor Schärli, an active participant and important contributor to the modern history of imperforate anus, tracks the ancient written history back to a 1600 B.C. Egyptian papyrus. Professor Schärli gives credit and recognition to those historical figures who conceived of and published suggestions for innovative operative approaches to imperforate anus as well as to those intrepid surgeons who had the courage to apply them.

The first major modern contribution to the surgical approach to the repair of imperforate anus was made in 1835 by J-Z Amussat[7] who described in *Gazette Médicale de Paris* a technique of perineal anoplasty which emphasized the importance of careful perineal dissection for the identification and mobilization of the rectal pouch so that the rectal mucosa could be sutured to the skin edges without tension. Amussat also was one of the first to suggest and carry out posterior saggital extension of the perineal incision when more exposure was needed.

The next major contribution to the management of imperforate anus was made in 1880 in the *British Medical Journal* by Edinburgh-trained Neil MacLeod[8] of Shanghai. In cases of perineal dissection failure (as he had experienced in a case) he suggested the use of laparotomy to identify and mobilize the high rectal pouch and the use of both incision wounds (perineal and abdominal) to achieve a pull-through of the distal hindgut for perineal suture without tension. This approach was modified in 1894 by Paul Delagenière[9] of Tours in a French surgical publication (*Arch. Prov. de Chir.*) in which he advocated and carried out (in four cases) initial abdominal incision for localization of the blind ending rectal pouch with subsequent utilization of a perineal incision for pull-through completion of the repair. His clinical approach had followed careful prior cadaver dissection of 6 stillborn imperforate anus infants (all died in the early postoperative period).

One of the most important and least remembered and appreciated contributions in the long history of imperforate anus appeared in the June 4, 1892 issue of the *British Medical Journal* (1:1197-1198) by Harrison Cripps[10] F.R.C.S. from St. Bartholomew's Hospital of London. It was titled "The Treatment of Imperforate Anus". Cripps reported the use of posterior saggital anoplasty in five infants, both male (3) and female (2), without mortality. Four of the five operations were carried out in the immediate post-natal period and with good results.

Distinguished American surgeons not ordinarily associated with pediatric surgery have made important contributions to our knowledge and care of imperforate anus. These have included Rudolph Matas,[3] Dwight E. Harken[11] and Jonathan E. Rhoads.[12] In 1897, Rudolph Matas[3] presented before the American Surgical Association an excellent and quite scholarly and detailed (100 pages) historical review of the development of operative techniques for the repair of imperforate anus. In 1942, Dwight E. Harken[11] made a most important contribution by calling attention to the overall gravity of the imperforate anus problem by pointing out the high nonsurgical mortality from additional congenital malformations.

In 1949, Jonathan Rhoads, with Pipes and Randall,[12] in a report of two cases in *Annals of Surgery* from the University of Pennsylvania at the Children's Hospital of Philadelphia effectively revolutionized the on-going management of imperforate anus by describing the successful use, at birth, of a combined abdominal and perineal approach to imperforate anus when it was apparent that the rectal pouch could not safely be reached from below. This dramatic report ended the overly long (69, 57 and 55 years) neglect of the important suggestions of MacLeod and Delagenière and particularly Cripps, cited above, and inaugurated the modern era of aggressive, studious and scientific management of imperforate anus.

I have had a long interest in imperforate anus as this topic was the subject of my first in-depth review of a major condition in clinical surgery,[13,14] as well as two of my most recent publications.[15,16] The first reviews were published in 1952 in *Surgery*[13] and in *Surgery, Gynecology and Obstetrics.*[14] The *Surgery* publication was at the Tenth Annual Meeting of the Society of University Surgeons which was held at the Johns Hopkins University in Baltimore, Maryland which also was the occasion of the celebration of the 100th anniversary of the birth of William Steward Halsted. This *Surgery* report[13] involved 120 cases of imperforate anus seen at the Indiana University Medical Center in a period of 25 years and included 11 cases managed in the previous three years without mortality by the combined abdominal-perineal approach at birth of Rhoads, Pipes and Randall as reported in 1949. This paper of the author was discussed by Robert E. Gross and C. Everett Koop, both of whom were quite enthusiastic about this approach of Rhoads and associates.

In his discussion of my *Surgery* paper, Gross described an experience with 70 cases of imperforate anus managed by the Jonathan Rhoads approach with only four deaths (a 5.7% mortality). He made four important observations in his discussion: "First, it is possible to pull down a rectal pouch no matter how high it is. Second, it is possible to form in all cases an anal opening devoid of stricture. Third, the fistula problem—which used to be so serious—has now completely disappeared, because fistulas in all these subjects can be permanently closed in one operation. Fourth, there is variability regarding the attainment of anal continence. Regarding the last point, our general impressions are about as follows: probably 70% of the children have good anal sphincteric action. There are about 15% who have been operated upon so recently that they can not be evaluated yet. There are a final 15% who apparently will never have any anal sphincter tone"—but nonetheless may be managed in later years by a constipating diet combined as needs with rectal lavage. This 82% success rate of cases operated upon long enough to permit evaluation is most impressive and far exceeds continence success rate of any of the more recent reports in which colostomy is carried out at birth and definitive repair is delayed until one year of age.

In his discussion of the author's *Surgery* paper, Koop refers to the origin of the Rhoads approach in their clinic at the University of Pennsylvania and their somewhat longer experience with this abdominal-perineal operation at birth. Of their 60 operations, 22 or 23 were done for a longer than 3 years and of these only 2 had completely patulous anoplasties (a 91% success rate)—again a most remarkable success rate in this at birth operative repair of imperforate anus.

My other major 1952 publication relating to imperforate anus[14] was published in *Surgery, Gynecology and Obstetrics* (95:281-288, 1952) and was the first publication in content and in title ("Congenital Malformations of the Rectum and Anus: II. Associated Anomalies Encountered in a Series of 120 Cases") to be devoted exclusively to the important role of additional and serious additional congenital malformations in the surgical management and clinical outcome of imperforate anus in the newborn.

An earlier, 1942, report in *Surgery* by Dwight E. Harken[11] had called attention to the gravity of the imperforate anus prob-

lem by pointing out the high nonsurgical mortality. At the time of my 1952 publication, only two other reports of more than 100 cases of imperforate anus had appeared in the world's literature. These were the 1934 report of 214 cases by Ladd and Gross[17] from the Children's Hospital of Boston in the *American Journal of Surgery* and the 1950 report of 165 cases from the Mayo Clinic by C. W. Mayo and Rice.[18] Although these 2 publications described a significant percentage of infants with additional malformations at 38% for Boston and 44% at the Mayo Clinic, those incidence of additional anomalies were substantially lower than the 72% encountered by me in the 120 cases from the Indiana University Medical Center in Indianapolis.

In my study, additional congenital abnormalities were encountered in 86 of the 120 cases of imperforate anus (72%) and in 33 of 34 patients upon whom careful post-mortem studies were carried out (97%). One hundred ninety associated anomalies in these 86 patients were encountered and a significant number of these ranged, at that time, from quite serious to being incompatible with life. These associated anomalies were found most frequently in the urinary tract (in addition to urinary tract fistulas which were considered a part of the ano-rectal formation). Fifty-four urinary tract anomalies, excluding recto-urinary tract fistulas, were found in 41 of the 120 patients (34%)-largely males. Malformations elsewhere in the alimentary tract were found in 27 of the 120 cases with the largest number involving the esophagus and the duodenum. Forty-one vertebral-neurological malformations were encountered with thoracic and lumber and sacral vertebral anomalies being the most common. The occurrence of 20 cases of congenital cardiovascular anomalies was cited and their recognition and potential cure received particular emphasis as this 1952 report was in the exciting early days of surgery for congenital heart disease. Fifteen patients had abdominal wall malformation and 10 had female genital tract malformations. Extremity malformations were encountered in 10 cases and included club foot (8) as well as supernumerary thumb and complete fusion of the lower extremities with an accompanying tail. A miscellaneous group of 13 additional malformations included bifid scrotum, hare lip, cleft palate, deformed or absent ears and deafness, strabismus and separation of pubic rami. As nearly one half of the deaths in this Indiana experience were associated with and were considered related to other congenital malformations, I stressed the importance of early recognition and treatment of these anomalies as an integral part of the imperforate anus "syndrome" (later called VATER, VACTERL, etc.). One bit of good news was that prematurity was infrequent.

A fall from grace in the operative management of imperforate anus began in the early 1960s as the emphasis shifted from neurophysiology (repair at birth for establishment of optimal brain-defecation neurocircuitry) to anatomy. During this period an avalanche of new reports of anatomical dissections by surgeons and new operations by the same surgeons hit the literature and attended glowing results. The alternating euphoria and gloom of this period has been expressed well by John Raffensperger[19] in his superlative textbook of pediatric surgery, "Each new operation, as it is enthusiastically introduced by its inventor, is hailed as a great step forward. Within 10 years, when the results are in, the operation is criticized, and the surgical community embraces a new operation."

With the increasing interest in the fine points of pelvic and ano-rectal anatomy, colostomy at birth was reintroduced almost universally with definitive repair deferred until one year of age or later so that a more precise anatomical repair could be carried out in the larger patient by the operating surgeons' preference of the many anatomical approaches and repairs on the surgeon's expanding "menu" of potential and suggested operative approaches.

Within quite recent years, there is increasing evidence that the timing (operation at birth without a colostomy) rather than exotic points of anatomy is the most impor-

tant factor in the successful outcome of imperforate anus repair with respect to the all-important issues of continence and avoidance of urinary tract contamination (in males).

CHALLENGES

1. The most important and critical challenge is when to do the definitive repair operation, at birth and without a colostomy or do a colostomy and wait a year (or longer or less).

I feel quite strongly that the operation should be carried out at birth and without a prior colostomy. My early experience with abdomino-perineal repair at birth ("à la Jonathan Rhoads et al"[12]) as reported at the 1952 meeting of the Society of University Surgeons and published in *Surgery*[13] with the excellent discussions and results of Gross and Koop have remained unequaled until the recent return to operation at birth without prior colostomy as reported by me[15,16] and by Professor A. P. R. Aluwihare[20,21] of Sri Lanka. It is of interest and coincidence that back-to-back reports on this issue by me and Professor Aluwihare appeared in the February 1990 issue of the *Journal of Pediatric Surgery*.[16,21] Earlier reports had appeared by both authors.

Professor Aluwihare's Hunterian Lecture[20] before the Royal College of Surgeons of England (Lincoln's Inn Fields, London) and published in 1989 in the *Annals of Royal College of Surgeons of England* is clearly one of the most important publications to appear regarding imperforate anus in this century (an instant classic in my opinion). In this important publication, Professor Aluwihare described 31 repairs of imperforate anus at birth in male newborn infants without colostomy. In all but 4 infants (13%) this repair was achieved by the perineal route alone. In these 4 newborn infants, the abdomen was entered because the rectum and fistula were considered to be too high.

These observations parallel my[16] experience as cited in my 1990 *Journal of Pediatric Surgery* publication and subsequent ones. Indeed in my 1990 publication, I had not as yet been required (in 6 years experience with at birth repair without colostomy) to enter the peritoneal cavity by an abdominal incision to complete the repair or to ligate the urinary tract fistula when present.

At the time of Professor Aluwihare's 1989 publication in the *Annals of the Royal College of Surgeons of England*,[20] 25 of his babies were over 2 years of age. Of these, 84% were continent for solid feces and 68% for liquid feces—a most remarkable result. These results again are similar to mine with a smaller number of male newborn infants operated upon at birth and without a colostomy.

I attended an excellent seminar put on by Alberto Peña and Pieter de Vries at the May 1983 meeting of the American Pediatric Surgical Association (APSA) at Hilton Head in South Carolina. The suitability of this approach in the newborn without colostomy was immediately apparent to me who long had considered colostomy as an invention of the Devil in cases of imperforate anus with its one year contamination of the urinary tract by unligated fistulas in males and one year of distal rectal pouch obstructive and peristaltic trauma resulting in an assuredly hypertrophied distal rectal pouch musculature (in the Peña and deVries approach[22,23] dealt with by "tapering" and in the puborectalis sling operation[24,25] by the blessing of a "blind" (out of sight) destruction of all pelvic floor levator muscle in the way of the traumatic "pull-through" of this hypertrophied rectal pouch monstrosity ("tapered" by Peña and deVries, but still a grotesque monstrosity).

I, at that point, felt a great liberation from the puborectalis sling operation with its detested colostomy-and-wait-a-year-for-definitive-repair "cross" to bear and resolved to do only this approach and only at birth and without a detested colostomy. My first opportunity came on August 8, 1983 and subsequently I have *never* done an imperforate repair except at birth, by the perineal route initially and without a colostomy (except in one case in which a severe cardiac malformation—A-V canal—demanded local anesthesia and transverse colostomy so that bowel obstruction would not complicate a severe cardiac malformation which ultimately proved fatal.

At a 1987 meeting of APSA, I cited my experience with this approach in the discussion of a paper relating to imperforate anus. In this discussion (printed in the *Journal of Pediatric Surgery* 1987;22:1167),[15] I emphasized the importance of one rather than three operations, the avoidance of rectal wall thickening and the need for tapering, the early elimination of urinary tract contamination from urinary tract fistulas and the facilitation of optimal early establishment of brain-anal control of defecation (misprinted as "basin-anal" control of defecation).

In my February 1990 publication[16] in the *Journal of Pediatric Surgery* titled "Advantages of Performing the Saggital Anoplasty Operation at Birth," the above points were again made and the major objectives in the management of imperforate anus were stated to be "relief of intestinal obstruction and restoration of anorectal continuity at birth, with optimal anatomic approximation, sphincteric function and the early postnatal establishment of the brain-defecation reflexes." In the summary/abstract of this publication, I stated that "it has been found that the saggital anoplasty can easily and preferably be carried out in the newborn period without the need for colostomy or 'tapering'." In the concluding sentence of the summary/abstract, it is stated that "this operation at birth relieves alimentary tract obstruction at birth, eliminates urinary tract contamination (when it exists) at birth, establishes anorectal continuity and maximum potential for 'normal' defecation reflexes at birth, and achieves all of this in one rather than three operations."

Professor Aluwihare's February 1990 publication[21] in the *Journal of Pediatric Surgery* is of particular importance and is concerned with primary perineal repair of high (supralevator) imperforate anus in female neonates. Of his 16 patients, 12 were operated upon as neonates without a colostomy. Two of these infants had no fistula and nine of the other infants had fistulas onto the perineum or into the vaginal vestibule. Of the 12 patients available for assessment two or more years after operation 92% were able to control solid stool and 75% did not soil at all.

A critically important series of observations were published in the May 1991 issue of the *Journal of Pediatric Surgery* by the highly respected and distinguished Professor Jan C. Molenaar of Rotterdam and his associate R.A.T.M. Langemeijer.[26] They reported the results of 40 posterior saggital anorectoplasty (PSARP) operations for imperforate anus as primary operations between one month and 5 years of age. All of these newborn infants had had a colostomy made within 72 hours of birth. The other 10 patients underwent "redo" PSARP operations as secondary procedures following a failed primary operation. All of these patients had high anorectal malformations and all were operated upon between June 1983 and May 1990. The concluding sentences of this monumentally important publication are as follows: "All patients are alive, and all but one are being evaluated regularly. Subjectively, the majority of patients were more or less incontinent, with soiling of pants at least once a day. On the basis of objective criteria, virtually all patients appeared to be incontinent, and in only one patient was the mechanism of defecation almost unimpaired after PSARP. From this study, we conclude that although PSARP provides a good aesthetic result, patients will never acquire normal continence." There is absolutely no substitute for care, candor and honesty in the reporting of results, surgical or otherwise!

An additional report of great significance was reported from the Great Ormond Hospital for Sick Children of London in the January 1989 issue of the *British Journal of Surgery* by A.J.L. Brain and E.M. Kiely.[27] It was titled "Posterior Saggital Anorectoplasty for Reoperation in Children With Anorectal Malformations." Their report concerned a prospective study in 12 consecutive patients to evaluate PSARP for the salvage of patients incontinent of feces after prior anorectal reconstruction in patients

ranging in age from 5 to 17 years of age. Their findings and conclusions from their summary/abstract are as follows: "Followup, between 4 and 46 months, revealed good fecal control in only two patients, with a significant improvement in two others. The rest remained incontinent although sensation was improved. These disappointing results, at variance with other published reports, lead us to conclude that posterior saggital anorectoplasty, when used as a secondary procedure, is good for correcting anatomical defects but not for improving fecal continence."

The crux of this problem rather clearly is that major attention and consideration should be paid to developmental neurophysiological matters affecting the establishment of activity-driven brain-anus neurocircuitry and reflexes at *birth* when it matters most importantly, rather than upon the fine points of one anatomical repair versus another.

Key observations relating to this matter derive from the Nobel Prize winning (1981) studies of David H. Hubel and Torsten N. Wiesel[28-34] during the 1960s and 1970s involving exploration of the primary visual cortex and influence of environment on the postnatal development of the visual cortex, studies which demonstrated the devastating effect (permanent blindness) of monocular deprivation in the early days and weeks of life. These studies were initially carried out at the Wilmer (eye) Institute at Johns Hopkins (1959-1962) and then at the Harvard Medical School. The initiation and design of these studies was influenced by the observation that children with congenital cataracts still have marked and permanent visual defects after removal of the cataract and proper refraction.

Their initial findings were that kittens with one eye occluded by lid suture during the first 3 months of life were blind permanently in the deprived and unused eye and that in the striate (visual) cortex the majority of cells responded only to stimulation of the normal eye. This defect appeared to be localized to the visual cortex and at the site of interaction between the lateral geniculate nucleus (LGN) afferents from the thalamus and the visual cortical cells. The results of these monocular deprivation experiments taken together with another series of experiments, which demonstrated that the properties of orientation specificity and binocularity are developed through innate mechanisms, indicated to these investigators that the neural connections present in early life can be modified by visual experience. Such neural plasticity was not observed in adult cats with one eye occluded for extended periods of time by lid suture (over one year), but existed only during the first 3 postnatal months.

Further studies by these investigators also demonstrated that the monkey was also susceptible to visual deprivation in the early postnatal period. When the newborn monkey's lid-sutured deprived eye is opened after months of deprivation, the animal is unable to see with it. As there are no obvious changes in the ocular media, the retina nor the lateral geniculate nucleus (LGN), the visual deficit which has occurred must be explained by marked changes at the level of the primary visual cortex, the striate cortex. As functional studies indicate that the geniculate cells are functionally normal and the cortical cells are altered in their properties, it must be concluded that some change in the effectiveness of the geniculocortical connections are responsible for those findings.

In 1991, in the *Annals of the New York Academy of Sciences*, Suzannah Tieman[35] of the State University of New York at Albany described additional structural changes encountered in monocularly deprived (MD) cats. She reported that the relay cells in the binocular segments of the deprived geniculate layers shrink and contain less of the excitatory amino acid neurotransmitter NAAG (N-acetylaspartyl glutamate). These changes appeared to be secondary to a loss of terminal arbor. Deprived geniculocortical cells projected to smaller dominance patches in layer IV of the visual cortex, where they made fewer and abnormal synapses. She concluded that the primary effect of monocular deprivation is disruption of the geniculocortical synapse, with the other changes, such as cell size and neurotransmitter content, being secondary. The full nature of the structural and molecular changes involved in the disastrous consequences (permanent blindness) in monocular deprived newborn animals remains to be elucidated.

In the same year as the awarding of the Nobel Prize to Hubel and Wiesel (1981), marked improvements in the surgical care of neonates with total monocular congenital cataracts, with good visual results, began to be reported and with emphasis on surgical repair very early in the critical postnatal period to prevent the appearance of any visual defect.[36]

In recent years, an important involvement at the molecular level of excitatory amino acids (glutamate and aspartate) and their receptors in activity-driven alterations in nervous system plasticity in both development and the laying down of learning and memory has been established. A number of studies of the developing visual pathways have indicated the NMDA (N-methyl-D-aspartate) glutamate excitatory amino acid receptor plays an important role in the consolidation of synapses and in the rearrangements in neural circuitry that occurs during normal brain development.

Chronic treatment with the NMDA receptor antagonist (APV) has been shown by Kleinschmidt, Bear and Singer[37] of Germany (*Science* 1987) to disrupt experience-dependent plasticity of kitten striate cortex by rendering this cortex resistant to the effects of monocular deprivation. In 1989, this group (Bode-Greuel and Singer)[38] reported that the development of APV-sensitive [³H] glutamate binding to NMDA receptors in the primary visual cortex of kittens parallels the time course of the critical post-natal period when the visual cortex is most susceptible to experience-dependent modifications. In 1991, Udin and Scherer[39] of Buffalo, New York presented evidence that the NMDA receptors play a key role in experience-dependent formation of binocular maps in the frog, *Xenopus laevis*, associated with metamorphosis. Eye movements near the end of the tadpole stage of life from a lateral facing, with little binocular overlap, to a more dorsal and frontal position with achievement of a binocular field. Their study system involved the ipsilateral visual projection to the optic tectum of *Xenopus* in which alterations in eye position can induce rearrangements in the ipsilateral tectal map during a critical period of post-metamorphosis development but not at later ages. They presented evidence that the NMDA receptor plays a key role in mediating the influence of vision on the connectivity of tectal maps. They also demonstrated that the normal loss of plasticity during the first few months after metamorphosis could be reversed by the chronic application of NMDA.

Swann and associates[40] (1991) have observed from studies on the memory-important mammalian hippocampus, in slice preparations, that the CA3 (Cornu Amonis 3) hippocampal neuronal network during a critical period early in neonatal life experiences a period of hyperactivity which coincides with a period when CA3-pyramidal cells possess an overabundance of recurrent excitatory axon collaterals. The CA3 area of the hippocampus is generally regarded as the pacemaker of the hippocampus. It is of interest the NMDA receptors in the hippocampus are present at times when the formation of recurrent excitatory synapses on CA3 hippocampal pyramidal cells appear to be taking place and when NMDA receptors in the developing hippocampus have been observed to have unique properties which distinguish them from those of the mature hippocampus.

Ben-Ari et al[41] of Paris reported in 1989 that in the early postnatal life, rat hippocampal CA3 neurons display spontaneous and evoked giant depolarizing (excitatory) potentials (GDPs) which are mediated by gamma amino butyric acid (GABA) and presynaptically controlled by NMDA receptors—a finding differing sharply from adult rats where non-NMDA glutamate receptors are involved.

A marked overexpression of NMDA glutamate receptors in the rat hippocampus during early postnatal development (postnatal days 4 to 13) has been found in comparison with adult rat levels.[42] A similar developmental pattern has been observed in developing human brain.[43] In the developing rat brain hippocampus this relative overexpression has been found to coincide with the development of afferent neuronal input and the elaboration of dendrites in this area.[44]

NMDA receptor binding in the CA3 area of the hippocampus in the immediate postnatal period develops more rapidly than in area CA1 which is consistent with the earlier development of afferent neuronal input to area CA3.[45,46]

It is of particular interest that the rapid and marked early postnatal increase in NMDA receptors in the hippocampus also coincides with the developmental onset (postnatal day 9) of long-term potentiation (LTP), a widely used electrophysiological model of learning and memory involving hippocampal stimulation. It also is of considerable interest that a greater capacity for the development of LTP has been observed during these early postnatal periods of nervous system development.[47,48]

In 1991, two important publications by Garthwaite and associates[49,50] of Liverpool (U.K.) brought nitric oxide into this picture of early brain development (hippocampus and cerebellum). They described NMDA receptor activation in the rat hippocampus to be through the L-arginine-nitric oxide (NO) pathway induction of cyclic GMP. They also reported an in-depth study of excitatory amino acid receptors coupled to the NO/cyclic GMP pathway in the rat cerebellum during development. The absolute cyclic GMP response to kinate glutamate receptor activation was maximally effective in both adult and immature tissues, remaining relatively constant throughout development, whereas NMDA produced very large accumulations of cyclic GMP in 8-day old animals (rats) with a striking reduction in cyclic GMP production during maturation.

It is important to recognize that excitatory amino acids act not only as neurotransmitters during central nervous system development but also function to regulate the development of neuronal connectivity circuitry and cytoarchitecture. They also play a major role in several forms of activity-dependent synaptic plasticity in early postnatal development including learning and memory and the stabilization and elimination of synaptic connections. They exert important trophic influences which affect neuronal survival, growth and differentiation during restricted developmental periods, particularly in the immediate and early (days) postnatal period.

Additional clinical pediatric surgical observations have identified the importance of early postnatal neuronal circuitry and reflex development in important functions at the other end of the alimentary tract and involving the development of appropriate swallowing mechanisms. In two clinical situations elimination of food swallowing has resulted in impaired nursing and swallowing. In long-gap esophageal atresia without fistula and without tracheoesophageal fistula to the lower esophagus, nutrition has been achieved by gastrostomy feedings for extended periods (up to a year and longer) until esophagus replacement with stomach or colon can be carried out. Control of saliva aspiration has been achieved by cervical esophagostomy. Failure to provide food to suckle and swallow during extended periods from the postnatal period on has resulted in severe nursing and swallowing difficulty once esophageal replacement has been achieved. This can be prevented by regular feedings of appropriate substances and volume—a bit messy at the cervical esophogostomy site, but effective with respect to establishing and maintaining normal nervous system circuitry and function with respect to nursing and swallowing. This nursing and swallowing problem also has been encountered in newborn babies who have to have greatly prolonged periods of total parenteral nutrition (TPN) for severe gut malformations, incapacitation or loss.

To return to the other (anal) end of the alimentary tract, comparatively recent data is accumulating relative to factors influencing continence and normal defecation following abdomino-perineal pull-through operations for Hirschsprung's disease. Early neonatal definitive repair operation without prior colostomy is rewarded by excellent defecation and continence results while the results of neonatal colostomy and wait 1 to 3 years for the definitive repair operation are wretched. The type of operation plays essentially no role in the outcome, although the major proponents of early (neonatal) operation without a prior colostomy tend to prefer the Swenson operation.

Professor Michel Carcassonne[51] of Marseille, France, the long-time and sadly ignored apostle of early neonatal definitive repair of Hirschsprung's disease (HD) without a prior colostomy, clearly presented the logic and rationale for this approach which he documented by his own personal and institutional excellent results in his classic publication with Morisson-Lacombe and Letourneau in the June 1982 issue of the *Journal of Pediatric Surgery* (17:241-243). This report is far and away the most important publication dealing with Hirschsprung's disease since Professor Orvar Swenson's original publications relating to his operation to cure Hirschsprung's disease by addressing its basic causative pathology (aganglionosis of the distal colon and rectum).

In this 1982 report,[51] Professor Carcassonne and his associates divided their results into 3 chronological periods based on their clinical approach to the management of Hirschsprung's disease. From 1965 to 1969, 54 of 67 patients were managed by Swenson's operation at ages ranging from 12 to 18 months after a preliminary colostomy. Thirteen of these 67 patients died between colostomy and a definitive operation (19.4%). From 1969 to 1977, the delay in carrying out corrective operations after colostomy was shortened to from 6 to 11 months of age in 69 patients. In doing so, mortality was eliminated. Nonetheless, the quality of functional results was compromised in 12 patients, by severe perianal dermalitis in 9 and partial incontinence in 3. At this point, the psychiatrist member of their team strongly advocated an earlier closure of the colostomy and a reduction in the number and length of hospital admissions. It was considered wise to establish as soon as possible normal and psychologic cortico-anal connections. In the last period, 1977 to November 1980, progress in the areas of immediate nursing and total parenteral nutrition (TPN) made colostomy unnecessary in 19 neonates and infants with severe Hirschsprung's disease in whom definitive repair without prior colostomy was carried out prior to three months of age with excellent results both in the quality of defecation and in the shortening of the total length of hospitalization (from a median of 188 to 40 days). At the time of their report, 10 patients were over 2 years following operation and all were completely continent.

In 1989, Professor Carcassonne and associates[52] presented in the October 1989 issue of the *Journal of Pediatric Surgery* (24:1032-1034) a most impressive up-dating of their approach to the repair of Hirschsprung's disease by early operation before three months of age and without elective prior colostomy in 32 infants with excellent results with respect to both mortality (zero) and defecation despite 7 of the 32 infants having total colonic aganglionosis. The seven patients with total colonic aganglionosis were alive and continent. Fifteen of the other 25 patients were more than 5 years old and all were continent with one to two stools per day. The remaining 10 patients were between 2 and 5 years old and were toilet trained and clean between bowel movements.

The discussion of their 1989 paper starts as following: "The results of this series prove that curative surgical treatment of HD is satisfactory in patients younger than 3 months of age and that preoperative decompression by a routine colostomy is not necessary. *Like other congenital malformations treated early and completely, HD benefits from logical, efficient, safe and complete management*" (italics added).

These results stand in stark contrast to the results of the colostomy and wait until 1 to 3 years of age before definitive operation standard approach which has functioned as "holy writ" for many years for the international pediatric surgery community where the principal controversy regarding Hirschsprung's disease has been riveted on which of the three major operative approaches to use (Swenson, Duhamel or Soave or a modification thereof).

Kottmeier and associates[53] in 1982 addressed the problem of failed operations for Hirschsprung's disease and observed that major complications after abdominoperineal pull-through operations (of all types) were more common than reported.

A report of major significance and refreshing candor by Mishalany and Woolley[54] of the Children's Hospital of Los Angeles appeared in the May 1987 issue of the *Journal of Pediatric Surgery* (22:443-446). They described the findings of a careful study of postoperative functional and manometric evaluation of 62 Hirschsprung's disease patients followed from one to 30 years following definitive operative repair. All of their patients had been operated on between 10 months and 6 years of age with a prior colostomy. In 39 patients the colostomy had been carried out in the newborn period. Fourteen patients had been operated upon by the Duhamel technique, 15 by the Swenson and 33 by the Soave. The functional results were quite disappointing. Less than half of the 47 patients with the Soave or Duhamel operations (49%) considered their stooling pattern to be normal, while only one quarter (26.6%) of those with the Swenson operation considered their stooling to be normal. The manometric results were ever worse. Resting external sphincter pressures were abnormally high and went even higher following rectal balloon inflation. The internal sphincter pressure showed a normal anorectal reflex in only 10% of the patients.

In 1990 in *Pediatric Surgery International* (5:446-448), an important and independent confirmation of the Carcassonne thesis appeared from Manchester (U.K.). The authors, L.K.R. Shanbhogue and A. Bianchi,[55] reported a 5 year experience (1984-1989) with 25 infants with Hirschsprung's disease (2 with total colonic aganglionosis) managed without mortality in the early neonatal period, as soon as the diagnosis was made and with the Swenson operation. The median age at presentation of their patients was 3 days (range 1-30 days) and the median age at operation was 14 days. All of their surviving patients were continent and had median stools of 2 per day (range 1-4). The authors conclude their discussion as follows: "Furthermore, it has been our experience that the primary reparative procedures are much preferred by parents and have the significant advantage of rapidly returning a relatively normal baby to the family after the first admission." These excellent results are a most impressive validation of the Carcassonne approach of early operation without a prior colostomy.

The most recent major publication on the importance of achieving early postnatal target area-brain cortical neurocircuitry appeared in the August 12, 1993 issue of *Nature* (364:623-626) by Schlaggar et al[56] of the Salk Institute and the University of Minnesota. Their findings demonstrated that the rat somatosensory cortex and primary visual cortex follow similar activity-dependent developmental rules. Their study was designed to test whether the developmental plasticity of somatosensory cortex (S1) is similar to that of the ocular dominance columns of the visual cortex (described earlier in this section of this chapter). Their study was based on prior observations that each "barrel" is the cortical representation of a large whisker on the rat's nose with each row of whiskers on the face represented by a row of barrels in the S1 area of the somatocortex. The "barrels" of the S1 somatosensory cortex are made up of discrete collections of layer 4 cortical neurons which are innervated by clusters of ventroposterior (VP) thalamocortical afferents. In the newborn rat VP afferents are diffusely distributed in S1. However, by the end of the first 24 hours postnatal they form discrete clusters in a well defined "barrel" pattern. It is of particular interest that this particular pattern

has been found to emerge after NMDA and non-NMDA gluatamate receptors are functional in the S1 somatosensory cortex at thalamocortical synapses. The experimental model of the Schlaggar et al study is based on 1973 observations of Van der Loos and Woolsey[57] that elimination of a row of whiskers on a mouse's face during the first week after birth prevents the development of the cortical "barrels" which would otherwise represent that row and permits adjacent "barrels" to expand into the territory of the damaged follicles. Schlaggar et al demonstrated that selective disruption of postsynaptic activation in the rat S1 somatosensory cortex by the chronic application of the glutamate NMDA receptor antagonist APV inhibits the rearrangements in the somatotopic patterning of thalamocortical afferents induced in untreated whisker row elimination animals as described above in the critical first postnatal week. They interpreted their findings as showing that postsynaptic activation has a prominent role in critical period plasticity in the S1 somatosensory cortex.

In summary, an impressive volume of clinical observations and basic neuroscience research appears to indicate clearly that, in the all important immediate postnatal "cortical space race", the bottom line is "use it or lose it". With respect to imperforate anus in the newborn, this means that the first order of business is to carry out definitive operative correction in the immediate postnatal period (initial 3 days) and without a colostomy. Without this, none of the other secondary challenges (coming) can be evaluated adequately.

SECONDARY (IN IMPORTANCE) CHALLENGES

As stated immediately above, evaluation of secondary challenges would be quite difficult without establishing appropriate ano-somatocortical neuroconnections and functioning neurocircuitry in the all important critical immediately postnatal period by prompt operative anatomical hook-up at birth and without a prior colostomy. Accordingly, these secondary challenges will be presented without any attempt to indicate their priority or relative importance.

2. Technical anatomic approach to repair (which operation and where to start)

The major anatomical approaches to imperforate anus repair in comparatively recent years and since the landmark introduction of the combined and simultaneous abdominal-perineal operation in the newborn by Rhoads et al[12] have been the puborectalis sling oriented sacro-perineal and sacroabdominoperineal operations (Stephens,[24] Kieswetter[25]), the endorectal pull-through procedures (Rehbein,[58] Roumaldi[59]), the anterior saggital approach (Mollard[60]) and the posterior saggital approach (Peña and de Vries).[22,23] With the passage of time, the posterior and anterior saggital approaches have become the most frequently employed.

The author of this book has preferred and employed only the posterior saggital approach. This exposure in the newborn is excellent, fistulas are easily identified and the rectal pouch is thin, supple and easily mobilized and brought to the skin of the anal dimple for mucocutaneous approximation without tension. Professor Aluwihare[20,21] of Sri Lanka has preferred the anterior approach in both males and females in neonatal operations. With the anterior approach, he has found it necessary to open the rectum to locate the fistula (to the urinary tract in the male) from within the rectal pouch in 8 patients in his total of 39 patients, with 31 operated upon at birth.

It is likely that the most important anatomical issue is the use of a midline saggital approach whether it be anterior saggital (a bit cramped) or the posterior saggital ("open book") approach. This anatomical issue and its historical background was presented quite well by Professor Martin Allgöwer[61] of Basel, Switzerland in his Guest Oration before the May 1982 annual meeting of the Society for Surgery of the Alimentary Tract. This excellent oration was published in the January 1983 issue of the *American Journal of Surgery* (145:5-7). He credits W.H. Cripps[62] (1880) for being the first to carry out deliberate splitting

of the sphincters in the posterior midline to approach rectal tumors (adults, but same basic anatomy) and also credits York Mason[63] in multiple publications from 1970-1974 with resurrecting Cripps' long-forgotten work and supported it by his own extensive personal experience. Allgöwer's lucid description of this matter and issue is as follows: "York Mason explained the dependable preservation of continence after splitting all sphincters, as well as the puborectal sling, in the posterior midline, by relating the fact that the vascular supply as well as the innervation enter all parts of the levator as well as the external sphincters strictly from the lateral side. One of his points was that the continence organ depends on two funnels, situated one within the other. The external funnel corresponds to the levator with its puborectal sling and the external sphincters at its lower end. The internal funnel is constituted by the muscular wall of the rectoanal channel. He thus dared to widely open the rectal canal like a book, in the posterior midline."

A June 4, 1892 report in the *British Medical Journal* (1:1187-1188) by Harrison Cripps[10] F.R.C.S. from St. Bartholomew's Hospital in London (presumably the same Cripps) and titled "The Treatment of Imperforate Anus" must clearly be accounted one of the most important forgotten gems and classics in the history of pediatric surgery literature. Cripps reported the use of posterior saggital anoplasty in five infants, both male (3) and female (2), without mortality. Four of the five operations were carried out in the immediate post-natal period. The antiquity of this important experience should enhance its significance. Reference to this classic, but forgotten, report was found by the author of this book in the superlative history of imperforate anus published in 1978 by Professor Alois Schärli[6] of Lucerne, Switzerland.

The challenge of *where* to start the operation is clearly the perineum, rather than the abdomen or elsewhere. This conclusion and approach is shared by both Professor Aluwihare and me. In the great majority of newborn infants, the imperforate anus repair can be carried out solely by the perineal route. Only 4 of Professor Aluwihare's[20] 31 newborn males required abdominal opening to complete the operative repair (13%) and only 2 of my 14 newborns (14%) did—none at the time of my 1990 report in the *Journal of Pediatric Surgery*.[16] I generally wait approximately 72 hours after birth to operate so that the thin-walled rectal pouch will, by distention, be pushed maximally toward the perineum.

3. The challenge of additional serious congenital malformations

The management of serious congenital malformations and overall improvement in care of the neonate in neonatal intensive care units has greatly reduced the hazards of these in the newborn infant with imperforate anus. Cardiac and tracheoesophageal malformations should be identified immediately after birth and cared for appropriately with prompt repair of the imperforate anus otherwise being given the top priority for immediate (within hours) repair. The relatively high incidence of urinary tract malformations and refluxes beyond the fistulas in males should not be forgotten and should receive early study once the anorectal and other matters are sorted out.

4. Matters such as frequency and duration of postoperative results and dilatations (Hegar), the use of skin flaps and the use or nonuse of fistulas in anorectal reconstruction.

These are comparatively secondary considerations which the test of time and experience should resolve once repair at birth has become established as a routine major aspect of the care of these infants, female as well as male. The author of this book does not use skin flaps, prefers prolonged, careful and atraumatic Hegar anorectal dilatations and does not consider the fistulas to be an important part of imperforate anus repair, but is quite prepared to permit these issues to be settled by time and experience.

5. Evaluation of results (clinical/"subjective" versus "objective"/manometric, etc.)

Few areas relating to imperforate anus provide more of a "challenge" than the evaluation of postoperative results. The most important recent study and publication in this area is the report of Professor John Raffensperger of Chicago and his associates[64] in the February 1993 issue of the *Journal of Pediatric Surgery*. They employed clinical evaluation, computed tomography (CT) and manometry in 25 patients. In comparing the objective criteria and clinical results, they found that no technique could predict continence. They also found no objective criteria that could evaluate the patient's clinical result or dictate therapy.

6. Laparoscopic potentials and challenges

Minimally invasive surgery by laparoscope or thorascope or both is one of the major temptations, lures and fascinations of contemporary surgery. Nothing is so exciting and exhilarating as seeing it on the "big screen" and, to top it off, send the patient home the next day and often with a video of the undertaking as a memento.

There are some real theoretical potentials of laparoscopy in the operative management of imperforate anus at birth. It might facilitate the intra-abdominal activities in the approximate 15% of cases of high imperforate anus which require a laparotomy in addition to the perineal dissection from the experiences of Professor Aluwihare and me as cited earlier in this chapter. It might also hasten the perineal dissection by mobilization and ligation of fistulas from above and in rectal pouch dissection/mobilization and "grabber" thrusting of the distal rectal pouch toward the sphincter area of the perineal dissection when the posterior saggital perineal approach is utilized. Simultaneous use of both approaches also is an intriguing possibility.

CONCLUSION

The overwhelmingly most important and significant challenge in the management of imperforate anus in the newborn is when to do the definitive reparative operation and with or without a prior colostomy. The weight of clinical and basic science research evidence presented in this chapter clearly and strongly indicates that definitive reparative operation should be performed in the immediate postnatal period (initial 72 hours after birth) and without a prior colostomy. This will make possible optimal activity-driven somatocortical neurocircuitry and neuroconnectivity between the peripheral target area (anorectal) and the somatic cortex of the brain and prevent the loss of cortical space by disuse deprivation in the all-important immediate postnatal "critical" period of neurodevelopment.

Resolution of other and secondary challenges must await their investigation in the neurocircuitry and neurofunction undamaged newborn with definitive operation prior to the termination of this quite brief and most "critical" period in postnatal neurodevelopment.

Other and secondary challenges are listed and discussed, including which anatomical operation to employ, and the author's tentative preferences (when they exist) are indicated. In this area, particular tribute and credit must be accorded Harrison Cripps[10] of London who published from St. Bartholomew's Hospital on June 4, 1892 an outstanding experience with posterior saggital anoplasty in five newborn infants, both male and female, without mortality and in four with operation in the immediate postnatal period and with good results. A more recent report (by 98 years) by Goon[65] from Kuala Lumpur (Malaysia) further confirms the value and safety of posterior saggital anoplasty for imperforate anus of the intermediate and high types in the newborn period by one operation and without prior colostomy. Twenty-eight of his 32 patients (87.5%) were operated upon within the first four days of life. There was no operative mortality. The functional results were good in 30 of the 32 (94%) and average in two. Goon found as did I, tapering to be unnecessary in the newborn operated upon within four days of birth.

This is one important neonatal malformation where the potentials of laparoscopic assistance in selected cases are real and worthy of careful exploration.

REFERENCES

1. Paulos V. Aegina. Pauli Aeginetae Totius Rei Medicae Libri Septum ad Perfektionem Parati, Lib. b, Caput 81. Basel, 1538.
2. Bodenhamer WH. A Practical Treatise on the Aetiology, Pathology and Treatment of the Congenital Malformation of the Rectum and Anus. New York, Wood, 1860.
3. Matas R. The surgical treatment of congenital ano-rectal imperforation considered in the light of modern operative procedures. Trans Am Surg Assoc 1897; 15:453-553.
4. Webster R. Historical review in: Stephes FD, Smith ED. Ano-Rectal Malformations in Children. Chicago: Yearbook Medical Publishers, 1971.
5. deVries PA. The Surgery of Anorectal Anomalies: Its Evolution with Evaluations of Procedures. Current Problems in Surgery. Vol 21, No 5, Chicago: Yearbook Medical Publishers, 1984.
6. Schärli AF. Malformations of the anus and rectum and their treatment in medical history. Prog Pediatr Surg 1978; 11:141-172.
7. Amussat J-Z. Histoire d'une opération d'anus artificiel pratique avec succès par un neuveau procédé, dans un cas d'absence congénitale d'anus. Gaz Méd de Paris 1845, 28 Nov.
8. MacLeod N. Case of imperforate rectum, with a suggestion for a new treatment. Br Med J 1880; 657-658, Oct 23.
9. Delagenière P. Du traitement de l'imperforation de l'anus. Arch Prov de Chir 1894; 3:405.
10. Cripps H. The treatment of imperforate anus. Br Med J 1892; 1:1197-1198.
11. Harken DE. Congenital malformations of the rectum and anus; An analysis of the embryological background, treatment and results in 25 patients. Surgery 1942; 11:422-435.
12. Rhoads JE, Pipes RL, Randall JP. A simultaneous abdominal and perineal approach in operations for imperforate anus with atresia of the rectum and rectosigmoid. Ann Surg 1949; 12:552-556.
13. Moore TC, Lawrence EA. Congenital malformations of the rectum and anus; I. Clinical features and surgical management in 120 cases. Surgery 1952; 32:352-365.
14. Moore TC, Lawrence EA. Congenital mal-

formations of the rectum and anus; II. Associated anomalies encountered in a series of 120 cases. Surg Gynec Obstet 1952; 95:281-288.

15. Moore TC. In: Lambrect W, Lierse W. The internal sphincter in anorectal malformations. J Pediatr Surg 1987; 22:1167 (discussion).

16. Moore TC. Advantages of performing the saggital anoplasty operation for imperforate anus at birth. J Pediatr Surg 1990; 25:276-277.

17. Ladd WE, Gross RE. Congenital malformations of the rectum and anus. Am J Surg 1934; 23:167-183.

18. Mayo CW, Rice RG. Anorectal anomalies. Surgery 1950; 27:485.

19. Raffensperger JG. Swenson's Pediatric Surgery, 5th ed. Norwalk: Appleton&Lange, 1990.

20. Aluwihare APR. Imperforate anus in male children: A new operation of primary rectourethroanoplasty. Ann Roy Coll Surg England 1989; 71:14-19.

21. Aluwihare APR. Primary perineal rectovaginoplasty for supralevator imperforate anus in female neonates. J Pediatr Surg 1990; 25:278-281.

22. de Vries PA, Peña A. Posterior saggital anorectoplasty. J Pediatr Surg 1982; 17:638-643.

23. de Vries PA, Peña A. Posterior saggital anorectoplasty: Important technical considerations and new applications. J Pediatr Surg 1982; 17:796-809.

24. Stephens FD, Smith ED. Ano-Rectal Malformations in Children. Chicago: Yearbook Medical Publishers, 1971.

25. Kieswetter WB. Imperforate anus: II. The rationale and technique of the sacro-abdominoperineal operation. J Pediatr Surg 1967; 2:106-110.

26. Langemeijer RATM, Molenaar JC. Continence after posterior saggital anorectoplasty. J Pediatr Surg 1991; 26:587-590.

27. Brain AJL, Kiely EM. Posterior saggital anorectoplasty for reoperation in children with anorectal malformations. Br J Surg 1989; 76:57-59.

28. Wiesel TN. Postnatal development of the visual cortex and the influence of environ-ment. Nature 1982; 299:583-591.

29. Hubel DH. Exploration of the primary visual cortex, 1955-1978. Nature 1982; 299:515-524.

30. Hubel DH, Wiesel TN. The period of susceptibility to the physiological effects of unilateral eye closure in kittens. J Physiol 1970; 206:419-436.

31. Wiesel TN, Hubel DH. Effects of visual deprivation on morphology and physiology of cells in the cat's lateral geniculate body. J Neurophysiol 1963:978-993.

32. Wiesel TN, Hubel DH. Extent of recovery from the effects of visual deprivation in kittens. J Neuorphysiol 1965; 28:1060-1072.

33. Wiesel TN, Hubel DH. Extent of recovery from the effects of visual deprivation in kittens. J Neurophysiol 1965; 28:1060-1072.

34. Dews PB, Wiesel TN. Consequences of moncular deprivation on visual behavior in kittens. J Physiol 1970; 206:437-455.

35. Tieman SB. Morphological changes in the geniculocortical pathway associated with monocular deprivation. Ann New York Acad Sci 1991; 627:212-230.

36. Beller R, Hoyt CS, Marg E et al. Good visual function after neonatal surgery for congenital monocular cataracts. Am J Ophthalmol 1981; 91:559-565.

37. Kleinschmidt A, Bear MF, Singer W. Blockade of "NMDA" receptors disrupts experience-dependent plasticity of kitten striate cortex. Science 1987; 238:355-358.

38. Bode-Greuel KM, Singer W. The development of N-methyl-D-aspartate receptors in cat visual cortex. Dev Brain Res 1989; 46:197-204.

39. Udin SB, Scherer WJ. Experience-dependent formation of binocular maps in frogs: Possible involvement of N-methyl-D-aspartate receptors. Ann New York Acad Sci 1991; 627:26-41.

40. Swann JW, Smith KL, Brady RJ. Age-dependent alterations in the operations of hippocampal neural networks. Ann New York Acad Sci 1991; 627:264-276.

41. Ben-Ari Y, Cherubini E, Corradetti R et al. Giant synaptic potentials in immature rat CA3 hippocampal neuron. J Physiol 1989; 416:303-325.

42. Tremblay E, Roisin MP, Repressa A et al.

Transient increased density of NMDA binding sites in developing rat hippocampus. Brain Res 1988; 461:393-396.

43. Repressa A, Tremblay E, Ben-Ari Y. Transient increase of NMDA-binding sites in human hippocampus during development. Neurosci Lett 1989; 99:61-66.

44. Pokorny J, Kamamoto T. Postnatal ontogenesis of hippocampal CA1 area in rats: I. Development of dendritic arborization in pyramidal neurons. Brain Res Bull 1981; 7:113-120.

45. Loy R. Development of afferent lamination in Ammon's horn of the rat. Anat Embryol 1980; 159:257 275.

46. McDonald JW, Johnson MV. Physiological and pathological roles of excitatory amino acids during central nervous system development. Brain Res Rev 1990; 15:41-70.

47. Harris KM, Teyler TJ. Developmental onset of long-term potentiation in area CA1 of the rat hippocampus. J Physiol 1984; 346:27-48.

48. Schmidt JT. Long-term potentiation during the activity-dependent sharpening of the retinotopic map in goldfish. Ann New York Acad Sci 1991; 627:10-25.

49. East SJ, Garthwaite J. NMDA receptor activation in rat hippocampus influences cyclic GMP formation through the L-arginine-nitric oxide pathway. Neurosci Lett 1991; 123:17-19.

50. Southam E, East SJ, Garthwaite J. Excitatory amino acid receptors coupled to the nitric oxide/cyclic GMP pathway in rat cerebellum during development. J Neurochem 1991; 56:2072-2081.

51. Carcassonne M, Morisson-Lacombe G, Letourneau JN. Primary collective operation without decompression in infants less than three months of age with Hirschsprung's disease. J Pediatr Surg 1982; 17:241-243.

52. Carcassonne M, Guys JM, Morisson-Lacombe G et al. Management of Hirschsprung's disease: Curative surgery before 3 months of age. J Pediatr Surg 1989; 24:1032-1034.

53. Velcek FT, Klotz DH, Friedman A et al. Operative failure and secondary repair in Hirschsprung's disease. J Pediatr Surg 1982; 17:779-785.

54. Mishalany HG, Woolley MM. Postoperative functional and manometric evaluation of patients with Hirschsprung's disease. J Pediatr Surg 1987; 22:443-446.

55. Shanbhogue LKR, Bianchi A. Experience with primary Swenson resection and pull-through for neonatal Hirschsprung's disease. Pediatr Surg Int 1990; 5:446-448.

56. Schlaggar BL, Fox K, O'Leary DDM. Postsynaptic control of plasticity in developing somatosensory cortex. Nature 1993; 364:623-626.

57. Van der Loos H, Woolsey TA. Somatosensory cortex: Structural alterations following early injury to sense organs. Science 1973; 179:395-398.

58. Rehbein F. Operation der Anal-und Rectumatresie mit Recto-Urethralfistel. Chirurg 1959; 30:417-418.

59. Roumaldi P. Eine aneue Operationstechnik fürdie Behandlung einiger Rectummissbildungen. Langenbecks Arch Klin Chir 1960; 296:371-377.

60. Mollard P, Marechal JM, Jaubert de Beaujeu M. Surgical treatment of high imperforate anus with definition of the puborectalis sling by an anterior perineal approach. J Pediatr Surg 1978; 13:499-504.

61. Allgöwer M. Sphincter splitting approach to the rectum. Am J Surg 1983; 145:5-7.

62. Cripps WH. Cancer of the Rectum. London: Churchill, 1880.

63. Mason AY. Transphincteric surgery of the rectum. Prog Surg 1974; 13:66-97.

64. Doolin EJ, Black CT, Donaldson JS et al. Rectal manometry, computed tomography and functional results of anal atresia surgery. J Ped Surg 1993; 28:195-198.

65. Goon HK. Repair of anorectal anomalies in the neonatal period. Pediatr Surg Int 1990; 5:246-249.

INVITED COMMENTARY

Jonathan E. Rhoads M.D.
Professor of Surgery and Former Chairman of the Department
University of Pennsylvania
President, American College of Surgeons 1971-1972
President, American Surgical Association 1972
Recipient, American Surgical Association Medallion for
Achievement 1979

In this chapter, Professor Moore has been extremely generous in his citation of the paper that I published with R.L. Pipes and J.P. Randall in 1949 when we reported two cases of imperforate anus with highly placed large bowel stumps treated by simultaneous abdominal perineal approach. This was followed a number of years later after I gave up pediatric surgery by a more extensive series from Dr. C. Everett Koop's service at the Children's Hospital of Philadelphia, "The Surgical Management of Imperforate Anus" published in *Surg Clin North Am.*[1] Our rationale was very simplistic compared with the rationale proposed by Dr. Moore which places the emphasis on carrying out the procedure during the first 72 hours rather than waiting a year after a temporizing colostomy. My information at the time (the 1940s) was that newborns who had colostomies did not do well and that a number of them did not live to grow up. Moreover, we had recently had a more extensive experience in adults being operated on for low lying large bowel carcinomas with the simultaneous abdominal perineal approach. This experience I reported orally at a joint meeting of the New York Surgical Society and the Philadelphia Academy of Surgery. We claimed shorter operating time and less blood loss when we used a double approach from the perineum and from the abdomen. This experience was reported in *Surgery.*[2] The experience taught us that the simultaneous abdominal and perineal approaches offered a significant advantage in allowing one to dissect alternatively from above or below, whereas, the conventional method at that time was to complete the abdominal procedure and then start the perineal procedure. When one followed this conventional procedure, one had to do all that he was going to do from the abdominal side before finding out whether it could be more quickly and conveniently done from the perineal side. With the simultaneous approach, it was easy to push the specimen up or down as proved to be most convenient. It was in the wake of this experience that we were confronted with the first of the two children with imperforate anus who seemed to require an abdominal approach. I would credit Dr. O. H. Wangensteen and Dr. C. O. Rice[3] with the simple device of putting a penny on the anal dimple or the perineum after the child had been born long enough to swallow some air and transmit it to the rectal stump and then take a lateral film in order to demonstrate the distance between the perineum and the end of the bowel. We used this technique in deciding how high the patent bowel was. One such patient I had the opportunity of following into her second decade. She had partial continence and was able to go to school but I later referred her to Dr. Harry Bishop at the Children's Hospital to see if he thought she needed an additional procedure. He thought she had a sufficient degree of continence so that with better dietary management, she would have an effective degree of continence and when I last knew, this had proved to be the case.

I can only thank Dr. Thomas Moore as I earlier thanked Dr. Robert Gross for giving such generous credit to our 1949 paper.

I am greatly intrigued by your concept that the early placement of the rectum in a normal position results in more normal development of the neurons concerned with the maintenance of continence. It would be nice if one could get the sort of experimental evidence for this which was obtained for the cats' vision but I imagine that will not be easy to obtain.

Congratulations on a very interesting chapter.

REFERENCES

1. Rhoads JE, Koop CE. Surg Clin North Am 1955; 35:1251-1257.
2. Rhoads JE, Schwegman CW. Surgery 1965; 58:600-606.
3. Wangensteen OH, Rice CO. Ann Surg 1930; 92:77-81.

Alfred A. deLorimer, M.D.
Professor of Surgery and Chief, Division of Pediatric Surgery
University of California, San Francisco
President, American Pediatric Surgical Association 1991-1992

Dr. Moore has described compelling arguments for repair of imperforate anus anomalies in the newborn period. The advantages are avoiding a colostomy, then a subsequent anorectoplasty, and finally a third operation for closure of the colostomy. In addition, Dr. Moore suggests that anorectoplasty in the newborn period allows the development of neural pathways which are required to achieve normal bowel control. He cites experimental work on the plasticity of the developing brain in which deprivation of sensory stimulation for a period of time after birth (such as covering one eye for three months) results in loss of sensory perception (for example sight). Another example of the "use it or lose it" principle are babies with long-gap esophageal atresia who have had a cervical esophagostomy, and if they had not been swallowing food from early infancy they lose the ability to swallow later on when continuity of the esophagus is established.

Pediatric surgeons should consider early repair of imperforate anus anomalies to determine whether there is improvement in bowel control compared to the current common practice of preliminary colostomy and then a pull through later. If the results are to be comparative, it is imperative that similar anomalies are analyzed and that the definition of continence is clearly defined. For example, an infant born with a very high rectal atresia and an absence of three or more sacral vertebrae should have a poorer outcome than an infant with a low anomaly and an intact sacrum. Objective criteria of bowel function should be defined. The literature is full of reports of an extraordinary number of patients who achieve "excellent" continence control. However, these "excellent" results could not be corroborated by other surgeons doing precisely the same operative repair. This is an issue where close, repeated follow-up over a period of many years is required, and the criteria of "continence" must be scored by objective observers. The scoring system should emphasize evidence of bowel control by objective symptoms and might be supplemented by manometric studies and defecograms. All too often, the reports of excellent results do not include factors such as laxatives, daily enemas, or age when control was achieved. We have had patients who have had a perineal colostomy without any apparent sphincter mechanism who achieved "control" without soiling after 15 or more years of grief. Therefore, the incidence of control should be related to age groups. When results are reproducible by a large number of pediatric surgeons, a true picture of what can be achieved by early vs late operative repair will become evident.

There are two major issues which concern the entity of continence. Sphincter control is obviously important, while colonic motility is equally a determinant of continence. It is my impression that 90% of children with all forms of anorectal anomalies (varying from congenital anal stenosis to high rectal atresia) have impaired colonic motility. Their colon does not develop a once-a-day mass evacuation. It remains as a passive conduit becoming engorged with stool which is pushed out like toothpaste from a tube by pressure generated by filling from the small bowel. This problem is well-recognized in patients with an intact anorectal mechanism, which we call functional constipation. These latter patients constantly soil whether their sphincters are competent or not. The question is will a sacroperineal pull through, when performed in the newborn period rather than in later life, influence the effectiveness of colonic peristalsis?

It is established that the perception of rectal fullness and discerning the presence of flatus versus stool is confined to a few centimeters from the anal canal. Are the nerves which are responsible for this sensory perception congenitally absent in the high anomalies, or do we transect them in the course of our operative procedures? Perhaps the plasticity identified in the brain also applies to the innervation of the anorectum. Therefore, pediatric surgeons should be encouraged to perform a definitive repair in the newborn period and then assess separately the components of sensory perception, sphincter contraction and colonic motility at least through the age of 10 years to provide meaningful results.

John G. Raffensperger, M.D.
Professor of Surgery, Northwestern University
Surgeon-in-Chief, Children's Memorial Hospital, Chicago
Editor, *Swenson's Pediatric Surgery*

There is very little to add to Dr. Moore's discussion of imperforate anus. He has made a case for the repair of imperforate anus during the neonatal period. Unfortunately, there are few long-term follow-up reports on patients who had neonatal repairs. This is despite the fact that during the 1950s many babies were operated upon in the newborn period. It is entirely possible that neither the timing nor the surgical technique are particularly important factors in determining the long-term result. Associated birth defects, particularly those of the spinal cord and the sacrum are the primary determinants of eventual outcome. One would not want to do a primary neonatal repair in an infant who has other major birth defects such as a tracheoesophageal fistula, congenital heart disease or major urinary anomaly. This leaves only those infants with an isolated, favorable lesion who would be candidates for early repair. These are the very patients in whom we would expect good results from almost any kind of operation, done at any time. My very best result in a child with imperforate anus was in a 12-year-old boy from the back woods of Wisconsin. A colostomy had been performed at birth. At 12 years of age I resected a small length of colon distal to the colostomy and then did an abdominoperineal pullthrough. He was totally continent within one month!

No matter which operation is performed, one must separate the rectum from the urinary or genital tracts. The bowel then must be tunneled immediately behind the urethra in boys or the vagina in girls. It should be brought through the center of the perineal musculature as determined by a nerve stimulator. It makes little difference whether this is done by an abdominoperineal approach, a perineal approach or a posterior saggital approach. Perhaps the most important aspect of the care of a child with imperforate anus is the detailed follow-up by the same interested surgeon who performed the operation. It is helpful if the parents of the child are highly motivated.

Jan C. Molenaar, M.D., Ph.D.
Professor of Pediatric Surgery
University of Rotterdam, The Netherlands
Surgeon-in-Chief, Sophia Children's Hospital, Rotterdam

The idea of early operation immediately after birth is not new. Professor Rehbein, in his book on "Kinderchirurgische Operationen" ("Pediatric Surgical Operations") published in 1976 by Hippokrates Verlag in Stuttgart, describes his experience with more than 100 patients with imperforate anus operated upon at birth using his surgical approach. In this book Professor Rehbein states that in his experience surgical repair is easier immediately after birth than it is later in neonatal or infant life (p. 380). The same is true for the timing of his operation for Hirschsprung's disease, which is done by him routinely at the age of 3 to 4 months, but preferably, if the child's condition does not forbid, at the age of 6 to 8 weeks.

Neill V. Freeman and M. Bulut (1986, *J Pediatr Surg*, 21, 218-220) advocate early operation based on experimental studies in the maturation of what has been called so nicely in the chapter the "activity-driven brain-anus neurocircuitry". There is very little understanding of what happens in that "neurocircuitry" when during the surgical procedure the rectum is mobilised to ligate the fistula and to pull through the neo-anus.

David L. Collins, M.D.
Pediatric Surgeon, Medical Group of San Diego
Clinical Professor of Surgery
University of California, San Diego

I agree with Dr. Moore completely that the ideal operation for this condition should be done at birth, so as to allow neuronal pathways to be established, facilitating fecal continence.

I also believe that the ideal operation should include the following principles:

1. Minimal dissection and freeing up of the rectum so as to retain its nerve supply, both motor and most importantly sensory.
2. Retention of rectal blood supply.
3. Division of the rectourethral fistula where present.
4. No cutting of the important puborectalis muscle.
5. Mobilization upwards of the perineal skin so as to produce a sensitive skin-lined neonanus, which is important in the development of continence.

All of the above principles are embodied in the operation first proposed by Nixon in 1968, published by him and Kiely in 1986,[1] and subsequently copied by Mollard, Aluwihare, and by Yazbeck.

The recent experience with this procedure was reported by Kiely at the 1993 meeting of the British Association of Paediatric Surgeons (BAPS) in Manchester, and will no doubt be published soon in the *Journal of Pediatric Surgery*.

My experience with this procedure consists of nine cases. So far, most of them are too young to assess continence very well, but those who are old enough, have continence that is approaching normal for their age, i.e., clean most of the time with occasional soiling at night. Two are perfectly continent.

Most procedures, even including abdomino-perineal pull-through procedures, will eventually achieve continence after the child passes through puberty. In many cases, they are condemned to wearing diapers through their formative and school years, which has been shown to have a seriously deleterious effect on their psychosocial adaptation.

This aspect of imperforate anus was also reported at the above mentioned BAPS meeting.

The procedure is done by Kiely at about one week of age, with a colostomy, but can also be done in the newborn without a colostomy after the surgeon has gained some experience with doing a few cases in older children.

REFERENCES

1. Kiely EM, Nixon HH. Anorectal agenesis: Neonatal correction by a minimal mobilization inversion proctodeaoplasty. Br J Surg 1986; 73:933-934 (November).

Professor Sidney Cwyes
Head, Department of Paediatric Surgery
Red Cross War Memorial Children's Hospital, Rondebosch
University of Cape Town, South Africa

The posterior sagittal anorectoplasty (popularized by Peña and De Vries) era is coming to maturity with the assessments of long-term results and continence being reported after 10 years. One needs to ask oneself whether there has indeed been a significant improvement. There is no doubt that the cosmetic results are very good, but it is disturbing to see several complications being reported—fistulae, neurogenic damage and urethral injuries. The major criticism has been leveled at the tapering, especially in rectobulbar fistula, where one cuts across the only bit of remaining internal sphincter. It is in these rectobulbar fistulae, without tapering, that the best results of full continence have been obtained. Many reports now echo the conclusions of Molenaar and his group. Thus it is not surprising that more and more surgeons are reverting to performing the definitive repair in the immediate postnatal period, without a prior colostomy and without tapering.

The question to be answered is as follows: can there ever be full normal continence with no internal sphincter at all, as is found in imperforate anus with high rectoprostatic or rectovesical fistulae no matter what procedure is performed? The current research area is motility, and dysmotility of the terminal portion of the rectum is being investigated. Other reasons for the incontinence are being looked at more critically. Research is being done on the embryology by Kluth and co-workers; more sophisticated imaging is being used for assessment of the anomaly and the musculature—all in search of new avenues to improve continence. Experimentally the antropylorus has been transposed on its mesentery to the anus in an attempt to control continence, with good results in the pig.

Undoubtedly the biggest advance in this field has been the management of fecal incontinence with once daily colonic irrigation by the patient him or herself in the morning or in the evening. It is simple, inexpensive, with good compliance producing completely controlled continence in about 90% of patients in the long-term. For children in developing countries where there are virtually no facilities for handicapped patients this form of controlled continence has been of the greatest benefit.

Professor Michel Carcassonne
Department of Pediatric Surgery
University of Marseille
Hôpital d'Enfants Timone, Marseille

Factors of a future fecal continence in high type lesions are the most important challenge to discuss. In 1953, Douglas Stephens emphasized the action of levator ani musculature and pubo-rectalis sling on continence. In 1980, DeVries and Peña provided evidence of the importance of external sphincter in fecal control. Kiesewetter stressed the sensation and proprioception factors to obtain a good continence. These important studies, with Mollard's, result in adjusting a careful technique that provides a good anatomic repair, from below, for 80% of high type malformations, without opening the abdomen. It does not appear anymore compulsory to wait six months or more with a colostomy, before performing the definitive procedure.

If the pubo-rectalis sling, as well as external sphincter, were found atrophic in the past because anal defecation was not obtained before six months, even now when the baby is operated upon at birth without colostomy or at one month with a primary colostomy, the external sphincter in particular, pubo-rectalis, is seldom found to be atrophic. Careful anatomic reconstruction is a necessary step to achieve continence. But it is not sufficient. The future fecal continence depends upon the anatomy of second to fifth sacral segments, particularly the third and fourth. As demonstrated by Stephens and later by us, high type ano-rectal anomalies are associated in 90% of cases with abnormal terminal cord, filum terminale or sacral roots, all types of dysraphism and partial or total sacral agenesis. Duhamel summarized this concept speaking of caudal regression. Quality of late continence depends upon uni- or bilateral loss of innervation from the second to the fifth sacral segment. Even after a perfect anatomic repair, if the nerve damage is high, wide or bilateral, continence will depend upon mother, family, social level, school and IQ.

Adrian Bianchi, M.D., F.R.C.S. (Eng. & Ed.)
Consultant Neonatal and Paediatric Surgeon
Royal Manchester Children's Hospital, England

The tragedy of incontinence, be it fecal or urinary or both is all too common to observe in most neonatal surgical follow-up clinics involved in the management of imperforate anus. The development of continence is all important to the quality of the child's life, his body image and the development of his personality. The emphasis in management should therefore shift from the imperforate anus to that of the "child" with an imperforate anus. Much emphasis has been placed on the development of surgical techniques and approaches for the reconstruction of the sphincteric mechanism—the motor unit. But perhaps less consideration has been given to the development of continence. It is clear that the "corticoanal neurocircuitry" is dependent for its establishment and subsequent function on the input of sensory stimuli passing from the anorectum and pelvic floor to the developing brain. It is evident therefore that interference with these stimuli by diversionary colostomy from the early postnatal period and extending over the first months of life, must result in an inevitable loss of basic patterns of recognition upon which eventual function depends. Indeed there is ample evidence for such impaired development from other systems (e.g. sight, hearing, swallowing and speech).

The relevant components for the development of continence, the ultimate aim in the management of imperforate anus, must therefore be the early establishment of a normal anatomy thus allowing normal phsyiological sensory stimuli to reach the brain at the appropriate moment for its development. This dependence on appropriate early brain stimulation must of necessity lead to the conclusion that neonatal reconstruction without a diversionary stoma is essential.

The technique of reconstruction of the motor unit (sphincter) has been the subject of great emphasis, with various and varied techniques proposed as "ideal", only to be found wanting at a later date. *The essential principle is the preservation, in as undamaged a state as possible, of all of the pelvic floor and the external sphincter musculature.* It is the anus which is imperforate and the anal canal which is essentially undeveloped. The first and crucial stage in reconstruction is to determine the position of the external sphincter complex by Peña muscle stimulation and to develop the central pathway through it, which is always present. For this an atraumatic transanal perineal approach is necessary turning the perianal skin inwards to line the anal canal. None of this highly precious sensory organ is extra, all is relevant and must be preserved.

The approach to the rectum and the fistula is variable. Whichever route is used, it is important that it in no way disrupts the pelvic floor, i.e. the levator ani and particularly the external sphincter complex. Scarring within this area will lead to major interference with sphincter function.

A well timed neonatal reconstructive procedure without a diversionary colostomy, thus enabling the development of appropriate corticoanal neurocircuitry will be of little value if the sphincteric mechanism in the pelvic floor is rendered useless by unnecessary scarring developed in the interest of a "wide and open" approach. Presently real, i.e. normal, continence levels, though better, remain unsatisfactory. More effort is required. It is clear that the final word has not as yet been written in the management of the child with an imperforate anus.

Professor A.P.R. Aluwihare, L.R.C.P. (Lond.), M.B., M.A., M.Chir. (Cantab.), F.N.A. Sci. (S.L.)
Department of Surgery, University of Peradeniya
Kandy, Sri Lanka
Hunterian Lecturer, Royal College of Surgeons of England, 1986

This exciting and challenging chapter is one I welcome, find easy to read and strongly support. It provides historical information which is useful both in itself and in highlighting the importance of significant current developments. The importance of very early operation for high imperforate anus is clear not only from the point of view of technical feasibility but also because of neurophysiological factors.[1] As regards technical feasibility, one has to pay tribute to the many authors who have stressed the importance of identifying muscles accurately, preserving nerves, and in males, tying the fistula securely. Without them our work might not have been so easy.

This chapter provides me the opportunity to point out that one still has the task of operating on patients in whom the nature of the anomaly was not recognized by the original surgeon.

It was the problems posed by this group of patients that for me opened up the idea of the primary recto-urethro/vagino-anoplasty.[2-4] I must point out that I still have on occasion to open the abdomen; but now do so extraperitoneally (going round the bladder) rather than transperitoneally to find and divide a very high fistula. Our results continue to be very acceptable as regards fecal continence, micturition and erections. Finally, I endorse the author's opinion that the timing of the operation for imperforate anus and what we have learnt from the results has relevance in deciding when to operate in neonates with diagnosed Hirschsprung's disease.

REFERENCES

1. Freeman NV, Burge DM, Soar JS, Sedgwick EM. Anal evoked potentials. Z Kinderchir 1980; 31:22-30.

2. Aluwihare APR. Correction of misdiagnosed supralevator imperforate anus in males. Proceedings of the 3rd Asian Congress of Paediatric Surgery. Bombay, India. 1976:49.

3. Aluwihare APR. Primary correction of suprlevator anal anomalies in the neonatal period. International Congress of Paediatric Surgery. Perth, Australia. Abstracts, 1984:Sect 7.

4. Aluwihare APR. Challenges in imperforate anus: I. Primary perineal rectourethroanoplasty for anatomical and functional correction in males with supralevator anomalies. Ann Acad Med Singapore 1987; 16:511-515.

Frank M. Guttman
Professor of Surgery, McGill Universiy
Director of General Paediatric Surgery
Montreal Children's Hospital, Canada

Important technical improvements have taken place in the treatment of imperforate anus, following a better understanding of the anatomy and physiology. It is now clear that all normal structures should be preserved in the repair, even if one thinks they are deficient. These structures include the rectum, the internal sphincter (around the site of the fistula), the puborectalis, the deep, superficial and subcutaneous portions of the external sphincter (circular and longitudinal fibers) and finally the anoderm.

Even if the repair is anatomically perfect, function is rarely perfect. It is hoped that earlier repair (before three months, ideally in the neonatal period) will be accompanied by better cortical integration of anorectal function. Not only do current techniques allow such an early neonatal repair, but it may in fact be easier. Whether primary neonatal repair without colostomy will prove superior to a staged repair completed in the neonatal period remains an open question.

═══ CHAPTER 2 ═══

HIRSCHSPRUNG'S DISEASE

INTRODUCTION

Hirschsprung's disease (aganglionosis of the colon and rectum) has long been one of the most fascinating and challenging of the clinical problems in infancy and childhood to confront the ingenuity of the pediatric surgeon. The identification of the cause and definitive cure (cut it out) of Hirschsprung's disease by Orvar Swenson[1] in the mid-1940s still stands as one of the great success stories and heroic events in the history and early development of pediatric surgery as a scholarly discipline and legitimate specialty within surgery.

Swenson rightly perceived the normal sized and innocuous appearing distal colon to be the culprit and villain (with its lack of ganglion cells in Auerbach's plexus) of this disorder rather than the grotesquely dilated "megacolon". His basic surgical approach of doing a sphincter-saving resection of the diseased distal colon and his pull-through reestablishment of intestinal continuity has stood the test of time and remains the definitive surgical approach to this problem despite a host of comparatively minor modifications which have in no significant way altered Swenson's basic and fundamental rationale and technical surgical approach.

I had the unique opportunity as a senior medical student at Harvard (1944-1945) during a clinical elective rotation in pediatric surgery at the Children's Hospital (Boston) to work with Swenson in his early studies as an active observer and minor participant (enema giver and retractor holder). These were the great "megacolon" days with the massive fecal impactions with incredibly foul smelling stools which rendered the enema givers socially unacceptable ("big barn smell") for prolonged periods of time.

The reader of this book is strongly advised to read Swenson's 1989 publication in the *Journal of Pediatric Surgery* (24:839-845) titled "My Early Experience with Hirschsprung's Disease" and his chapter with John Raffensperger (chapter 70) titled "Hirschsprung's Disease" in the 1990 5th Edition of *Swenson's Pediatric Surgery* to capture the flavor and excitement of these early heady days of experience, discovery and innovation.[2,3]

Although many of the key features of Hirschsprung's disease have long been known, this intriguing disorder has been slow to yield up all of its secrets and mysteries. In several important areas it has remained a malformation of paradoxes. With an incidence in patients and siblings of only about 1%, it is not truly a "familial" disease, yet there are families with a high incidence of Hirschsprung's disease.[4] Although there is a strong male predominance of approximately 80% in the most common extent of aganglionosis into the sigmoid colon, this differential diminishes in the approximately 10% of patients in which the aganglionosis involves the entire colon. Other alimentary tract malformations in the newborn such as esophageal, duodenal and anorectal atresias have a high incidence of additional congenital malformations including other segments of the alimentary tract. Hirschsprung's disease patients are remarkably free of other congenital malformations, including those of other segments of the alimentary tract. The principal additional malformation, Down's trisome, 21, occurs in only about 4% of the patients.

Hirschsprung's disease is generally considered to be a congenital malformation. Nonetheless, it may also be "acquired". In 1979, I and my associates[5] reported in the *Journal of Pediatric Surgery* (14: 158-161) the occurrence of Hirschsprung's disease discordant in one of monozygotic twins. The effected twin weight 1290 g at birth and developed necrotizing enterocolitis in the early postnatal period in association with mild respiratory distress syndrome and umbilical artery catheterization. This was managed nonoperatively with short term success until recurrent abdominal distention and vomiting led to further study and the identification of aganglionosis which was managed successfully by colostomy and one year later a Soave-type pull-through. The other and larger twin had no such problems. In 1983, Slipovich et al[6] of Israel reported two additional cases of Hirschsprung's disease discordant in monozygotic twins. In one it also was associated with neonatal asphyxia, umbilical artery catheterization and necrotizing enterocolitis and in the other with neonatal gut perforation and peritonitis. Acquired Hirschsprung's aganglionosis also has been reported to be associated with pull-through operations for imperforate anus and for Hirschsprung's disease.[7-9]

Although the aganglionosis has long been known, even before Swenson identified this feature as the cause of the symptoms and the vehicle (resection) to achieve a "cure", the precise nervous system malfunctioning at the molecular and cellular level remain a mystery—despite an avalanche of studies of all sorts to solve these riddles.

Even the most serious complication, enterocolitis, has a Janus face to it. Despite its frequent occurrence (up to 30% of cases) and one-time high lethality, enterocolitis in the immediate and early postnatal period, with failure to pass meconium and abdominal distension, has contributed to the early diagnosis and care of Hirschsprung's disease with the potential and enhanced safety for immediate postnatal definitive surgical resection of diseased colon without prior colostomy and within the immediate and early postnatal "critical" period for the development of somatocortical neurocircuitry and function (discussed in detail in chapter 1).

Intestinal perforation (colon, appendix, ileum) is quite infrequent (3-5%) in Hirschsprung's disease. When it appears in the early postnatal period it may point to the presence of total colonic aganglionosis (about one half of the cases).[10]

The brilliant and superlative in-depth studies of Professor Michel Carcassonne and associates[11-13] of Marseille, France have revolutionized the surgical care of Hirschsprung's disease and clearly rank as the most important contribution to the management of Hirschsprung's disease since the original work of Swenson more than 40 years ago. They have demonstrated both the safety and effectiveness of early postnatal surgery and without a prior colostomy. They also have shown the effectiveness of this approach, not only for the commoner forms of aganglionosis (sigmoid colon), but also for total colonic aganglionosis. Details of Professor Carcassonne's work and that of others and the rationale for this early postnatal initiation of definitive surgical therapy are presented in chapter 1 on imperforate anus where the fundamental challenges are quite similar with respect to the urgent need for early/immediate postnatal establishment of appropriate and functioning somatocortical neurocircuitry.

CHALLENGES

1. The most important and critical challenge is when to do the definitive repair operation, at birth/diagnosis and without a colostomy or do a colostomy and wait one to three years for the definitive repair.

As with imperforate anus (chapter 1), I feel quite strongly that definitive operation should be carried out as soon after birth and early diagnosis (with emphasis on the earliest postnatal diagnosis) as possible and without a colostomy. The details supporting this approach, clinical as well as basic science, are presented in this (Challenges) section of chapter 1.

From my first exposure to Professor Carcassonne's lucid and persuasive 1982 publication[11] to the present, he has followed Professor Carcassonne's approach and done all Hirschsprung's disease cases on diagnosis and without a prior colostomy. Initially, the Soave-Boley approach was continued but without a prior colostomy. Early serious trouble led to a quick change to the Swenson operation which was almost exclusively employed by Professor Carcassonne. One infant developed a fulminant and rapidly fatal enterocolitis four months after a Soave-Boley operation without a prior colostomy and another infant was found on rectal examination several months following operation to have a very tight and spastic feeling endorectal "sleeve". At this point, I feel that the newborn endorectal "sleeve" has too much spastic and contractile "vigor" to be left behind as in the Soave and Duhamel approaches.

Professor Carcassonne has employed both the Swenson and Duhamel operations early and with success in total colonic aganglionosis cases, but not the Martin operation of colonic onlays to small intestine. For technical and space reasons he has deferred Martin modification of the Duhamel with spur crushing/cutting until the infants have reached six months of age.

The important and confirming 1990 report of Shanbhogue and Bianchi[14] from Manchester, England concerned 25 infants managed successfully during a five year period (1984-1989) with no mortality and limited morbidity. The medium age of their patients was three days (range 1-30 days) and the median age at operation (Swenson) was 14 days. These authors emphasized the importance of dissecting within the leaves of the mesentery for rectum mobilization and the value of keeping very close to the bowel wall as well as the use of bipolar diathermy for dissection to minimize blood loss (and blood-blurring of the operative field). They found that they could provide sufficient tension-free length by dividing the inferior mesenteric pedicle in these newborn infants with careful preservation of the marginal vessel. By these measures, including cauterizing all blood vessels under direct vision, they were able to keep their blood loss per operation between 8 and 15 ml. Enterocolitis, an assist in the early postnatal diagnosis, was found in 32% of their patients but was rapidly controlled by a combination of systemic antibiotics, bowel deflation and colonic washouts. Of particular importance was their observation that all surviving patients were continent.

Also in 1990, Cass[15] of Westmead Hospital, Westmead, New South Wales, Australia in *Pediatric Surgery International* described his use of the endorectal technique in a neonatal one stage repair of Hirschsprung's disease with no deaths and a low complication rate in 13 neonates. His last seven patients (1988 and 1989) were operated upon at 5, 6, 6, 7, 8, 8 and 11 days of age. During the 1985 to 1989 period, 79% of Hirschsprung's disease at this hospital were diagnosed in the first week of life. These last seven patients were managed by definitive repair at the next available operating time.

The endorectal technique use without colostomy also was reported by So et al[16] in 1980. This report involved multiple authors (5), 20 cases, multiple hospitals (7) in multiple countries (2). The follow-up of these cases was limited. Ten cases were done in three hospitals in the Philippines between 1968 and 1974 and 10 were done in 4 New York hospitals between 1976 and 1979. TPN was not employed in this experience.

In the July 1991 issue of the *Journal of Pediatric Surgery* W-T Hung[17] of Taipei, Taiwan reported a 25 year experience with the use of a modified Duhamel operation in 248 patients with Hirschsprung's disease. From April 1984 to January 1990 all patients were managed by the pull-through operation (Duhamel modification) without colostomy, even in neonates. During this period, 18 infants less than two months of age were managed by this approach. All patients survived the operation without any significant complications. They cite the Carcassonne experience in their discussion.

The recent publications cited above suggest that the Carcassonne message is beginning to take hold. Both the functional and economic advantages of the one stage early neonatal repair without a colostomy are of sufficient magnitude that they cannot be ignored much longer by the national and international pediatric surgery community.

2. The question of which operation or its multiple modifications to do has long dominated the challenges and controversies arena involving Hirschsprung's disease.

This question must now be relegated to a secondary role and be resolved with reference to which approach is best in the early postnatal newborn. If leaving behind hyperexcitable aganglionic gut as in the Soave[18] and Duhamel[19] operations and their modifications proves to be undesirable in the early postnatal period, the basic Swenson[1] operation will likely become the operation of choice. Time and experience will provide answers.

3. Other secondary challenges include enterocolitis (reduced in frequency and gravity by early postnatal operation without colostomy), where to place the colostomy (nowhere), the question of neuronal intestinal displasia (a malformation or a complication) and the molecular and *cellular causes of Hirschsprung's disease gut malformation.*

The molecular and cellular causes of Hirschsprung's disease functional pathology will continue to fascinate and stimulate investigators who may find more pertinent answers in the study of neonatal aganglionic gut which has been spared the ravages of prolonged (years) bypassing by colostomy and by repeated episodes of enterocolitis of varying degrees of severity.

4. A very major challenge is provided by the extremely rare occurrence of total intestinal aganglionosis.

Until recently this condition was uniformly fatal.[20,21] In 1987, Ziegler, Ross and Bishop[22] of the Children's Hospital of Philadelphia reported an ingenious new multiple myotomy technique for prolonged survival in a case of total intestinal aganglionosis.

5. Laparoscopic potentials and challenges

Laparoscopic biopsy of Auerbach's myenteric plexus in the newborn with the first suggestive symptoms of Hirschsprung's disease might hasten definitive diagnosis and earlier effective one-stage surgical repair. This would bypass the more cumbersome and time consuming suction biopsy of mucosa and the more invasive and extra-rectal contaminating full-thickness biopsy through the ano-rectal opening. An additional challenge would be to do a sequential or simultaneous laparoscopy assisted resection of the aganglionotic colon and Swenson-type pull-through and anastomosis in the early postnatal newborn period.

CONCLUSION

As with imperforate anus, the overwhelmingly most important and significant challenge in the management of Hirschsprung's disease is to do the definitive repair in the early postnatal period and without a colostomy. This involves early postnatal diagnosis which is achievable and is being achieved with greatly increased frequency as recent published reports indicate. The clinical and basic science evidence in support of this approach is presented in greatest detail in chapter 1 and involves the attainment of activity-driven somatocortical neurocircuitry and functional neuroconnectivity in the early postnatal "critical" period of development of the nervous system.

It appears to be more important to resect all defective aganglionic colon and rectum in the early postnatal period than after one to three years of colostomy diversion as in the "traditional" and happily soon to be abandoned approach. This would make the Swenson operation the approach of choice. Professor Carcassonne has employed the Swenson operation in the neonatal period without prior colostomy with great success[11-13] and others[14] have followed his lead, including me who switched from the Soave endorectal approach to the Swenson after some disastrous results which appeared to result from hyperactive spasticity of the aganglionic endorectal "sleeve" in these neonatal infants.

Other serious management challenges such as the enterocolitis problem seem to be diminished both in frequency and severity by early postnatal repair without colostomy.

The potentials of laparoscopy in early definitive Auerbach's myenteric plexus biopsy and frozen section and in resection of aganglionic bowel and pull-through alimentary tract reconstruction in the early postnatal period are rather exciting and should be explored clinically in the not too distant future.

Recent reports in *Nature* and *Nature Genetics*[23-27] mapping a gene for Hirschsprung's disease to chromosome 10 and its co-localization and close relationship to the human RET protooncogene are exciting new findings with immense new challenges for the study of Hirschsprung's and related diseases at the molecular and genetic levels.

REFERENCES

1. Swenson O, Bill AH. Resection of rectum and rectosigmoid with preservation of the sphincter for benign spastic lesions producing megacolon. Surgery 1948; 24:212-220.

2. Swenson O. My early experience with Hirschsprung's disease. J Pediatr Surg 1989; 24:839-845.

3. Swenson O, Raffensperger JG. Hirschsprung's disease. In: Raffensperger JG, ed. Swenson's Pediatric Surgery. 5th ed. Norwalk: Appleton & Lange, 1990.

4. Cohen IT, Gadd MA. Hirschsprung's disease in a kindred: A possible clue to the genetics of the disease. J Pediatr Surg 1982; 17:632-634.

5. Moore TC, Landers DB, Lachman RS et al. Hirschsprung's disease discordant in monozygotic twins: A study of possible environmental factors in the production of colonic aganglionosis. J Pediatr Surg 1979; 14:158-161.

6. Slipovich L, Carmi R, Bar-Ziv J et al. Discordant Hirschsprung's disease in monozygotic twins. J Pediatr Surg 1983; 18: 639-640.

7. Ehrenpreis T. Hirschsprung's Disease. Chicago: Year Book Medical Publishers, 1970:48-50.

8. Cogbill TG, Lilly JR. Acquired aganglionosis after Soave's procudure for Hirschsprung's disease. Arch Surg 1982; 117:1346-1347.

9. West KW, Grosfeld JL, Rescoria FJ et al. Acquired aganglionosis: A rare occurrence following pull through procedures for Hirschsprung's disease. J Pediatr Surg 1990; 25:104-109.

10. Stringer MD, Drake DP. Hirshsprung's disease presenting as neonatal gastrointestinal perforation. Br J Surg 1991; 78:188-189.

11. Carcassonne M, Morisson-Lacombe G, Letourneau JN. Primary corrective operation without decompression in infants less than three months of age with Hirschsprung's disease. J Pediatr Surg 1982; 17:241-243.

12. Carcassonne M, Delarue A. Management of Hirschsprung's disease. The definitive operation: which, when, why and how. Aust NZ J Surg 1984; 54:435-438.

13. Carcassonne M, Guys G, Morisson-Lacombe G et al. Management of Hirschsprung's disease: Curative surgery before 3 months of age. J Pediatr Surg 1989; 24:1032-1034.

14. Shanbhogue LKR, Bianchi A. Experience with primary Swenson resection and pull-

through for neonatal Hirschsprung's disease. Pediatr Surg Int 1990; 5:446-448.

15. Cass DT. Neonatal one-stage repair of Hirschsprung's disease. Pediatr Surg Int 1990; 5:341-346.

16. So HB, Schwartz DL, Becker JM et al. Endorectal "pull-through" without preliminary colostomy in neonates with Hirschsprung's disease. J Pediatr Surg 1980; 15:470-471.

17. Hung W-T. Treatment of Hirschsprung's disease with a modified Duhamel-Grob-Martin operation. J Pediatr Surg 1991; 26:849-852.

18. Soave F. Hirschsprung's disease: A new surgical technique. Arch Dis Child 1964; 39:116-124.

19. Duhamel B. A new operation for the treatment of Hirschsprung's disease. Arch Dis Child 1960; 335:38-39.

20. Caniano DA, Ormsbee HS III, Poito W et al. Total intestinal aganglionosis. J Pediatr Surg 1985; 20:456-460.

21. Rudin C, Jenny P, Ohnacker H et al. Absence of enteric nervous system in the newborn: Presentation of three patients and review of the literature. J Pediatr Surg 1986; 21:313-318.

22. Ziegler MM, Ross HJ III, Bishop HC. Total intestinal aganglionosis: A new technique for prolonged survival. J Pediatr Surg 1987; 22:82-83.

23. Lyonnet S, Bolino A, Pelet A et al. A gene for Hirschsprung disease maps to the proximal long arm of chromosome 10. Nature Genet 1993; 4:346-350.

24. Angrist M, Kauffman E, Slaugenhaupt SA et al. A gene for Hirschsprung disease (megacolon) in the pericentromeric region of human chromosome 10. Nature Genet 1993; 4:351-356.

25. Romeo G, Ronchetto P, Luo Y et al. Point mutations effecting the tyrosine kinase domain of the RET proto-oncogene in Hirschsprung's disease. Nature 1994; 367:377-378.

26. Edery P, Lyonnet S, Mulligan LM et al. Mutations in the RET proto-oncogene in Hirschsprung's disease. Nature 1994; 367:378-380.

27. Schuchardt A, D'Agati V, Larsson-Blomberg L et al. Defects in the kidney and enteric nervous system of mice lacking the tyrosine kinase receptor Ret. Nature 1994; 367: 380-383.

INVITED COMMENTARY

John G. Raffensperger, M.D.
Professor of Surgery, Northwestern University
Surgeon-in-Chief, Children's Memorial Hospital, Chicago
Editor, *Swenson's Pediatric Surgery*

Dr. Moore has given credit to Dr. Orvar Swenson for his original work in the treatment of Hirschsprung's disease. At the Children's Memorial Hospital in Chicago we continue to follow Dr. Swenson's teaching. In the newborn period, when Hirschsprung's disease is suspected, we carry out a barium enema in order to determine the length of the aganglionic segment and the diagnosis is confirmed with a rectal suction biopsy. When the parents are cooperative and reliable and the mother is willing to breast feed, we will forego a colostomy and treat the infant with daily rectal irrigations until he is about one year of age. If the infant is unstable or remains distended despite rectal irrigations, we will carry out a colostomy placed in the bowel where ganglion cells are found by frozen section. We continue to wait until the child is about one year of age before doing the pull-through procedure. It certainly could be done at an earlier age but we see no advantage since most parents accept either the colostomy or rectal irrigations with equanimity. At the time of the pull-through operation, the level of aganglionosis must again be ascertained with a frozen section biopsy. The pulled through intestine must have normal ganglion cells, a good blood supply and the anastomosis must be tension free. We perform the anastomosis within about 1 cm from the dentate line. I, personally, now remove the appendix and leave the catheter in the cecum and ascending colon for decompression. Postoperative abdominal distention or constipation is usually corrected with a vigorous dilatation of the internal sphincter under general anesthesia. Total colon aganglionosis may be treated in a number of ways. I continue to follow some of Dr. Swenson's patients who had a straight ileal pull-through. These patients are now in their 20s, have normal bowel control and 4-5 stools a day. One young mother with total colon Hirschsprung's has recently had a baby who also had Hirschsprung's disease. At this time, for long segment aganglionosis, we prefer the Kimura operation in which a patch of the aganglionic cecum and ascending colon is sutured side to side to the small intestine, which does contain ganglion cells. At a later date, this bowel is pulled through according to the Swenson procedure. Many years ago I tried both the Duhamel and the Soave operation. Neither provided as good long term results as the Swenson operation. I suspect the surgeons who originally learned with the Swenson operation gave it up in favor of the other procedures because they either did not understand the principles of the Swenson operation or else when they did the rectal dissection, they did not stay exactly on the muscular wall of the bowel. At this time, we utilize bipolar electrocoagulation for hemostasis when dissecting on the muscular wall of the rectum. This makes the operation go quickly and easily and there is no risk to the pelvic nerves. In all of our long term follow-ups, we have never seen bladder or sexual dysfunction following the Swenson pull-through.

Within the past year, we have tested the feasibility of performing the Swenson pull-through laparososcopically in dogs. With the aid of the harmonic scalpel, we were able to dissect directly on the rectal wall and the dogs appeared to have normal rectal function in the postoperative period. We have used the laparoscopic technique and the harmonic scalpel on one child who had been managed with rectal irrigations for one year. This operation went very smoothly and the child, at this time, appears to have a normal postoperative course. In a second patient, we were unable to manipulate the hugely dilated sigmoid with the laparoscopic instruments and had to convert the operation to an open procedure. In the future, with more experience, a laparoscopic Swenson pull-through should be perfectly feasible.

Professor Michel Carcassonne
Department of Pediatric Surgery
University of Marseille
Hôpital d'Enfants Timone, Marseille

The necessity of performing the definitive operation as soon as possible after birth without colostomy is actually a challenge accepted by a majority of pediatric surgeons. However this statement requires some discussion.

A sure diagnosis of an aganlionosis is obtained in a majority of trained pediatric surgery centers, but unfortunately not everywhere. It may need some days to be ascertained. On another hand, it is good if the mother can feed her baby, or at least know him. Therefore there is no need to rush: colonic decompression is easily obtained using a daily rectal finger, careful isotonic enemas +/- parenteral fluids. For the last 17 years either occlusive or enterocolic problems were corrected without colostomy and the baby maintained in optimal condition to be operated on from 4 to 8 weeks of age.

At this age, I demonstrated the operation of choice was Swenson's, easy to perform, safe, and the only curative one. Since my last published report, 102 infants less than 2 months old were operated on using the original Swenson technique without mortality or morbidity requiring surgery. The quality of the late results confirm our first conclusions (text not yet been published).

Since Swenson recognized Hirschsprung's disease for what it was, research has been focused on enteric nervous system's development troubles. Acquired, often ischemic pseudo-Hirschsprung's disease, has now been separated from the true malformative aganglionosis. But beside aganglionosis which appears to be the most complete malformation of ganglion cells numerous abnormalities have been demonstrated espeacially by J.C. Molenaar[1] and P. Donahoe[2] using histochemical investigation combined with immunocytochemical technique. Their studies on neurocrestopathies led to an important step forward in the knowledge of gut innervation related motility disorders. Beside the quantitative anomalies of ganglion cells, they focused on secretion disorders of apparently normal ones.

What may inhibit normal maturation of neurogenic precursors process is not yet clear. But their studies using the monoclonal antibodies is probably the pathway to the solution. Marked elevation of class II major histocompatibility antigens in the aganglionic area may indicate an underlying auto-immune mechanism in the etiology of Hirschsprung's disease to be only a type of innervation related motility disorders.

REFERENCES

1. Molenaar JC, Tibboel D, Van der Kamp AW et al. Diagnosis of innervation-related motility disorders of the gut and basic aspects of enteric nervous system development. Prog in Ped Surg 1989; 24:174-185.
2. Hirobe S, Doody DP, Ryan DP, Kim SM, Donahoe P. Ectopic class II major histocompatibility antigens in HD and neuronal intestinal dysplasia. J Ped Surg 1992; 27:357-363.

Adrian Bianchi, M.D., F.R.C.S. (Eng. & Ed.)
Consultant Neonatal and Paediatric Surgeon
Royal Manchester Children's Hospital, England

The basic concept underlying the management of Hirschsprung's disease in the neonate is now beyond question. It is clear that the aganglionic bowel together with a proportion of the dilated ganglionic colon just proximal to the transition zone, require resection. The ganglionic colon is then advanced (pulled through) to the perianal margin. The type of procedure, be it Swenson, Soave, Duhamel, or another must achieve full resection/release of the aganglionic muscle and the internal sphincter if it is to be successful. The aim of management is to render the child of "normal" bowel habit and therefore continent as well. It is evident that continence is a learnt activity which is dependent on the development of the "somatocortical neurocircuitry". Observation of normal childhood development and physiological research indicated that this process of essential basic brain programming occurs during the early weeks and months after birth. It is evident and also borne out by clinical experience, that major interference with this delicate mechanism, as occurs by elimination of the sensory anorecto-pelvic floor component by a diversionary colostomy, must inevitably impact on the long term ability to achieve full continence, particularly at night time. Once the "window of early learning" has closed the ability to achieve continence is never the same again.

It is relevant therefore to attempt to preserve normal learning by allowing normal stimuli from the anorecto-pelvic floor, a concept that disallows the use of a diversionary stoma for any significant period. It appears crucial for continence therefore that the definitive curative procedure for Hirschsprung's disease be undertaken as soon after birth as possible. The advantage to the child and his family of one rather than three operations, avoiding the weeks of stoma morbidity from prolapse, bleeding, skin irritation, etc. are more than obvious. Following a single neonatal operation a "normal" child is returned to the family, allowing them to develop normal relationships and interactions, as though "there had never been a problem".

A single stage neonatal resection and pull-through under frozen section control and without a stoma is the treatment of choice. However the conditions required to achieve this (i.e. neonatal intensive care, expert neonatal anaesthesia and intraoperative pathology) are not easily achievable everywhere.

The overriding principle in all neonatal surgical management must remain the "safety of the child". It is evident that a perfect operation in a dead child is of little value indeed.

Professor A.P.R. Aluwihare, L.R.C.P. (Lond.), M.B., M.A.,
M.Chir., (Cantab.), F.N.A. Sci. (S.L.)
Department of Surgery, University of Peradeniya
Kandy, Sri Lanka
Hunterian Lecturer, Royal College of Surgeons of England, 1986

It is of importance that in this informative and provocative chapter Professor Moore has named all but one of the operations for Hirschsprung's disease. The one is a long segment internal sphincterectomy with excision of a contiguous strip of lower rectal muscle. This procedure is sometimes necessary for definitive histological diagnosis in patients with ultrashort segment disease and cures some of these patients. It is also useful to be able to do a frozen section of colonic muscle especially if operating on referred patients.

Our experience with Hirschsprung's disease involves patients of all ages presenting with various complications and also without any! I endorse the policy of operating on patients with Hirschsprung's disease at as young an age that the diagnosis can be made, but tempered by the experience of the surgeon, an assessment of the skills and experience of the anaesthetic and nursing staff, and an evaluation of the facilities available in the hospital concerned. I make this point since I am sure that the facilities in all the hospitals in the various countries in which this book will be read will vary considerably. I also cannot emphasize too strongly the importance of any surgeon dealing with Hirschsprung's disease having the ability to do any and all of the operations available as sometimes one has to change one's plans during an operation, especially in referred and complex patients, however good the preoperative workup may be.

REFERENCE

1. Aluwihare APR. Adaptations for developing countries in the surgery of congenital anomalies and Hirschsprung's disease. Sri Lanka J Surg 1975; 2:55-60.

CHAPTER 3

GASTROSCHISIS

INTRODUCTION

My interest in gastroschisis has been both long and challenging and has been associated with 11 scientific publications during the past 40 years—the first in 1953 and the most recent in 1992.[1-11]

I encountered my first case of gastroschisis on May 15, 1951 while completing a chief residency in surgery in Indianapolis. The patient was a newborn female first child of a 17-year-old mother and a 19-year-old father who had been born five weeks prematurely and weighed 4 pounds and 1 ounce. Labor had lasted 20 hours. The patient was mildly cyanotic and a very large mass, composed of loops of darkly discolored intestine of leathery consistency embedded in a sizable amount of firm gelatinous-type material, was found to be protruding from an over four-centimeter long defect in the anterior abdominal wall to the right of a normal appearing umbilical cord stump which was not involved in the evisceration. There was no membranous sac covering the mass and the margins of the defect were rounded and smooth. Multiple areas of small intestinal atresia were identified on careful examination of the mass. However, the number and extent and precise location of the atresias could not be determined due to the dense and firm matrix ("peel") in which the intestinal loops were embedded. No other malformations were encountered.

The infant was taken immediately to the operating room where limited dissection of the mass readily revealed the inadvisability of this approach as the atresias were so extensive and the loops of intestine so embedded in the firm, gelatinous matrix ("peel") that injury to both the intestine and its blood supply would be difficult to avoid. It was concluded that covering the mass should be the primary objective with an attack on the atresia deferred until a later date. Enlargement of the abdominal wall superiorly and inferiorly revealed a peritoneal cavity which was markedly diminished in size. It was clear that covering the huge and rigid mass could only be achieved by widely dissected skin flaps and the creation of a large ventral hernia. It was done with dissection of skin flaps around to the back on both sides.

The patient was managed postoperatively by nasogastric suction and parenteral fluid, electrolytes and dextrose. Visible peristaltic activity under the skin flaps was first noted 18 days following operation. Contrast X-ray studies the next day showed the distal portion of the large intestine to be patent with a portion of it in the hernia sac. Several air-filled dilated loops of small intestine also were seen. A day later, the infant was returned to the operating room and the incisional wound was reopened. The findings were most remarkable. The undersurface of the skin flaps had become endothelialized and were easily separated from the contained and perfectly normal appearing intestines. The huge and rigid gelatinous matrix/"peel" in which the intestines had been embedded had completely disappeared without a trace. At that time I speculated that the gelatinous mass had been metabolized (a sort of auto-"hyperalimentation"). The small intestine was found to be distended to the point of atresia in the ileum. The atresias were found to extend to the mid-colon. A side-to-side ileocolostomy was carried out with two layers of 5-0 "arterial" silk sutures, bypassing the area of atresias. The stoma was judged to be adequate and the incision was closed. Stool was passed on both the first and second days following operation signifying successful reestablishment of alimentary tract continuity. The patient did well until the fourth postoperative day when an acute respiratory distress occurred and appeared to be associated with a fluid overload and within a short period of time the infant died. The pulmonary pathology was confirmed at autopsy. Beyond the area of bypassed atresias and the associated malrotation, no other congenital abnormalities were found.

Three months later, on August 10, 1951, a second newborn infant with gastroschisis was admitted to the hospital. The mother was 21 years old, pregnancy had been of normal duration and labor had lasted five hours. There were two normal siblings and no family history of malformations. The thickened and discolored loops of leathery consistency were matted together with a gelatinous firm substance similar to that of the first case but smaller in amount. There were no other malformations.

The defect was similar in size and appearance to that of the first case and the abdominal insertion of the umbilical cord was normal with no sac or ruptured remnants present. The patient was taken to the operating room by the new chief resident, G.E. Stokes. I, a new junior faculty member in surgery, was consulted. A photograph documenting the classical experience of the mass of thickened and discolored intestines without a sac or remnants and the normal insertion of the umbilical cord was obtained. As in the first case, enlargement of the defect superiorly and inferiorly revealed an abnormally small peritoneal cavity. Also, as in the first case, the mass was covered by necessity with widely dissected skin flaps. Two days following operation rapidly developing respiratory distress led to the death of the infant. At autopsy, the gelatinous matrix and thickened and discolored appearance of the intestines remained. There was no intestinal atresia and no other anomalies were encountered. Microscopic study of the thickened intestine and photomicrographs revealed the thickened and leathery consistency of the small intestinal wall to be due to a thick layer of granulation on and external to the serosal wall of the intestine with no intrinsic intestinal wall change. I postulated in the published report of this case that this thickening had resulted from prolonged extracorporeal immersion of this intestine in amniotic fluid and debris—a judgment I now question.

A careful search of the literature at that time revealed only 5 cases which appeared similar to these two cases. Two of these have subsequently been dropped. That of Krauss[12] because of inadequate description and that of Bernstein[13] because recent review of this publication, description and photographs showing a large segment of eviscerated liver to reclassify this case as a ruptured omphalocele and likely as a case of syndrome omphalocele of the upper midline syndrome type (Cantrell et al[14]).

The literature search was quite fascinating because of the large number of terms in use and based largely on theorized embryological sequences conjured up to explain each reported case and monstrosity.

I decided to publish my case with that of Stokes and to present a practical and logical terminology and classification of anterior abdominal wall defects. The opening paragraph of this paper which appeared in the January 1953 issue of *Surgery*[1] is as follows:

An understandable confusion exists in the literature concerning congenital eviscerations through anterior abdominal wall defects due to the lack of a clear and established classification of these anomalies. Furthermore, the large number of descriptive names applied to these malformations has served to hinder the accumulation of a coherent and organized body of reported experience with them. This is especially true with respect to gastroschisis.—This relatively disordered state of the literature pertaining to gastroschisis has prompted us to formulate a clinical classification of congenital eviscerations through abdominal wall defects which we hope will prove to be of some practical assistance in the future grouping of these cases (Table 3.1).

Three types of congenital eviscerations through anterior abdominal wall defects in the newborn period were presented in Table 3.1 of this publication. Omphalocele was presented as an umbilical cord anomaly featuring a herniation of viscera into the base of the umbilical cord. A covering membranous sac or its ruptured remnants were present with the umbilical cord inserting into the sac. Gastroschisis was classified as an extraumbilical abdominal wall anomaly with a large eviscerated matrix. The defect was extraumbilical with the

Table 3.1. Occurrence of necrosis/gangrene, perforation, atresia and stenosis in reported cases of gastroschisis not managed by preterm and prelabor cesarian section

Author	Year	No. Cases Gastroschisis	Necrosis/ Gangrene	Perforation	Atresia	Stenosis	More than one	Total of cases with one or more	Percent of Cases with one or more
Moore & Stokes[1]	1953	2			1			1	50
Lewis et al[23]	1973	31	6		2			8	26
Hollabaugh & Boles[24]	1973	47		1	6			7	15
Amoury et al[50]	1977	46	1				5	6	13
Pokorny et al[51]	1981	22	1		5			6	27
Luck et al[49]	1985	106	3	3	7	3		16	15
Tibboel* et al[41]	1986	6			1	2		3	50
Bond* et al[36]	1988	11	2		2			4	36
Gornall[52]	1989	22			4		1	5	23
Moore[11]	1992	8	1		1			2	25
Totals		301	14	4	29	5	6	58	19.3

*Antenatal ultrasound diagnosis

insertion of the umbilical cord into the abdominal wall being flush with it (not into a sac) and normal. There were no covering sacs or ruptured remnants.

Gastro ("belly") and schisis ("cleft") appeared to be appropriate and consistent with uncovered dorsal torso defects (cranioschisis and rachischisis). Omphalocele (rather than examphalos or other terms then in use) was selected as most appropriate in description and consistent with covered dorsal torso defects (encephalocele, meningocele, myelomeningocele).

In searching for the appropriate terms, I consulted the Shorter *Oxford English Dictionary*[15] (then residing in the library of my father's home—and now in my own). In addition to the umbilical cord, omphalos also referred to a stone in Greece, the Omphalos Stone. It was located at Delphi at the site of the Delphic Oracle ruins. The original now is in the Museum at Delphi at the Oracle site and a reproduction is at the site of discovery within the Oracle compound. This was the source of great prestige for the Delphic Oracle. According to widely believed legend, Zeus, king of the Greek gods, being somewhat of a scientist, wished to discover the center of the earth. He released two eagles, which flew at the same rate of speed, from each of the two corners of the world. They met over Delphi which clearly marked it as the center of the world. I, on my first visit to Greece, made a point of visiting Delphi to see this Omphalos Stone which marked the spot of the eagles' meeting. The site high on Mount Parnassus and overlooking the Ionian Sea is one of incredible beauty and the Omphalos Stone (original and reproduction) look exactly like an omphalocele.

From the vantage point of 40 years of retrospective wisdom, the 1953 *Surgery* publication[1] was a most remarkable one. Among the reasons are as follows:

1. It established the terminology, classification and differentiation for gastroschisis and omphalocele which have withstood the test of time.
2. It described for the first time the association of prematurity with gastroschisis.
3. It recorded for the first time the association of gastroschisis and very young mothers.
4. It identified for the first time the occurrence of intestinal atresia (large as well as small intestine) in gastroschisis babies.
5. It was the first report of the use of skin flaps to cover gastroschisis eviscerated intestine and the occurrence of very small peritoneal cavities in gastroschisis babies (Fig. 3.1).
6. It was the first report of the use of biological covering and "watchful waiting" to manage intestinal atresias in gastroschisis.
7. It described the first use of intestinal anastomosis (ileocolic) in the management of gastroschisis intestinal atresia and successful reestablishment of alimentary tract continuity (the passage of stools in the first two postoperative days).
8. It identified and illustrated (photomicrograph) for the first time the histological cause of the bowel wall thickening ("peel") and leathery consistency to be acute granulation tissue external to the serosa with normal appearing bowel wall under the serosa. These findings have been duplicated and confirmed by the important and in-depth histologic studies of ten gastroschisis bowel specimens from 105 gastroschisis neonates by Amoury et al[16] in 1988. These studies have concerned both light microscopic and ultrastructural findings as well as the use of special stains. They found that the serosal "peel" was by far the most consistently abnormal element in the intestinal wall. Their observations indicated that the peel is primarily deposited on the serosal surface rather than in the subserosa. This was further confirmed to them by the basically normal histological appearance of the serosa following resolution of the peel in two of their patients. Ischemic damage to the intestinal wall was encountered only in

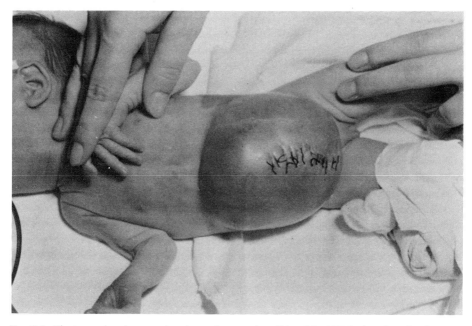

Fig. 3.1. Photograph taken at the time of operation (May 25, 1951) showing the first use (published) of skin flaps to cover a gastroschisis at birth in a newborn infant. The mass was quite large and with multiple atresias. The infant was born five weeks prematurely and weighed 4 pounds and 1 ounce. The gastroschisis defect was enlarged inferiorly and superiorly and widely mobilized skin flaps were required to cover this large mass. This infant was operated upon by me.

those neonates with complicating atresia. These are all particularly important observations concerning cause, prevention and management of intestinal thickening and "peel" (Fig. 3.2).

9. It described for the first time the rapid (2 week) disappearance of the bowel wall thickening and large and firm gelatinous matrix under the biological covering (skin flaps).

10. It also correlated for the first time the duration of labor with the size of the matrix/"peel"—huge with 20 hours of labor and much smaller with five hours of labor.

11. It reported for the first time the fortuitous use of gelatinous matrix and bowel wall thickening ("peel") for metabolic support (auto-"hyperalimentation") during the prolonged (18 day) postoperative period of "watchful waiting".

12. This was the first report of a "series" of gastroschisis cases (2 cases).

13. The report of two cases of gastroschisis

within the short period of three months doubled the world's reported authentic cases of gastroschisis and raised the question that gastroschisis might be more frequent than indicated by the reported cases.

14. It suggested for the first time that the bowel wall thickening/"peel" and gelatinous matrix might have resulted from prolonged immersion of eviscerated intestine in amniotic fluid (probably wrong).

In 1963, after a hiatus of 10 years, I revisited gastroschisis with the report of an additional case in *Annals of Surgery* and a review of the budding literature which had accumulated.[2] The literature, including the new case being reported, had expanded to 32 cases with 14 infants being treated successfully by surgery, all single case reports. In five of the successfully managed cases, the large skin flap closure creating a large ventral hernia approach had been utilized. Prematurity was encountered in one half

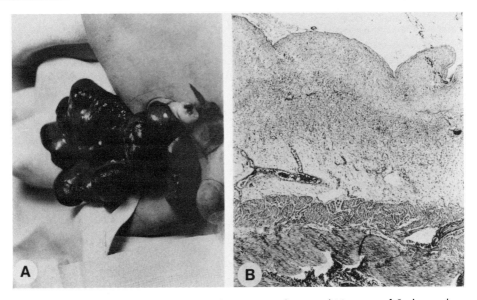

Fig. 3.2. Photograph and photomicrograph from Case 2 of gastroschisis paper of Stokes and me (Surgery 1953; 33:112-120). The appearance of the gastroschisis protrusion with discoloration, rigidity and thickening ("peel") is shown in (A) and the thickening/"peel" identified as granulation tissue external to the musculature and serosa is shown in (B).

of the cases in which this information was available. Intestinal atresia, the only serious malformation encountered, was reported in three cases.

The author's new case was the first born child of young parents and had a massive and particularly rigid herniation which included the urinary bladder as well as all of the large and small intestine. Large skin flaps clearly could not cover the huge and rigid eviscerated mass. During this period, the author had carried out a number of decortications of inflammatory granulation "peel" entrapped lungs. The "peel" decorticated in these cases bore a resemblance to the extraserosal bowel wall thickening granulation tissue found histologically in Case 2 of the author's 1953 gastroschisis publication. Decortication seemed to be the only way to reduce the size and rigidity of the mass sufficiently to cover it with large skin flaps. Complete decortication of both the intestinal and urinary bladder masses was carried out by careful dissection and in much the same manner of a pulmonary decortication with the much the same sort of "peel" and with normal appearing intestine underlying the removed "peel". This was a difficult and

tedious dissection. Considerable edema fluid was encountered under the "peel" and had helped exaggerate the size of the prolapsed intestinal mass. Most of the edema was removed during decortication and later by compression. Following decortication, the large and small intestine were essentially normal in appearance (except for a few punctate serosal hemorrhages) and normal in pliability. Despite the abnormally small peritoneal cavity, the decorticated intestines could easily be covered by dissected skin flaps with ventral hernia creation. The postoperative course was quite uneventful. A meconium stool was passed the day after operation. Good bowel sounds were heard on the third postoperative day—a remarkable occurrence in a case of gastroschisis. Oral feedings were started the next day, skin flap sutures were removed 16 days following operation and the infant was home on the next day. The ventral hernia was repaired at seven months of age. At 18 months following operation the child had grown and developed normally and the mother had given birth to another normal infant. The very important and critical observation in this case was that the intestine under the decorticated "peel" was normal both in appearance and function and that intestinal malfunction in gastroschisis is largely "peel"-generated and is decortification-reversible.

In 1964, I contributed a chapter on "gastroschisis" to the new and scholarly book on *Hernia* edited by L.M. Nyhus and H.N. Harkins[3] and published by J.B. Lippincott and in 1965 published in *Surgery* (with Judd and Wince)[4] reports of two gastroschisis infants treated successfully with the skin flap closure method first used by me in 1951.

In 1963, Professor Peter Rickham of Liverpool (U.K.) published a report in *Archives of Diseases of Childhood*[17] involving 13 patients with ruptured omphalocele and gastroschisis with only two survivors (85% mortality). No distinction between the two groups was made and the number of cases of gastroschisis in this experience is not known. Nonetheless, this was a substantial experience compared with the largely single case reports up to this time and pointed to both the frequency and gravity of these conditions.

Gastroschisis attracted little attention through the middle and late 1960s. The number of reports and the number of cases per report remained quite small and the mortality remained high. Prillewitz and deBoer[18] reported three cases in 1968 in the Netherlands surgical literature and also in 1968 Denes et al[19] reported 5 cases in *Surgery* from Budapest, Hungary. The mortalities were 33 and 40%. During the next year, 1969, Rangarathnam, Lal and Swenson[20] in the *Archives of Surgery* reported 8 cases of gastroschisis seen at the Children's Memorial Hospital in Chicago during the previous two and a half years. Only four of their patients survived (50% mortality). They were able to find only 50 recorded cases of gastroschisis in the world's literature. In 1971, the mortality in seven cases of gastroschisis from South Africa was 57%. Also in 1971, eight cases of gastroschisis were recorded from the Adelaide (Australia) Children's Hospital by Savage and Davey.[21] One was minimally eviscerated and easily repaired. Four had substantial evisceration

and all died. Three additional cases were managed successfully by the creation of transverse ventral hernias by transverse incision through all abdominal layers with skin flap closure only.

In the early 1970s a veritable explosion occurred in the number of cases of gastroschisis reported. In 1972, Gilbert et al[22] reported 17 cases from Miami while, in 1973, Lewis et al[23] reported 31 cases from St. Louis and Hollabaugh and Boles[24] 47 cases from Columbus, Ohio. The mortality, however, remained high. It was 47% in the Miami experience, 49% for Columbus and 32% for St. Louis. In the more recent cases mortality statistics had improved to 30% in Columbus and 25% in St. Louis.

The Columbus experience illustrated quite well the sudden and marked increase in the incidence of gastroschisis. In the 20 year period up to 1967, the incidence of gastroschisis was one case per year (20 cases). In the five year period from 1967 to 1972, they had 27 cases of gastroschisis (5.4 cases per year) for a 5.4 fold increase in the incidence during this short period of time. A rather similar (5.6 fold) marked increase in gastroschisis incidence was found by Nur and me in Scandinavia during this period in a review of an international survey of 490 cases of gastroschisis and omphalocele published in *Pediatric Surgery International* in 1986.[7] A 1980 update of the Columbus (Ohio) Children's Hospital experience by King, Savrin and Boles[25] increased the yearly incidence of gastroschisis (64 cases in 9 years) to 7.1 cases per year. A further updating of the gastroschisis experience in 1990 by Caniano et al[26] placed the yearly incidence of gastroschisis (80 cases in 7 years) at 11.4 cases per year—a 11.4 fold increase from the prior-to-1967 experience. This is highly significant and should spur the search for the teratogenic agent or agents involved in gastroschisis and associated efforts at prevention. A 1984 report in *Pediatrics* by Sarda and Bard[27] clearly indicated maternal alcohol consumption to be one of those teratogenic agents.

The Lewis et al[23] experience included six cases of intestinal necrosis and two of intestinal atresia in their 31 cases (26%). They attributed their improved results to the recent availability of "hyperalimentation" (total parenteral nutrition, TPN), to improved respiratory ventilatory assist devices and to the availability of silastic sheets (silon) with dacron mesh impregnation which could be used for prosthesis construction for the enlargement of the abnormally small peritoneal cavities of these infants to contain the large and firm eviscerated masses of intestine with their "peels" and gelatinous matrices of various degrees of severity.

Within a period of three months in late 1968 and early 1969, Gilbert et al[28] and Allen and Wrenn[29] had reported the successful use of Dow Corning Silon-dacron mesh prostheses for gastroschisis repair. The Gilbert et al studies were published in the December 1968 issue of the *Journal of Pediatric Surgery* and included 20 animal studies (15 dogs and 5 pigs) as well as six patients (one with gastroschisis). They considered one sheet of dacron covered on both sides by silicon rubber to be the best prosthesis. Their prosthesis was constructed to resemble a hernia-type of mound.

Allen and Wrenn[29] in the February 1969 issue of the *Journal of Pediatric Surgery* reported the use of Dow Corning sacs made from dacron coated with silastic for temporary covering of eviscerated intestines in two cases of gastroschisis and two cases of ruptured omphalocele with one death (their first case). They employed a long and comparatively narrow "silo" shape which permitted both gravity and progressive heavy ligature/tube narrowing of the sac from the top down to induce eviscerated intestines to return to the peritoneal cavity which hopefully was slowly increasing in size.

The 1972 Gilbert et al[22] 17 case gastroschisis report and the 1971 Touloukian and Spackman[30] studies from Yale cast some interesting light on the bowel thickening and apparent shortening problem in gastroschisis and its duration. Gilbert et al[22] measured bowel length at the initial sur-

gical procedure in 12 babies with gastroschisis and found marked shortening with the small bowel length averaging 76 cm and the small and large bowel combined averaging 113 cm. These figures may be compared with the 267 cm and 317 cm measurements for 26 neonates with no intra-abdominal disease studied by them at postmortem. They also recorded that this "short bowel" was not an irreversible problem. One of their patients was reexplored at one week due to a leak at the gastrostomy site. The thick greenish exudate had disappeared and the bowel length had increased by one third. Another baby was reexplored at one months for bowel obstruction. Again the thickening exudate had disappeared and the small bowel had tripled in length from the original 50 cm to 158 cm.

The 1971 publication of Touloukian and Spackman[30] in the *Journal of Pediatric Surgery* provided particularly important information relative to the fate of the thickened, "shortened" and discolored intestine in gastroschisis in five of six surviving of 10 patients. All six of the surviving patients were found to have normal growth and development. Barium studies in five patients showed normal small intestinal lengths and mucosal patterns in all five despite initial operation estimation of intestinal "shortening" to by one third to one half of normal length. They concluded that the shortening and severe inflammatory thickening of the eviscerated intestines are reversible following gastroschisis repair in surviving patients. Their report also was of interest that, in two of their four nonsurviving patients, intestinal necrosis and gangrene (ileocolic volvulus and midgut volvulus) co-existed with intestinal atresia. This finding suggests a continuum of these two conditions and of comparatively recent onset (possibly labor stimulated?) and an incidence of these complications in 20% of their gastroschisis patients.

As indicated above, ongoing (necrosis and gangrene) or terminated (atresia and meconium peritonitis) intrauterine intestinal necrosis or both present major problems in the care of newborn infants with gastroschisis. In the larger reported series, these problems occur in from 15 to 25% of the cases and represent major challenges. They will be considered in detail in the challenges section.

The great breakthrough in survival and mortality statistics occurred in the 1974 report of Raffensperger and Jona[31] in the February issue of *Surgery, Gynecology and Obstetrics* (138:230-234). In a three-year period (July 1970-July 1973) they treated 24 infants with gastroschisis (8 cases per year) and achieved the remarkable mortality of only 16% despite six infants (25%) with atresia (2), perforation (2) (1, Meckel's) or gangrene (2 with 1 total). They attributed those remarkable results to the large number of patients in a short period of time which permitted them to develop a management plan which took advantage of new anesthetic and ventilation techniques and intravenous hyperalimentation (total parenteral nutrition, TPN) and their intensive care unit. All infants were admitted directly to their intensive care unit where hypothermia was readily corrected with heat lamps and warming mattresses (the average time between hospital admission and operation was one and a quarter hour) and antibiotic therapy was initiated. Cyanosis of the infants on admission disappeared with warming. They also avoided excessive fluid administration which may have contributed to the deaths of my two patients with gastroschisis in his 1953 report. The three operative approaches employed were skin without fascia closure in 15 cases (62.5%), a Silon prosthesis in 5 (20.8%) and closure of both skin and fascia in 4 (16.7%). An early and disastrous (fatal) experience with gastrostomy under widely unmined skin flaps (Moore operation) led to the abandonment of both. They wisely speculated that, of the almost simultaneous introduction of hyperalimentation (TPN) and silastic prostheses, the improved mortality rates reported by them and others were most likely due to improved nutrition.

The availability of these and new modalities such as silastic prostheses, hyperalimentation (TPN) and improved postoperative ventilator support with muscle paralysis triggered a vigorous "contest" between the "do-it-yourself prosthesis" advocates and the "fascial-closure-or-bust" proponents. Actually serious flaws existed with both approaches. Surgeon-at-the-operating-table constructed silastic silo prostheses with multiple (minimum of 3) suture lines which were water and bacteria tight in neither direction were recognized early on as presenting hazards of sepsis and bowel perforation and intestinal fistula formation. The fascial-closure-or-else approach ignored the serious potential of excessive and necrosis producing intestinal compression while the lungs were being spared by improved ventilatory techniques and methodology. These matters will be considered in more detail in the Challenges section as well as the "surprise" winner, the Shermeta bag [32] and the Shermeta application technique[33] (stay tuned!).

In 1975, a surprise suggestion appeared that gastroschisis and omphalocele were not separate and uniquely different disease/malformations but rather the same and that, indeed, gastroschisis was a "myth".[34] This undocumented assertion led to an expansion of knowledge of gastroschisis and omphalocele by its refutation in a 1978 publication in the February issue of the *Journal of Pediatric Surgery* by Noordijk and Bloemsma-Jonkman[35] of the Sophia Children's Hospital in Rotterdam (the Netherlands) in an article entitled "Gastroschisis: No Myth" and by me in an article in the November 1977 issue of *Surgery* entitled "Gastroschisis and Omphalocele: Clinical Differences".[5]

The Noordijk and Bloemsma-Jonkman[35] report involved the careful and in-depth study of the family histories of 37 patients with omphalocele and 14 patients with gastroschisis. They found that the number of congenital abnormalities in families of omphalocele patients was considerably larger than in the families of gastroschisis patients. They concluded that the difference was so significant that they could assume that genetic factors play a role in the origin of omphalocele, whereas this is not the case in gastroschisis. They advocated genetic evaluation and counseling for the parents of children with omphalocele but not for those of parents of children with gastroschisis. They also concluded that there appeared to be little contraindication for another pregnancy in the case of gastroschisis.

The 1977 article by the author of this book[5] considered the clinical differences encountered in a review of 236 cases of omphalocele and 278 cases of gastroschisis largely from the recent literature. Multiple, marked and significant differences were encountered and chronicled in detail in this publication.

The matter of the sameness or difference of these conditions is of considerably more than of theoretical or "passing" interest and significance in the era of antenatal ultrasound diagnosis of gastroschisis and omphalocele and their unique ultrasound differences. The tragic "termination" of seven gastroschisis pregnancies recorded in two recent (1988 and 1989) publications[36,37] should render beyond question the importance of a recognition of these two malformations, gastroschisis and omphalocele, as quite different conditions in every important respect and that incipient parents should be so notified.

The development of alpha-feto-protein (AFP) screening for neural crest malformations and the fortuitous associated antenatal ultrasound diagnosis of gastroschisis has also had an "up" (favorable) side in providing an opportunity for preterm and prelabor management of gastroschisis by Cesarian section. This will be considered in greater detail in the Challenges section as the most important challenge of all relating to gastroschisis.

CHALLENGES

1. *The most important challenge by far is whether or not to do a preterm and prelabor elective Cesarian section once lung maturity is established by biochemical testing of amniotic fluid in cases of antenatal ultrasound diagnosis of gastroschisis.*

If elective preterm and prelabor Cesarian section delivery of gastroschisis babies once lung maturity has been established will eliminate not only the dreadful bowel thickening, "peel" and matrix formation but also the occurrence of the serious acquired antenatal complications of intestinal atresia/stenosis necrosis/gangrene and perforation as early observations by a limited number of others and me suggest, the answer is an emphatic *yes*!

Virginal, "peel"-free and normal appearing bowel achieved by preterm and prelabor Cesarian section can readily be inserted back into the peritoneal cavity and the relatively small defect closed with umbilicus preservation in a matter of minutes (10 to 15). The simplicity and speed of this undertaking render its use as an outpatient procedure or at most an overnight admission quite within the realm of reason and practicality. This approach is in stark contrast to the dreadful problems with the typical gastroschisis thickened and rigid bowel mass with frequent (20%) atresia, perforation or necrosis/gangrene, significant mortality and morbidity and prolonged (multi-month) hospitalization with its phenomenal monetary, as well as other, costs.

An important report by Lenke and Hatch[38] of Seattle, Washington appeared in the March 1986 issue of *Obstetrics and Gynecology*. It concerned 24 cases of gastroschisis referred to the Children's Orthopedic Hospital of Seattle between 1982 and 1984. Seventeen had been delivered by the vaginal route and seven (four at the University of Washington Hospital) were delivered by Cesarian section. All infants born by section were repaired by primary closure without mortality or complications. In all of these cases the operative reports indicated "no peel" or "easy to repair". Of the 17 vaginal delivery patients, two had intestinal necrosis or perforation at birth and three died with one additional expected death from total bowel necrosis and resection induced by too tight a primary closure (24% mortality). One of the deaths resulted from post-primary closure necrotizing enterocolitis. An updating of this Seattle experience appeared in *Obstetrics and Gynecology* in 1988[39] and included only infants born at the University of Washington Hospital. Of the 14 infants, three had induction of labor and attempted vaginal delivery and three required more than one surgical operation, one for resection of ischemic bowel after primary closure. One had a two-stage repair involving silo use. It was not indicated which patients (attempted vaginal delivery and induced labor or otherwise) required additional operations. This report lacked the clarity of the initial one.

In 1988, I[9] published in *Pediatric Surgery International* the details of a most remarkable personal experience with gastroschisis. Two consecutive cases of gastroschisis diagnosed in utero by AFP induced ultrasound were delivered by elective preterm and prelabor Cesarian section and were found to have no bowel thickening or "peel". The normal appearing bowel was readily and easily replaced in the peritoneal cavity with primary closure of all layers with no tension at all. This was the first time in 36 years of personal experience that I had encountered a case of gastroschisis without the "standard" bowel thickening, rigidity, discoloration and "peel". I speculated that the trauma of labor and delivery might be a factor in the serious bowel damage routinely encountered in gastroschisis and recommended this elective preterm and prelabor approach for the management of antenatal diagnosed cases of gastroschisis.

Also in 1988, Professor Sture Hagberg and associates[40] reported from Gothenburg University in Sweden an experience with gastroschisis which virtually mirrored mine as cited above. They compared a four-year (1984-1988) experience with 11 cases of gastroschisis with an earlier (1971-1980) experience with 27 cases. In the 1984-1988 experience, seven cases of gastroschisis were diagnosed by ultrasound and all seven were delivered by elective Cesarian section. There was a total lack of bowel thickening, edema and "peel" in all seven cases and all were repaired primarily, easily and

with umbilicus preservation. There was no mortality and hospital stay was shortened significantly in comparison with the earlier experience. Nine of the 27 cases in the earlier experience had been delivered by acute, labor-induced Cesarian section and 18 by the vaginal route. Eight of these infants were managed by primary closure and 19 by secondary closure. The mean hospital stay for the former group was 50 days and that for the latter group was 81 days. The mean period for total parenteral nutrition (TPN) was 18 days for the primary closure group and 44 days for the secondary closure group. There were two deaths (7.4%) in this earlier group of 27 patients. The authors of this important publication speculated that labor trauma was the most likely cause of the bowel thickening.

In a 1986 publication of a joint Rotterdam and Glasgow experience[41] with 50 cases of gastroschisis, there were 13 deaths (26%) and 10 newborn infants were found to have associated atresias of the small intestine (20%). Twenty-two of their patients (44%) required silastic sacs before secondary closure of the defects. Six patients (all Glasgow) were diagnosed and followed prenatally by ultrasound. The prenatal care did not involve Cesarian section. At delivery three of these six patients were found to have atresias or stenosis (50%) and five died (33%).

A 1990 report from Ohio State University and the Children's Hospital of Columbus by Caniano et al[26] presented an awesome picture of the "costs" on multiple levels of the "traditional" forms of delivery of babies with gastroschisis. Their report concerned 80 gastroschisis patients referred to them between 1979 and 1986. Ten of the 80 patients had intestinal atresias (12.5%) and were classed as "complicated" cases. Their report was concerned largely with the costs in time and gold, as well as results, in the 70 "uncomplicated" cases and their operative management with or without silo prosthetic repairs. For the silo group of patients the cost in hospital days was 56 days and in money was $39,900. This group constituted approximately one half of their "uncomplicated" group. The cost for the nonsilo group was 47 hospital days and $32,800. The cost in money for the 10 "complicated" cases with intestinal atresia was not given. Two of the 10 died and four additional patients experienced multiple complications and the short bowel syndrome with initial hospital stays ranging from eight months to three years. The four lucky "complicated"/atresia patients who escaped death or the short bowel syndrome did not escape all complications and had an average hospital stay of 65 days. A prior report from this hospital concerning atresia or intestinal perforation in seven newborn infants with gastroschisis had reported seven deaths (100% mortality).[24]

In 1992, I[11] published in *Pediatric Surgery International* (7:256-259) an article entitled "The role of labor in gastroschisis bowel thickening and prevention by elective preterm and prelabor cesarian section". This report concerned 12 consecutive cases of gastroschisis seen during the prior three-year period. Four were managed by elective preterm and prelabor Cesarian section as soon as lung maturity could be established by biochemical means and eight by delivery after the onset of labor, four by vaginal delivery and four by Cesarian section. There was no intestinal thickening or "peel" in any of the four infants born by elective preterm and prelabor section. All were quickly and easily repaired (the last two with umbilicus preservation) with no associated atresias, stenosis, necrosis/gangrene or antenatal intestinal perforation and with minimal lengths of hospitalization which easily could have been even shorter. The eight cases delivered after the onset of labor all had marked intestinal thickening, two (25%) had severe and extensive intestinal necrosis (40% of small intestine) or severe atresias ("apple peel"), and one died (12.5%). All had prolonged and complicated hospital stays with multiple operations. I strongly recommended the routine use of elective preterm and prelabor section in all cases of gastroschisis diagnosed prenatally by the alpha-feto protein (AFP)

screening and ultrasound. The concluding paragraph of this 1992 article is as follows:

> The debilitating and severely compromising bowel thickening of gastroschisis, its awesome cost in financial resources as well as in morbidity, mortality and associated necrosis and atresia and its preventability by elective preterm and prelabor section as soon as lung maturity has been established provide very strong support for this approach to the improved care of gastroschisis and for the routine use of AFP screening and ultrasound studies in all cases of human pregnancy.

2. The second most important challenge with respect to the management of gastroschisis is which operative approach to use in cases of bowel thickening, rigidity and "peel" formation associated with "traditional" delivery after onset of gut-traumatizing labor (vaginal delivery or emergency/nonelective Cesarian section).

The major options for these difficult-to-manage cases are primary closure with large skin flaps only (Moore operation[1]), small skin flaps only (Raffensperger operation[31]) or both fascial and skin closure and the use of prosthetics in the form of silo sacs fashioned at the operating table from dacron mesh impregnated silastic sheets with multiple suture lines or the seamless Shermeta bag[32] with the Shermeta placement technique.[33]

The silo sac introduced by Allen and Wrenn[29] was a major advance in its time with wide use and popularity. The silo sac operation introduced in 1969 made obsolete the decortication operation introduced by me[2] in 1963 for management of the eviscerated masses of intestine which were too huge and rigid to be managed by large skin flap closure. Silo sac problems with sepsis and gut necrosis and fistula formation were encountered early on and proved increasingly troublesome with the passage of time. Reports of difficulty with the Silon pouch approach by Rubin and Ein[42,43] in the mid and late 1970s triggered an unfortunate rush to the primary fascia and skin operation. Their 1976 report in the *Journal of Pediatric Surgery*[42] recorded a mortality of 35% with silon pouches in 23 newborn infants with gastroschisis.

Pouch difficulties and the availability of new and improved ventilating support supplemented by muscle paralysis turned the rush to primary fascial closure into an avalanche.[44-46] Experience and time have indicated that the risks of excessive pressure on viscera with primary fascia closure was underestimated in the initial enthusiasm for this operation.

Recent (1988) reports by Ein et al[47] of Toronto and Gainesville of severe and extensive bowel necrosis after primary fascial closure and by Oldham, Coran, Wesley and associates[48] of Ann Arbor (University of Michigan) recording a surprisingly high (45%) incidence of necrotizing enterocolitis after primary fascial repair should temper enthusiasm for this clearly hazardous and risky approach even when supplemented by "stretching".

The sound and non"trendy" approach of the Raffensperger group[31,49] of Chicago over the years and with many (106) patients with gastroschisis, with the use of short skin flaps only in over one half of their patients, has produced consistently better results with respect to both mortality and morbidity (complications) that have been achieved by the exclusive use of silastic pouches and silos or primary fascial closure.

However, at the present time (1993), for the grand prize the author's vote for the preferred and best management approach to the thickened, rigid bowel "peel" problem goes to the Shermeta bag[32] and Shermeta bag placement technique.[33] The original publication and introduction of this bag in its original version appeared in the December 1975 issue of the *Journal of Pediatric Surgery* (10:973-975) in an article by Dennis Shermeta and Alex Haller of Johns Hopkins.[32]

The Shermeta bag is an ingenious device. It is a seamless and transparent silicone rubber bag of a silo shape with a firm yet pliable circular enlargement at the base. A steel coil inside the base silicone ring

enlargement provides the firmness and pliability which are ideal for placement of the thickened eviscerated gut within the bag and the placement of the bag base ring within the peritoneal cavity at the evisceration site (Fig. 3.3). A single heavy ligature purse-string through the skin at the margins of the defect secures the base ring and the gut-containing bag without the need for any skin-bag sutures whatsoever (Shermeta bag placement technique[33]). The top of the bag has a silicone extension with a hole to permit upward bag tension and contents elevation. The entire operation requires at most five minutes and provides a sterile and skin-to-bag sutureless environment for bag elevation to facilitate gut return and peritoneal cavity enlargement both by gravity and progressive bag size diminution by repeated umbilical tape-type heavy ligature placement around the bag in a downward direction. This bag and the purse-string technique of its placement make obsolete all other approaches to the management of this most difficult "peel" gut thickening and rigidity problem in "traditional" delivery cases of gastroschisis.

3. The third most important challenge involves the management of the very serious atresias, gut necrosis/gangrene and gut perforation which occur with relative frequency (15 to 25%) in association with gut thickening, rigidity and "peel" formation in "traditional" delivery gastroschisis. The "peel" thickening and rigidity greatly complicate the management of these complications.

The use of biological tissue covering and "watchful waiting" (18 days) in the author's first case in his 1953 report resulted in total disappearance of the huge matrix and "peel" formation with normal appearing bowel resulting to permit a comparatively easy atresia bypassing by ileocolic anastomosis. Despite the passage of 40 years and extensive experience with other approaches, this still remains the best and safest approach, particularly with the availability of TPN and effective sump tube chronic naso-gastric suction decompression.

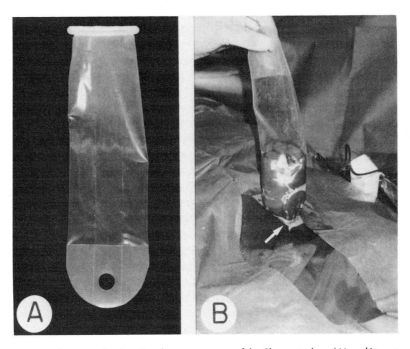

Fig. 3.3. Photographs showing the appearance of the Shermeta bag (A) and its use in a case of gastroschisis employing the Shermeta bag placement technique (B). The bag is a transparent and seamless silastic bag with a silastic covered metal coil at the base for combined mild rigidity and plasticity for ease of intra-abdominal placement and a mesh reinforced top with a hole for suspension of bag for gravity assistance in controlled gastroschisis gut return (also assisted with progressive bag shortening with externally applied tape, ligature, etc.). The intra-abdominal base coil is secured in place by a heavy purse-string suture through the skin at the slightly enlarged gastroschisis defect margin (arrow). This permits mild upward tension on the bag. The transparent silastic provides excellent visual monitoring of the "peel" thickened gut. The placement of the gastroschisis gut in the sterile Shermeta bag and its securing with the heavy purse-string suture require a maximum of five minutes (Shermeta bag placement technique). The bag may be obtained from the Mentor Company, 5425 Hollister Ave., Santa Barbara, CA 93111. Phone (805) 967-3451.

In the 1973 report of Hollabaugh and Boles[24] from the Columbus (Ohio) Children's Hospital 7 of 47 gastroschisis infants had atresia (6 patients) or gut perforation (1 patient) and were managed by atresia resection at birth in the presence of gut thickening and "peel" formation. All 7 (100%) died.

The first publication to address the problem of atresia complicating gastroschisis both in content and in title was the 1977 report in the September issue of *Surgery* by Armoury, Ashcraft and Holden[50] from Kansas City, Missouri. This report, given before the Central Surgical Association, must be accredited one of the great classic publications in pediatric surgery. It

is a classic for its excellence in every way; lucid case reports, perceptive comments, excellent illustrations and drawings and a scholarly review of the literature. Here, for the first time, a continuum in gastroschisis infants of intestinal necrosis/gangrene, intestinal perforation and intestinal atresia or atresias, including the coexistence of two or all of these related problems and complications of gastroschisis in patients born by "traditional" delivery methods is presented. These problems occurred in six of their 46 patients (13%) with a mortality of 67%. Atresia, necrosis/gangrene and perforation occurred in two patients, multiple atresias and gangrene in one, single atresias and marginal viability or necrosis remnants in two and necrosis only in one with atresia developing post-intestinal anastomosis one cm proximal to a still patent anastomosis. At this time, the salvage of two of six so severely compromised gastroschisis patients was a remarkable achievement. Their review of the literature presented clear evidence of the hazard and multiple occurrence of atresia, necrosis/gangrene and perforation in gastroschisis cases in the period prior to 1973 when the marked increase in the incidence of gastroschisis occurred. Ten cases of atresia with gastroschisis had appeared in nine published reports. In only three of the ten (30%) did atresia alone occur. Six had atresia plus necrosis/gangrene (60%) and one had atresia with perforation and necrosis/gangrene (10%). Nine of the ten died for a mortality of 90%.

A major breakthrough in the management of atresia and associated complications in gastroschisis occurred in the June 1981 issue of the *Journal of Pediatric Surgery* (16:261-263) in a paper by Pokorny, Harberg and McGill[51] from Houston, Texas. The basic principles of their approach were proximal gut decompression (ileostomy in all cases) and delay of two to four weeks in definitive anastomic reconstruction to permit "peel" and intestinal thickening to disappear. One infant with proximal colon atresia was managed by cecum resection and end ileostomy with definitive repair deferred to 10 months of age. Two of these patients had single atresias, one multiple atresia, one atresia with necrosis/gangrene and one with necrosis/gangrene only. All five of their patients were managed successfully without mortality (0%). In all of their four cases managed by delayed anastomosis (14, 22, 24, and 28 days) the "peel", thickening and related problems had disappeared with normal appearing intestine which could be managed by primary single layer anastomosis as with intestinal atresia in the newborn without gastroschisis and its related problems. These observations concerning "peel" and thickening disappearance within 14 to 28 days after eviscerated gut cover-

age reconfirmed the significance and importance of earlier observations by me in my first case in the 1953 publications[1] and of Gilbert et al[22] in two cases reexplored at 14 and 28 days.

The continuing hazard of atresia-perforation-necrosis with primary anastomosis (100% mortality in 7 cases in 1975 reported by Hollabaugh and Boles[24]) was little changed in the 1989 report of Peter Gornall[52] from Birmingham, England. Four of his five patients had atresia only (multiple atresias in one) and one had atresia with perforation. All three with primary anastomosis had multiple operations associated with stricture stenosis and one died. Of the other two cases, one with a proximal colon atresia was managed by colostomy and closure at eight months and the other by mass coverage after mass dissection abandonment. The mass-covered infant was reexplored at 32 days. By this time, a jejunal atresia had produced massive dilation of proximal intestine which require extensive tapering which resulted in chronic obstruction and ultimately in a most severely handicapped child. This result illustrates the inadvisability in delaying reexploration so long.

Shah and Woolley,[53] of the Children's Hospital of Los Angeles, reported in 1991 the successful use of closure and delayed resection and anastomosis in two cases at one week and 20 days after the initial closure.

For the extensive necrosis/gangrene patient with a genuine hazard of serious short bowel difficulties, the use of large skin flaps with extensive peritoneal Penrose drain drainage and TPN, as found in Case 1 in my 1991 paper,[10] involving the "patch, drain and wait" approach (illustrated in article photographs) may facilitate maximum bowel salvage and the avoidance of serious short bowel difficulties.

The management of atresia and its associated complications (necrosis/gangrene, perforation and stenosis) represents a major problem in gastroschisis care as its incidence approximates 20% with a 15 to 25% range (Table 3.1). In this setting, prevention must also be considered an important component of management. In the 1992 publication, I[11] also suggested that preterm and prelabor Cesarian section might eliminate atresia-necrosis complications as well as the serious "peel" and thickening problems. If one is to compare the incidence of atresia and associated complications in ultrasound antenatal cases of gastroschisis managed either by "traditional" delivery (Table 3.1—reports of Tibboel et al[41] and Bond et al[36]) and by preterm and prelabor Cesarian section (Table 3.2—reports of Lenke and Hatch,[38] Moore[9,11] and Hagberg et al[40]), the results are rather dramatic. The incidence of atresia et al complications in "traditional" delivery in 17 cases was 7 (41%) and that in preterm and prelabor section in 18 cases was 0 (0%).

In summary for this challenge, the experiences of the author in 1953,[1] of Pokorny et al[51] in 1981 and Shah and Woolley[53] in 1991 would clearly indicate the use of coverage and delay of resection and intestinal anastomosis. As for the period of delay, it most likely should be about two weeks and delay beyond 30 days, being associated with marked and serious proximal bowel dilation[52] should be avoided. As to the best method of "coverage" and, although its use in this situation has not been reported, the author of this book would prefer the Shermeta bag [32] and Shermeta application

technique[33] (discussed in prior challenge section).

4. A fourth major challenge and elusive one is to determine the teratogenic cause or causes of gastroschisis so that preventative measures may be taken.

The issue of possible teratogenic factors was addressed in my 1986 publication[7] of data from an international survey which collected data on relative incidence in both time and geography, local and international, maternal age and pregnancy factors and drug (legal and illegal) and environmental factors. A marked increase in gastroschisis in the 1970s was noted. This also was a period of Vietnam War-induced increase in international tensions and drug use. The high incidence of gastroschisis in very young mothers also was noted and this also raised the question of drug use including contraceptives. Environmental factors were more difficult to elicit. As a follow-up to this survey, an International Registry of Gastroschisis and Omphalocele has been established in the author's research laboratory at the Harbor-UCLA Medical Center in Torrance, California. At present (1993) insufficient data has been accumulated to shed any light on this important teratogen challenge.

An important publication in this area appeared in *Pediatrics* in 1986 by Sarda and

Table 3.2. Occurrence of necrosis/gangrene, perforation, atresia and stenosis in reported cases of gastroschisis managed by preterm and prelabor cesarian section*.

Author	Year	No. Cases Gastroschisis	Necrosis/ Gangrene	Perforation	Atresia	Stenosis	More than one	Total of cases with one or more	Percent of cases with one or more
Lenke & Hatch[38]	1986	7	0	0	0	0	0	0	0
Moore[11]	1988 1992	4	0	0	0	0	0	0	0
Hagberg et al[40]	1988	7	0	0	0	0	0	0	0
Totals		18	0	0	0	0	0	0	0

*All antenatal ultrasound diagnosis

Bard[27] (74:94-96) concerning the appearance of gastroschisis in both of dizygotic twins born to an alcoholic mother who had consumed large amounts of alcohol in the first trimester of pregnancy. In addition to gastroschisis, both children had various stigmata of fetal alcohol syndrome.

CONCLUSION

By far the most important challenge in gastroschisis is the prevention of the serious thickening, "peel" and rigidity problem and the often associated and likely related necrosis/gangrene, perforation and atresia/stenosis complications which regularly accompany "traditional" delivery (vaginal or emergency labor-triggered Cesarian section). There is substantial information and clinical data suggesting that both of these critical challenges ("peel" thickening and atresia etc.) may be met successfully and prevented by elective preterm and prelabor Cesarian section once lung maturity has been established by biochemical means. The ultimate and most effective use of this approach will require antenatal ultrasound monitoring of all pregnancies.

In the all-too-frequent nonsection protected gastroschisis neonates with the customary and expected intestinal thickening, "peel" and rigidity, the use of the Shermeta bag [32] and Shermeta placement technique[33] clearly is the quickest, most effective and safest method of managing this dreadful and costly (morbidity, mortality, money) problem.

As for the management of the atresia/stenosis problem, prompt covering of the eviscerated mass and atresia/stenosis, nasogastric suction decompression, total parenteral nutrition (TPN) with a Broviac catheter and 10 to 15 days of "watchful waiting" to permit disappearance of the "peel"[1,9,11,16,22,51,53] to permit resection of atresia/atresias or stenosis and reestablishment of intestinal continuity using normal appearing and histologically normal intestine is clearly the approach of choice. Primary resection of atresias and anastomosis at birth are to be avoided at all cost.[24,52]

For the necrosis/gangrene and perforation cases, with or without atresia/atresias or stenosis, the proximal enterostomy and prompt (10-15 day) reexploration approach of Pokorny et al[51] would appear to be the safest. In the case of extensive necrosis where the hazard of short bowel syndrome is a genuine threat, my large skin flap closure and "patch, drain and wait" approach as described in Case 1 of my 1991 publication[10] would permit maximum salvage of compromised intestine.

The sorting out of etiologic and teratogenic factors will involve substantial international effort and cooperative data collection studies. The elimination of gastroschisis, if possible, is a number one priority but, unfortunately, one not likely to be achieved anytime soon. Nonetheless there is no reason not to make major efforts in this important area.

REFERENCES

1. Moore TC, Stokes GE. Gastroschisis: Report of two cases treated by a modification of the Gross operation for omphalocele. Surgery 1953; 33:112-120.
2. Moore TC. Gastroschisis with antenatal evisceration of the intestines and urinary bladder. Ann Surg 1963; 158:263-269.
3. Moore TC. Gastroschisis. In: Nyhus LN, Harkins HN, eds. Hernia. Philadelphia: Lippincott, 1964:334-337.
4. Judd DR, Wince LL, Moore TC. Gastroschisis: Report of two cases with survival. Surgery 1965; 58:1033-1036.
5. Moore TC. Gastroschisis and omphalocele: Clinical differences. Surgery 1977; 82: 561-568.
6. Moore TC, Nur K. An international survey of gastroschisis and omphalocele (490 cases): I. Nature and distribution of additional malformations. Pediatr Surg Int 1986; 1:46-50.
7. Moore TC, Nur K. An international survey of gastroschisis and omphalocele (490 cases): II. Relative incidence, pregnancy, and environmental factors. Pediatr Surg Int 1986; 1:105-109.
8. Moore TC, Nur K. An international survey of gastroschisis and omphalocele (490 cases):

III. Factors influencing outcome of surgical management. Pediatr Surg Int 1987; 2:27-32.

9. Moore TC. Elective preterm section for improved primary repair of gastroschisis. Pediatr Surg Int 1988; 4:25-26.

10. Moore TC. Management of midgut volvulus with extensive necrosis by "patch, drain and wait" in early infancy and childhood. Pediatr Surg Int 1991; 6:313-317.

11. Moore TC. The role of labor in gastroschisis bowel thickening and prevention by elective preterm and prelabor cesarian section. Pediatr Surg Int 1992; 7:256-259.

12. Kraus F. Zwei seltene Missbildungen. Deutche Med Wehrschr 1936; 62:258.

13. Bernstein P. Gastroschisis, A rare teratological condition in the newborn. Arch Pediatr 1940; 57:505-513.

14. Cantrell JR, Haller JA, Ravitch MM. A syndrome of congenital defects involving the abdominal wall, sternum, diaphragm, pericardium and heart. Surg Gynecol Obstet 1958; 107:602-614.

15. Shorter Oxford English Dictionary, Oxford: Clarendon, 1936; 1368.

16. Amoury RA, Beatty EC, Wood WG et al. Histology of the intestine in human gastroschisis—relationship to intestinal malfunciton: Dissolution of the "peel" and its ultrastructural characteristics. J Pediatr Surg 1988; 23:950-956.

17. Rickham PP. Rupture of exaomphalos and gastroschisis. Arch Dis Childh 1963; 38:138-141.

18. Prillewitz HW, deBoer HMM. Gastroschisis. Arch Chir Neerl 1968; 20:141.

19. Denes J, Leb J, Lucasc FV. Gastroschisis. Surgery 1968; 63:701-705.

20. Rangarathnam CS, Lal RB, Swenson O. Gastroschisis. Arch Surg 1969; 98:742-748.

21. Savage JP, Davey RB. The treatment of gastroschisis. J Pediatr Surg 1971; 6: 148-152.

22. Gilbert MG, Mencia LF, Puranik SR et al. Management of gastroschisis and short bowel: Report of 17 cases. J Pediatr Surg 1972; 7:598-606.

23. Lewis JE, Kraeger RR, Danis RK. Gastroschisis: Ten year review. Arch Surg 1973; 107:218-222.

24. Hollabaugh RS, Boles ET. The management of gastroschisis. J Pediatr Surg 1973; 8:263-270.

25. King DR, Savrin R, Boles ET. Gastroschisis update. J Pediatr Surg 1980; 15:553-557.

26. Caniano DA, Brokaw B, Ginn-Pease ME. An individualized approach to the management of gastroschisis. J Pediatr Surg 1990; 25:297-300.

27. Sarda P, Bard H. Gastroschisis in a case of dizygotic twins: The possible role of maternal alcohol consumption. Pediatrics 1984; 74:94-96.

28. Gilbert MG, Mencia LF, Brown WT et al. Staged surgical repair of large omphaloceles and gastroschisis. J Pediatr Surg 1968; 3:702-709.

29. Allen RG, Wrenn EL. Silon as a sac in the treatment of omphalocele and gastroschisis. J Pediatr Surg 1969; 4:3-8.

30. Touloukian RJ, Spackman. Gastrointestinal function and radiologic appearance following gastroschisis repair. J Pediatr Surg 1971; 6:427-434.

31. Raffensperger JG, Jona JZ. Gastroschisis. Surg Gynecol Obstet 1974; 138:230-234.

32. Shermeta DW, Haller JA. A new preformed transparent silo for the management of gastroschisis. J Pediatr Surg 1975; 10: 973-975.

33. Shermeta DW. Personal communication.

34. Shaw A. The myth of gastroschisis. J Pediatr Surg 1975; 10:235-244.

35. Noordijk JA, Bloemsma-Jonkman F. Gastroschisis: No myth. J Pediatr Surg 1978; 13:47-49.

36. Bond SJ, Harrison MR, Filly RA et al. Severity of intestinal damage in gastroschisis: Correlation with prenatal sonographic findings. J Pediatr Surg 1988; 23:520-525.

37. Lafferty PM, Emmerson AJ, Fleming PJ. Anterior abdominal wall defects. Arch Dis Child 1989; 64:1029-1031.

38. Lenke RR, Hatch EI. Fetal gastroschisis: A preliminary report advocating the use of Cesarian section. Obstet Gynecol 1986; 67:395-398.

39. Fitzsimmons J, Nyberg DA, Cyr DR et al. Perinatal management of gastroschisis. Obstet Gynecol 1988; 71:910-913.

40. Hagberg S, Hokegard KH, Rubenson A et

al. Prenatally diagnosed gastroschisis: A preliminary report advocating the use of elective Cesarian section. Z Kinderchir 1988; 43:419-421.

41. Tibboel D, Raine P, McNee M et al. Developmental aspects of gastroschisis. J Pediatr Surg 1986; 21:865-869.

42. Rubin SZ, Ein SH. Experience with 55 silon pouches. J Pediatr Surg 1976; 11:803-806.

43. Ein SH, Rubin SZ. Gastroschisis: Primary closure or silon pouch. J Pediatr Surg 1986; 15:549-552.

44. Bower RJ, Bell MJ, Ternberg JL et al. Ventilatory support and primary closure of gastroschisis. Surgery 1982; 91:52-55.

45. Filston HC. Gastroschisis—primary fascial closure: The goal for optimal management. Ann Surg 1983; 197:260-264.

46. Canty TG, Collins DL. Primary fascial closure in infants with gastroschisis and omphalocele: A superior approach. J Pediatr Surg 1983; 18:707-712.

47. Ein SH, Superina R, Bagwell C et al.

Ischemic bowel after primary closure for gastroschisis. J Pediatr Surg 1988; 23: 728-730.

48. Oldham KT, Coran AG, Drongowski RA et al. The development of necrotizing enterocolitis following repair of gastroschisis:A surprisingly high incidence. J Pediatr Surg 1988; 23:945-949.

49. Luck SR, Sherman JO, Raffensperger JG et al. Gastroschisis in 106 consecutive newborn infants. Surgery 1985; 98:677-682.

50. Amoury RA, Ashcraft KW, Holder TM. Gastroschisis complicated by intestinal atresia. Surgery 1977; 82:373-381.

51. Pokorny WJ, Harberg FJ, McGill CW. Gastroschisis complicated by intestinal atresia. J Pediatr Surg 1981; 6:261-263.

52. Gornall P. Management of intestinal atresia complicating gastroschisis. J Pediatr Surg 1989; 24:522-524.

53. Shah R, Woolley MM. Gastroschisis and intestinal atresia. J Pediatr Surg 1991; 26:788-790.

INVITED COMMENTARY

J. Eugene Lewis, Jr. M.D.
Professor Emeritus of Pediatric Surgery
St. Louis University

The modern era of the management of gastroschisis begins with the report of Dr. Moore in 1953. This chapter is a superb review. Whether the increased incidence is real or reflects increased surgical attempts at correction cannot be determined. I am confident that in earlier years many infants died without surgical referral.

Stretching of the abdominal wall with reduction and primary closure remains the ideal treatment. The use of skin flaps, plastic silos or the Shermeta bag have increased salvage. In addition, the use of total parenteral nutrition, ventilatory assistance and antibiotics have played a major role.

The management of atresias is improved by low ostomies. Correction of proximal atresias with peels are best deferred for 2 to 3 weeks. The emphasis on avoiding long delays before final anastomosis seems wise.

There are conflicting results on the benefits of Caesarean section.

The reports from Sweden are very encouraging. Further trials and investigation seem worthwhile. There does seem to be good evidence of a reduced peel in those avoiding vaginal delivery.

The use of "patch, drain and wait" in extensive necrosis and gangrene is intriguing. It seems to offer an opportunity for salvage in an almost certain fatal or crippling condition.

Further review of preterm, prelabor Caesarean delivery seems wise. It is a feasible approach and may improve morbidity and mortality in the treatment of this mechanical problem.

Most of us worked for years preaching prompt diagnosis of newborn surgical problems. Now we are urging antenatal ultrasound monitoring for diagnosis before birth! Time marches on!

Raymond A. Amoury, M.D.
Katherine Berry Richardson Professor of Pediatric Surgery
University of Missouri, Kansas City
Surgeon-in-Chief, Children's Mercy Hospital, Kansas City, MO
President, American Pediatric Surgical Association 1993-1994

Gastroschisis was first reported in the English literature by James Calder of Glasgow in 1773.[1] It remained a medical curiosity until the classic and precise description of the anomaly by Moore and Stokes in 1953.[2] The authors emphasized the abnormal appearance of the eviscerated mass of gut, noting that it is often embedded in a thick, rigid, gelatinous matrix. In 1963 Moore[3] first referred to this matrix as a "peel". These two contemporary publications proved timely, as a sudden increase in the incidence of gastroschisis made it a major newborn anomaly beginning in the 1970s.

One of the greatest problems with recovery following repair of this anomaly is intestinal hypoperistalsis. Various authors have speculated on the pathogenesis of delay in onset of intestinal function. As Doctor Moore has noted, we examined the histology of the intestine in human gastroschisis and related it to intestinal malfunction so commonly seen.[4] By far and away, the most abnormal layer of the intestine was the serosal "peel" which consisted chiefly of fibrin and collagen. Using electron microscopy we found that the ultrastructural characteristics of collagen showed striations which were consistent with Type I collagen. I would like to speculate on the origin of the collagenous "peel" by proposing that it is produced when high molecular weight fibrinogen molecules leave the intestinal capillary bed and pass transmurally to the serosal surface of the prolapsed intestine, which acts as a dialyzing membrane. Fibrinogen adheres to the serosal surface of the intestine, is converted to fibrin, and then serves as a lattice onto which migrating fibroblasts can colonize. The fibroblasts then elaborate collagen in a "layered" configuration. This process evolves over a period of time as evidenced by the appearance of squames at different levels in the "peel". The origin of the fibroblasts in this hypothesis is uncertain, however, Haller et al[5] made an isolated observation which showed that there was a depletion of submucosal fibroblasts in their model. It is possible that migration of fibroblasts from the submucosa through the intestinal wall could occur and populate the fibrin matrix on the serosa. An alternative possibility would be that migrating, differentiated fibroblasts or undifferentiated mesenchymal cells in the amnion could establish themselves in the lattice and lay down collagen.

The disappearance of the "peel" is a fascinating, biological phenomenon. The mechanism(s) is unknown. I detail the "peel" further in order to explain the occurrence of necrotizing enterocolitis (NEC) following repair of gastroschisis. In 1980 we reported for the first time on necrotizing enterocolitis following a variety of operations in the neonatal period.[6] Three of the neonates described in this initial report had gastroschisis. A high incidence of postoperative NEC was also noted by Mollitt and Golladay,[7] and Oldham et al.[8] A mechanisms(s) was proposed to explain this association.[9] It was hypothesized that *"The intestinal wall in gastroschisis may be predisposed to NEC because of a higher than normal tissue pressure (requiring a higher perfusion pressure for an adequate microcirculation) due to: (1) the "peel" that invests it, (2) increased intraluminal pressure due to kinks and partial intestinal obstruction. Postoperative NEC could results from stress(es) causing a relative, or absolute low flow state in the intestine."* For example, contraction of the infant's blood volume (secondary to dehydration, fever, hyperosmolar feedings, etc.) could lead to selective circulatory shunting away from the gut, resulting in hypoperfusion of this "stiff" intestinal wall, and the onset of NEC. These same pathophysiologic disturbances might be better tolerated in a more compliant intestine, where the "peel" has partially resolved, especially if these were transitory insults and/or reversed by early intervention(s). In these cases the "peel" may no longer be as diffuse and the NEC may be short-lived, and appear "benign". Persistence of the "peel" relatively late into the postoperative period could account for later onset of NEC seen in the patients described by Oldham et al[8] in whom the complication appeared independent of the method of repair of the anomaly. This association between gastroschisis and postoperative NEC deserves attention as the diagnosis can be difficult to make. If the patients are managed aggressively with restoration of an adequate intestinal perfusion, they can be restarted on oral feeding early, without the necessity of a prolonged course of total parenteral nutrition and survival in most instances.

REFERENCES

1. Calder J. Two examples of Children born with preternatural conformations of the guts. In: Medial Essays and Observations. Vol.1, 3rd. ed. Edinburgh:W. T. Ruddimans, 1733:203-206.

2. Moore TC, Stokes GE. Gastroschisis: Report of two cases treated by a modification of the Gross operation for omphalocele. Surgery 1953; 33:112-120.

3. Moore TC. Gastroschisis with antenatal evisceration of the intestines and urinary bladder. Ann Surg 1963; 158:263-269.

4. Amoury RA, Beatty EC, Wood WG et al. Histology of intestine in human gastroschisis—relationship to intestinal malfunction: Dissolution of the "peel" and its ultrastructural characteristics. J Pediatr Surg 1988; 23:950-956.

5. Haller JA Jr., Kehrer BH, Shaker IJ et al. Studies of the pathophysiology of gastroschisis in fetal sheep. J Pediatr Surg 1974; 9:627-632.

6. Amoury RA, Goodwin CD, McGill CW et al. Necrotizing enterocolitis following operation in the neonatal period. J Pediatr Surg 1980; 15:1-8.

7. Mollitt DL, Golladay ES. Postoperative neonatal necrotizing enterocolitis. J Pediatr Surg 1982; 17:757-763.

8. Oldham KT, Coran AG, Dron Jowski RA et al. The development of necrotizing

enterocolitis following repair of gastroschisis: A surprisingly high incidence. J Pediatr Surg 1988; 23:945-949.

9. Amoury RA. Postoperative necrotizing enterocolitis. Letter to the Editor. J Pediatr Surg 1989; 24:513-514.

John G. Raffensperger, M.D.
Professor of Surgery, Northwestern University
Surgeon-in-Chief, Children's Memorial Hospital, Chicago
Editor, *Swenson's Pediatric Surgery*

Dr. Moore has described the evolution of the treatment of infants born with gastroschisis over the past 40 years. He deserves credit for his initial description of the lesion and for his persistence in differentiating gastroschisis from omphalocele. Prior to Dr. Moore's description of gastroschisis, all those babies were diagnosed as "a ruptured omphalocele". In fact, the 1953 edition of "The Surgery of Infancy and Childhood", showed the photograph of an infant with gastroschisis labeled as "ruptured omphalocele". I treated my first infant with gastroschisis in 1960 by widely undermining skin flaps. The infant survived, even without intravenous hyperalimentation and later we closed the huge ventral hernia with a silastic patch.

There was a veritable epidemic of infants born with a gastroschisis during the 1970s and early 1980s. Initially, I used the "silo" but found that by irrigating all the meconium from the intestine with 1% acetylcysteine and stretching the abdominal wall, it is possible to close the abdominal skin in almost all cases. The skin is undermined for not more than 1 cm on either side. It is closed with subcuticular sutures and large steri strips. The infant is then left paralyzed and ventilated for 2-3 days, until the abdomen commences to soften. The fascia is not closed but, in fact, by one year these infants often have only a very minimal midline ventral hernia, which in some cases, does not require closure. When there is a coexisting intestinal atresia, the dilated intestine can often be resected and an anastomosis made at the time of the initial closure. We monitor intra-abdominal pressure by having the anesthesiologist observe airway pressures and, in addition, a Doppler monitor on the leg will give indication of diminished circulation to the lower extremities. If we do see evidence of increased abdominal pressure after attempted replacement of the bowel and peritoneal cavity we will back off and sew on a small silastic patch.

I would never recommend elective cesarean section following a prenatal diagnosis of gastroschisis. The infants are already small for gestational age and I see no advantage to delivering them earlier. Not all infants born vaginally have a thick intestinal peel. In fact, we also have seen infants with gastroschisis in which the bowel was nearly normal and could be easily dropped back into the peritoneal cavity.

Michael D. Klein, M.D.
Professor of Surgery, Wayne State University
Chief, Pediatric General Surgery
Children's Hospital of Michigan, Detroit

If one believes that it is the condition of the bowel which is responsible for morbidity and mortality in gastroschisis, one should therefore attempt delivery and repair prior to these events.

After some cogitation and much political difficulty, I arranged for a program of delivery room repair at the Detroit Medical Center. The attending pediatric surgeon and pediatric surgery fellow, the attending pediatric anesthesiologist and pediatric anesthesia fellow, the scrub nurse and the circulating nurse, are all from the Children's Hospital of Michigan, and travel less than a mile to reach Hutzel Hospital where the delivery service is located. We use one of the delivery rooms as an operating room, and the patient is delivered by cesarean section across the hall in another delivery room. The patient is then carried immediately to the prepared operating room where the vernix caseosa is removed, the patient is intubated, an intravenous line is begun, and monitoring devices are applied. By the time the traditional prep and drape is appropriate, the surgeon and assistant have reduced the massive bowel, and all that is necessary is a fascial closure.

The most important finding in this approach was entirely serendipitous. In watching the cesarean section and photographing events from the moment of delivery onward, I have noticed that although these children are born at term (37 to 40 weeks), the bowel is very seldom, if ever, thickened, edematous or possessed of fibrinous exudate. It is the normal soft and pliable bowel, although certain portions may be more distended than others. It is usually quite easy to reduce. I believe we have now operated on approximately fifty patients in this manner.

What I have learned from this experience is that it can be important for pediatric surgeons to participate in antenatal and perinatal care.

David L. Collins, M.D.
Pediatric Surgeon, Medical Group of San Diego
Clinical Professor of Surgery
University of California, San Diego

I agree with Dr. Moore completely. He deserves great credit for first really defining this condition, separating it from ruptured omphalocele, and identifying the major principles of management. This includes the fact that the dense firm matrix which sometimes envelops the bowel will dissolve if the bowel is reduced en mass with future manipulations regarding anastomosis, etc. postponed until later.

I also agree that the greatest new development in managing this condition is its identification by intrauterine ultrasound, and early caesarean delivery as soon as the lung profile shows maturity.

I have so far managed three cases this way, and found bowel to be of normal consistency with shiny serosa, and completely normal pliability permitting an easy primary repair.

Charles E. Bagwell, M.D.
Professor of Surgery and Pediatrics
Chairman, Division of Pediatric Surgery
Medical College of Virginia, Richmond

Until resolution of the interesting questions raised by Dr. Moore regarding the lessened bowel thickening and induration in infants with gastroschisis born by planned C-section prior to the onset of labor, problems with management of this condition will continue to involve resuscitation of the infant and prompt operative intervention to reduce or cover the exposed viscera. Typically this is performed in the operating theater by stretching the abdominal cavity, evacuating the gut (using both nasogastric and colonic tubes) and reducing the abdominal contents (or, if unsuccessful, proceeding with silo placement). Some authors have attempted to quantitate tight closure by measurement of intra-abdominal pressure as a guide to vascular compromise of the viscera.[1,2] Most clinicians, however, use increased ventilatory pressure at the time of reduction, the presence of discoloration of the lower extremities or of the viscera as an indication to retreat from attempts at primary closure and employ staged methods by constructing a prosthetic silo.

Management of associated atresias should best be left until the thickened and indurated bowel has returned to normal. One case of an obvious atresia in a baby with gastroschisis and thickened bowel loops with a clearly demonstrable mesenteric defect can be recalled which allowed primary closure of the abdomen; while awaiting an operative date to reexplore the infant and repair the atresia, the baby began passing meconium per rectum and continued to do so without further difficulties. Obviously what was felt to be an atresia was, in fact, an area of edematous or folded induration of the foreshortened intestine illustrating the occasional risks of such a diagnosis even to experienced observers.

With the increased incidence of gastroschisis defects over the past two decades documented by the author is a concomitant decline in the number of infants with omphalocele defects. Elucidation of the suspected teratogenic or other agents responsible for these abdominal wall defects would be of enormous benefit in understanding the epidemiology of embryonic and congenital malformations at various sites.

REFERENCES

1. Yaster M, Scherer TLR, Stone MM et al. Prediction of successful primary closure of congenital abdominal wall defects using intraoperative measurements. J Pediatr Surg 1989; 12:1217-1220.
2. Lacey SR, Bruce J, Brooks SP et al. The relative merits of various methods of indirect measurements of intraabdominal pressure as a guid to closure of abdominal wall defects. J Pediatr Surg 1987; 12:1207-1211.

Edwin I. Hatch, Jr., M.D.
Children's Hospital and Medical Center, Seattle
Clinical Associate Professor of Surgery
University of Washington

Thank you for asking me to comment on your chapter on gastroschisis. As you know, this has been a longterm interest of mine and my opinions are based mainly on our institutional experience here in Seattle at the Children's Hospital where we have treated over 200 children with gastroschisis over the last 15 years since my arrival in 1979.

Whatever the cause of the initial event, the consequences of gastroschisis and what we see at birth definitely are different from omphalocele. My belief is that the fetus with gastroschisis has a relative decrease in the size of the umbilical defect with more peel resulting from lymphatic obstruction, then venous obstruction, and ultimately arterial obstruction with loss of bowel, or atresia related to this.

I feel that early delivery is important to prevent this ongoing process in the last three to four weeks of pregnancy. My present recommendation based on this is that serial ultrasounds be followed during the last eight weeks of the pregnancy of the mother of the fetus with gastroschisis, and, if and when this peel begins to become obvious based on thickness of bowel and bowel dilatation then move to delivery. The essential component of this is to make sure that the lungs are mature so that you do not have a baby with respiratory problems in addition to gastroschisis. By moving to early delivery, we very often end up with a C-section and our results with babies who have been delivered early by C-section have been outstanding.

The next area of controversy is whether to close all gastroschisis babies primarily, or place all gastroschisis babies in a silo and close them in a delayed fashion. There is no science to this because of the spectrum of gastroschisis. There are those babies who can be closed primarily that another surgeon would place in a silo for reasons of safety. The babies with less peel do great where the babies with atresia and thickened peel do relatively poorly. Unfortunately, no one institution has a large enough experience to get adequate scientific data.

CHAPTER 4

OMPHALOCELE

INTRODUCTION

Omphalocele is a major abdominal wall defect of the newborn of fairly constant incidence and a seriously compromising high incidence of other congenital malformations which have contributed to a continuing high level of complications, morbidity and mortality. Omphalocele was classified as different from gastroschisis by Stokes[1] and me in a 1953 publication. It was characterized as having a covering sac or its ruptured remnants with the umbilical cord arising from the sac. Large sacs were liver-containing. This classification has permitted the development of separate and distinctive literature in the past 40 years pertaining to these quite separate and distinct newborn malformations.

The relative incidence of small or "simple" and large or "giant" omphalocele has varied widely in different reports. In 1979, Gough and Auldist[2] reported a ten year experience with 87 cases of omphalocele from the Royal Children's Hospital, Parkville, Victoria, Australia. Seventeen of their patients were classified as giant omphalocele (19.5%). These patients had defect diameters measuring more than 5 cm. A 1980 report by Towne, Peters and Chang[3] from the Children's Hospital of Denver included 30 cases of omphalocele with seven (23%) being classified as small or "simple" and 23 (77%) classified as large or "giant". These 30 patients were seen within a three year period (1975 to 1978). A 1981 report from Columbus, Ohio by Knight, Sommer and Clatworthy[4] identified 22 of 43 omphaloceles (51%) to be small and 21 to be large. In 1985, Hershenson, Raffensperger and associates[5] of Chicago classified 29 of 51 omphaloceles as small (57%) and 22 as giant. In the Columbus Children's Hospital experience[4] the 22 small omphaloceles experienced a greater mortality (33%) than the large omphaloceles (20%). The number and nature of additional malformations made the difference as 26 infants with isolated omphalocele (no additional malformations) had only one death (4%) with nine small and 17 large omphaloceles in this group. Forty percent of their patients had "syndrome" omphalocele (33%) or trisomy 13, 18 or 21 (7%).

In 1963, Peter Jones[6] reported an experience with 44 cases of omphalocele from the Royal Children's Hospital of Melbourne, Australia. Thirteen of their patients (30%) had large omphaloceles (over 5 cm in diameter) and the mortality in this group was 77%. The overall mortality for the group of 44 patients was 50%. In 1966, Pohl and Schnierer[7] reported 45 cases of omphalocele from Czechoslovakia with an overall mortality of 48%. The mortality in the 45% of their cases with additional malformations (20 cases) was 80%. They treated giant omphaloceles (7 cases) conservatively with a mortality of 57%.

A 1971 report by Firor[8] from Cape Town, South Africa, was concerned with a recording of 47 cases of omphalocele and an appraisal of therapeutic approaches to the management of omphalocele. He cites the high mortality in omphalocele series in six, then recent, publications of 40, 44, 48, 48, 50 and 56%. He reports an overall mortality of 36% (17 cases) which includes seven untreated babies (15%) who died in the initial 24 hours of multiple major malformation. His most notable success was with the use of nonoperative, "conservative" therapy employing the sac painting method of Grob with two percent aqueous solution of mercurochrome. With this method he achieved a survival of 14 of 15 patients (93%). This contrasted with a survival of only 3 of 8 patients (37.5%) managed by the skin flap closure of Gross.[9]

Stringel and Filler[10] in 1979, recorded 79 cases of omphalocele from the Hospital for Sick Children of Toronto (Canada) with an overall mortality of 33%. Here again the overwhelming cause of mortality was the presence of additional serious malformations. The mortality without additional malformations in 42 patients was 12% (5 cases) whereas that for the 37 patients with additional malformations was 57% (21 cases). Trisomy with multiple anomalies was encountered in 8 cases (10%) and all died. The trisomies were 13 (2 cases), 18 (5 cases) and 21 (1 case). Ten of their 13 babies managed by the painting method died (77%), all of additional malformations.

The last report of a major series of omphalocele (55 cases) appeared in a 1985 publication by the Raffensperger group[5] of Chicago. Their overall mortality was 29% (16 cases). For the giant omphalocele group of 22 cases, the mortality was 50% and for the small omphalocele group of 29 cases

it was 10.4% (3 cases). Forty-six percent of their giant omphalocele group had congenital heart disease (10 cases) as did 10% of their small omphalocele group. In addition, "syndrome" omphalocele was encountered in 24% of their cases (13 patients) and trisomy in 5.5% (3 cases). Of the "syndrome" omphalocele cases, upper midline syndrome (Cantrell, Haller and Ravitch[11]) was found in three, the lower midline syndrome (cloacal extrophy, vesicointestinal fissure) in four and the Beckwith-Wiedemann syndrome[12,13] (macroglossia, gigantism) in six. They considered small, narrow thoraces and possible pulmonary hypoplasia to be serious problems in cases of giant omphalocele.

The decreasing frequency of reports of significant series of omphalocele likely reflects the continuing dismal results associated with the high incidence of very serious and life-threatening additional, often multiple malformations.

As the awesome incidence and high lethality of additional malformations in omphalocele patients is a major component of the clinical differences between gastroschisis and omphalocele, I undertook two in-depth studies of this problem in the mid-1970s and mid 1980s. The first was a review of the usable data in the major published series which yielded 236 cases of omphalocele and the second was the use of an international survey by questionnaire which yielded 287 cases of omphalocele.

The 1970s literature review was published by the author of this book[14] in the November 1977 issue of *Surgery* (82:561-568). Additional malformations were encountered in 88 of 236 cases of omphalocele (37%) and all but 1% were at nonjejunoileal locations, in contrast to 14% in this area in 278 cases of gastroschisis. Congenital heart disease was found in 46 of the 236 cases of omphalocele (20%) and "syndrome" omphalocele in 31 cases (13%). The breakdown of the "syndrome" omphalocele cases showed 11 with upper midline syndrome, 16 with lower midline syndrome and four with the Beckwith-Wiedemann syndrome.

"Syndrome" omphalocele has been defined as recognized syndromes in which omphalocele occurs in 70% or more percent of the cases.[14] Omphalocele is a constant feature of the Beckwith-Wiedemann syndrome and occurs in 68% of cases of complete upper midline syndrome and in 89% of cases of lower midline syndrome.[14]

The 1980s international questionnaire survey results were published in a series of three articles in *Pediatric Surgery International* in 1986 and 1987.[15-17] The first of these three articles in *Pediatric Surgery International* (1:46-50) was concerned with the nature and distribution of additional malformations in 490 cases of gastroschisis and omphalocele.[15] The incidence of additional malformations in 287 cases of omphalocele was 54% (155 cases). In 74% of these 155 cases with additional malformations, the additional malformations were both serious and multiple. "Syndrome" omphalocele cases were encountered in 41 of the 287 cases of omphalocele with seven being upper midline, 20 lower midline and 14 Beckwith-Wiedemann. In addition, there were 12 cases of trisomy 13, 18 or 21 (4.2%). Sixteen percent of these 287 omphalocele patients had congenital heart disease (45 cases).

CHALLENGES

1. The most serious and difficult challenge in cases with antenatal diagnosis of omphalocele is whether or not to terminate the pregnancy.

The awesome incidence and gravity of additional malformations, as chronicled in the Introduction to this chapter must give pause and serious consideration to both physicians and parents. Further information of value may be obtained by amniocentesis. It is extremely important to differentiate clearly and unambiguously between gastroschisis and omphalocele and this is possible. Protrusion of liver through the defect on antenatal ultrasound indicates omphalocele.

2. The most important and challenging surgical problem in the newly born infant with omphalocele is the management of giant omphalocele, when it occurs.

Giant omphalocele is generally defined as a defect in excess of 5 cm in diameter. As in gastroschisis and congenital diaphragmatic hernia, the abdominal cavity has not received normal growth stimulus due to the extracoelomic location of abdominal viscera during intra-uterine life and is abnormally small. The presence of a significant amount of noncompressible liver in the large and giant omphalocele sac further complicates the problem of viscera replacement and abdominal wall covering even with large hernia creation, including the skin flap closure of Gross.[9]

Often the chest wall in the giant omphalocele patient is abnormal. It may have a cylindrical rather than a bell-shaped configuration. The sternum is short and the costal margin and the diaphragm are cephalad in position. The Raffensperger group,[5] as cited earlier in the Introduction section, has postulated an associated pulmonary hypoplasia to further complicate the management of these patients. The suprahepatic inferior vena cava is often displaced anteriorly in these infants and damage may occur to it as well as to the hepatic veins. The distance from the sternum to the vena cava hiatus in the diaphragm is very short and at times these vessels appear to be adherent to and intimately associated with the upper part of the omphalocele sac as it seems to blend with the diaphragm.

DeLorimer, Adzick and Harrison[18] in 1991 reported in the *Journal of Pediatric Surgery* (26:804-807) a remarkable experience in which six infants with giant omphaloceles, all over 7 cm in diameter, were managed successfully without fatality by an amnion inversion technique. They characterized their undertaking not only as a challenge but as an "extreme" challenge. The amnion was left intact and it was progressively inverted into the abdominal cavity by using the silastic silo. Their patients were kept intubated and paralyzed postoperatively and the silastic silo was squeezed once or twice a day to reduce the viscera.

I have quite recently used the Shermeta bag [19] and the Shermeta placement technique[20] in a case of rupture of a large liver containing epigastric omphalocele of the upper midline syndrome type in which there was also a diaphragmatic hernia (pleura-covered) and downward displacement of the heart. The Shermeta bag with its silo shape and seamless nature and its ready placement potential would render it particularly useful in the sort of amnion inversion advocated by deLorimer et al[18] and used with such success by them.

3. Cases of syndrome omphalocele may provide major surgical challenges.

The Beckwith-Wiedemann syndrome (BWS) is challenging in two rather divergent areas, surgery and genetics. The principal surgical challenge involves the decisions of whether and when to surgically reduce the size of the macroglossia (greatly enlarged tongue) which appears to have no tendency to diminish in real or relative size with patient growth or the passage of time.

On the genetic side, BWS in addition to the regular appearance of omphalocele is a fetal overgrowth disorder which is characterized by a predisposition to tumors including Wilms' tumor.[21,22] This predisposition to Wilms' and other tumors in BWS patients appears to involve a relaxation or loss of genomic imprinting of the insulin growth factor 2 (IGF2) and H19 genes.[23,24] These genes are a pair of physically linked, reciprocally imprinted loci on mouse chromosome 7 and in humans map to chromosome 11p15, a region that frequently is inherited as two paternal copies in patients with BWS. The phenomenon of genomic imprinting is the preferential expression of the maternally or paternally inherited allele. Recent findings indicate imprinting to have importance and bearing in such diverse areas as gene expression (phenotypic consequences), development, cancer and evolution. It had been speculated that human IGF2 was synonymous with the BWS gene because of its effects on growth and its paternal-specific expression.[25,26] Recent studies reported in *Nature Genetics* (4:93-97 and 98-101, 1993) show that IGF2 is paternally expressed in human fetuses and parentally imprinted in a perinatal BWS patient.

In the upper midline syndrome, cardiac malformations provide a major challenge. The use of the Shermeta bag by the me in a recent case is cited in the prior Challenge section.

The lower midline syndrome presents a host of complex challenges including imperforate anus and the absence of all colon except the cecum. I, together with Castagna,[27] have reported in the *Journal of Pediatric Surgery* (8; 331, 1973) the use of the appendix as a colon substitute in a case of lower midline syndrome omphalocele. In addition, the author has found sac painting may be the only option when a large omphalocele coexists with a urinary bladder extrophy and a vesicointestinal fissure.

CONCLUSION

There are few sadder, more intractable or more disheartening malformations of the newborn than omphalocele. The high incidence, multiplicity and grave nature of additional malformations and the awesome technical surgical challenge of the giant omphalocele present "extreme" and seemingly insoluble challenges in multiple ways. The use of the Shermeta bag and Shermeta placement technique in the deLorimer et al[18] amnion inversion approach may offer a small ray of hope in some cases of giant omphalocele uncompromised by multiple additional life threatening malformations.

REFERENCES

1. Moore TC, Stokes GE. Gastroschisis:Report of two cases treated by a modification of the Gross operation for omphalocele. Surgery 1953; 33:112-120.
2. Gough DCS, Auldist Aw. Giant exomphalos—conservative or operative treatment. Arch Dis Child 1979; 54:441-444.
3. Towne BH, Peters G, Chang JHT. The problem of "giant" omphalocele. J Pediatr Surg 1980; 15:543-548.
4. Knight PJ, Sommer A, Clatworthy HW. Omphalocele:A prognostic classification. J Pediatr Surg 1981; 16:599-604.
5. Hershenson MB, Brouillette RT, Klemka L et al. Respiratory insufficiency in newborns

with abdominal wall defects. J Pediatr Surg 1985; 20:348-353.

6. Jones PG. Exomphalos (syn. Omphalocele). Arch Dis Child 1963; 38:180-187.

7. Pohl V, Schnierer M. Analysis of experience in the therapy of omphalocele over the period of the last 15 years. Cs Ped1966; 21:426-430.

8. Firor HV. Omphalocele—an appraisal of therpeutic approaches. Surgery 1971; 69:208-214.

9. Gross RE. A new method for surgical treatment of large omphaloceles. Surgery 1948; 24:277-292.

10. Stringel G, Filler RM. Prognostic factors in omphalocele and gastroschisis. J Pediatr Surg 1979; 14:515-519.

11. Cantrell JR, Haller JA, Ravitch MM. A syndrome of congenital defects involving the abdominal wall, sternum, diaphragm, pericardium and heart. Surg Gynec Obstet 1958; 107:602-614.

12. Wiedemann HR. Complete malformatif familial avec hernie ombilicale et macroglossie—un "syndrome neuveau"? J Génét Humaine. 1964; 13:223.

13. Beckwith JB, Wang CI, Donnell GN et al. Hyperplastic omphalocele fetal visceromegaly with macroglossia, omphalocele, cytomegaly and other abnormalities. Newly recognized syndrome. Proceedings of the American Pediatric Society. Seattle, WA, June 16-18, 1964 (Abstr. No. 41).

14. Moore TC. Gastroschisis and omphalocele: Clinical differences. Surgery 1977; 82: 561-568.

15. Moore TC, Nur K. An international survey of gastroschisis and omphalocele (490 cases): I. Nature and distribution of additional malformations. Pediatr Surg Int 1986; 1:46-50.

16. Moore TC, Nur K. An international survey of gastroschisis and omphalocele (490 cases):II. Relative incidence, pregnancy and environmental factors. Pediatr Surg Int 1986; 1:105-109.

17. Moore TC, Nur K. An international survey of gastroschisis and omphalocele (490 cases): III. Factors influencing outcome of surgical management. Pediatr Surg Int 1987; 2:27-32.

18. deLorimer AA, Adzick NS, Harrison MR. Amnion inversion in the treatment of giant omphalocele. J Pediatr Surg 1991; 26: 804-807.

19. Shermeta DW, Haller JA. A new preformed transparent silo for the management of gastroschisis. J Pediatr Surg 1975; 10: 973-975.

20. Shermeta DW. Personal communication.

21. Davies K. Imprinting makes its mark. Nature 1993; 363:94.

22. Emergy LG, Shields M, Shah NR et al. Neuroblastoma associated with Beckwith-Wiedemann syndrome. Cancer 1983; 52:176-179.

23. Rainier S, Johnson LA, Dobry CJ et al. Relaxation of imprinted genes in human cancer. Nature 1993; 362:747-749.

24. Ogawa D, Eccles MR, Szeto J et al. Relaxation of omphalocele insulin-like growth factor II gene imprinting implicated in Wilms' tumor. Nature 1993; 362:749-751.

25. Henry I, Bonaiti-Pellie C, Chehensse V et al. Uniparental paternal disomy in a genetic cancer predisposing syndrome. Nature 1991; 351:665-667.

26. Little M, Van Heyningen V, Hastie N. Dads and disomy and disease. Nature 1991; 351:609-610.

27. Castagna JT, Moore TC. Use of the appendix as a colon substitute in vesicointestinal fissure. J Pediatr Surg 1973; 8:331.

INVITED COMMENTARY

Alfred A. deLorimer, M.D.
Professor of Surgery and Chief, Division of Pediatric Surgery
University of California, San Francisco
President, American Pediatric Surgical Association 1991-1992

Dr. Moore has made a real contribution in identifying a classification between syndromic versus nonsyndromic omphaloceles. Infants with associated anomalies have a much greater morbidity and mortality. I find that omphaloceles which are less than 5 cm in diameter, centrally located on the abdominal wall, with the umbilical cord at the apex of the sac (hernia into the umbilical cord) have few associated anomalies and the primary operative repair is readily attainable with excellent outcome. Problems begin with larger omphaloceles where the umbilical cord is at the perimeter of the sac. When the defect is centrally located, the survival remains very good.

When the defect extends into the epigastrium, associated cardiac anomalies are common. The heart should be evaluated shortly after birth for septal defects, Tetralogy of Fallot and endocardial cushion defects. These anomalies will result in congestive failure and poor tissue perfusion, and repair of large defects in these circumstances results in wound infection and dehiscence and death from sepsis. In these instances, repair of the cardiac defect takes priority. Pediatric cardiac surgeons today have excellent results in repairing cardiac defects in the newborn period, and correction of impaired tissue perfusion is essential for healing of the abdominal wall repair.

In the very large omphaloceles, there is no reason to remove the amnion sac in the course of the operative repair. The major concern about leaving the amnion is the presumed difficulty in sterilizing the sac and avoiding infection when inverting it into the abdominal cavity. In addition, the sac does add bulk to the abdomen when the abdominal capacity is already deficient. However, I have not had any infections and the amniotic membranes completely resorb. How soon resorption occurs is not clear, but when I have had to re-operate several months later for fundoplication, the remnants of the sac are gone. To remove the sac invites major causes for morbidity: peritonitis, bowel fistula and torsion of the liver on its vascular pedicle.

A highly successful method for repair of large defects is to use the silo, similar to gastroschisis. A silicone rubber sheet is formed into a tube which is sutured to the ring at the skin-amnion junction. The skin flaps should not be raised at this stage to suture the silo to a fascia. This is because during the subsequent staged repair, the linea alba becomes very soft and does not hold sutures very well. The infant is maintained intubated for ventilation and he is paralyzed to facilitate stretching of the abdominal wall and to reduce the viscera into the abdomen. After pushing the bowel into the abdomen, the apex of the silo is tied or sutured to maintain the intra-abdominal pressure and expand the abdominal cavity. Once the edges of the abdominal wall defect have been closely approximated (preferably within 5 to 7 days before the sutures pull through the skin), the infant is returned to the operating room to close the abdominal defect by approximating the linea alba. If excessive tension is present during this suture closure, a prosthesis, such as teflon or gortex mesh, is used to bridge the gap. This is usually the problem with epigastric omphaloceles where the fascia is so widely separated, closure would require approximating the costal arches. The inverted amnion protects the bowel from adhering to the prosthetic patch. The skin flaps are then mobilized to cover the patch.

Nonoperative management has a place for those patients with huge defects and severe associated anomalies. The objective is to convert the amnion cover over the defect into a tough, granulating membrane which would stimulate wound contraction and ingrowth of skin. Unfortunately, an inordinate length of intensive hospitalization is required before the defect has healed. We use silver sulfadiazine to maintain sterility of the amnion because of the potential toxicity with mercury or iodine when using mercurochrome or iodinated antiseptics.

John G. Raffensperger, M.D.
Professor of Surgery, Northwestern University
Surgeon-in-Chief, Children's Memorial Hospital, Chicago
Editor, *Swenson's Pediatric Surgery*

The number of infants born with "giant omphalocele" appears to be decreasing at least in Chicago. Most likely, after prenatal diagnosis, parents are wisely choosing the option to abort the malformed fetus. When the liver is outside the peritoneal cavity, the lower chest wall and lungs are underdeveloped. Any further elevation of the diaphragm by increased intra-abdominal tension, or even a general anesthetic and endotracheal tube, can lead to respiratory failure and long term ventilator support. Furthermore, any surgical manipulation such as excision of the sac and its replacement with silastic carries the risk of damage to the liver with bleeding or obstruction of the inferior vena cava and hepatic veins. The technique of painting the sac with mercurochrome allows gradual reduction of the abdominal contents but at the risk of systemic mercury poisoning. I suspend the umbilical cord and sac from the top of the isolette and paint the sac with Betadine or silvadene ointment. The sac is then wrapped with a bandage and left to gradually reduce. This process may be hastened by applying multiple ligatures at the apex of the sac, just beneath the umbilical cord. This will gradually reduce the contents into the abdominal cavity. If the sac is ruptured, it can be sutured at the baby's bedside and this therapy continued. This process avoids a general anesthetic and the risk of long term ventilator dependence, it allows for complete evaluation of the infant and it achieves reduction of the omphalocele over a period of several weeks. Unfortunately, many of these infants have major associated congenital defects. Children who survive long term are unhappy with this body image and often return to their surgeon years later to request scar revisions.

CHAPTER 5

MIDGUT ATRESIAS
AND MECONIUM PERITONITIS

INTRODUCTION

This is the first of three chapters which will deal with the problems, consequences, lessons and challenges provided by catastrophic intestinal necrosis and gangrene in utero and in the early postnatal period. The midgut, the part of the large and small intestine supplied by the superior mesenteric artery, is the most frequent target of these gut "extinction" catastrophes.

In utero, these catastrophes occur in a sterile environment and overall total-body nutrition is maintained by the mother and her placental circulation. The spectrum of consequences of in utero necrosis and gangrene may, in a sense, provide "lessons of nature" pertaining to necrosis, gangrene and perforation of midgut in the early postnatal period associated with such devastating conditions as necrotizing enterocolitis and midgut volvulus.

I have had a long interest in these problems with publications dating from 1953 to the present.[1-14] These interests have had a broad spectrum ranging from the multiple and important differences between midgut and duodenal atresias,[1-3] to meconium peritonitis and giant cystic meconium peritonitis,[4-6] to the unique challenges of colonic atresia,[7] to the midgut "extinction" atresia,[8] to atresia in gastroschisis patients,[9-13] and to ileal atresia with and without meconium peritonitis and pneumoperitoneum resulting from in utero intussusception.[14]

My 1953 report in *Surgery, Gynecology and Obstetrics*[1] was a review of a 25-year experience at the Indiana University Medical Center with 40 consecutive cases of atresia or stenosis of the small intestine, 23 involving the duodenum and 17 involving the jejunum and ileum. Early in the evaluation of this experience, it was apparent that there were marked differences between duodenal atresias and stenoses and those involving the jejunum and ileum. The incidence of serious additional malformations (greater in duodenal obstructions), of multiple atresias including the colon (greater with jejunal and ileal obstructions) and results of operative management (better with duodenal obstructions, a mortality of 33% versus 89%). Prematurity was encountered in 5 of the 23 duodenal obstruction cases (22%) and in 7 of the 17 jejunoileal cases (41%). These findings led to a publication which considered these obstructions under two separate headings, duodenal and jejunoileal. I divided jejunoileal atresias into those with a diaphragm, those with a fibrous cord connecting patent bowel ends and those with a discontinuity between proximal and distal segments which often were associated with a gap in the mesentery, a classification later designated by Louw as types I, II and III.

One of the most important and significant publications in all of pediatric surgery, and certainly of those relating to midgut atresias, appeared in the November 19, 1955 issue of *Lancet*.[15] It was by J.H. Louw and C.N. Barnard of Cape Town, South Africa and was titled, "Congenital intestinal atresia; Observations on its origin".

The origins of this remarkable study which revolutionized the understanding and care of newborn infants with midgut atresia(s) derived from astute earlier clinical observations by the senior author, J.H. Louw. Four years earlier, Professor Louw had carefully reviewed a series of cases of intestinal atresia at the Great Ormond Street Hospital for Sick Children in London (U.K.). He was impressed by certain features of these malformations which suggested that some atresias might be due to interference with the blood supply to the fetal gut.

These features which were present in most cases of midgut atresias which presented with "blinds ends" were reported by Louw in 1952 in the *South African Journal of Clinical Science* and included the following:

1. Anomalous vascular supply to the atretic portion. In about 40% there was a V-shaped defect in the mesentery. In one case, personally operated upon, it was noted that the anastomotic arcades in the mesentery between the blind ends were deficient, and in two others there was thrombosis of the vessels.

2. Early necrosis of the proximal blind end. This occurred quite apart from a complicating volvulus in 20% of the cases as well as a further 30% with a volvulus. In more than half of the cases the infant was less than 48 hours old.

3. Postoperative atony and ileus in apparently healthy blind ends anastomosed to the distal bowel. This was a common complication in cases treated by primary anastomosis. It was suggested that the cause was primary impairment of the blood-supply rather than distension alone.

In his 1955 classic *Lancet* article, Louw went on to state that the above observations had been confirmed by him in subsequent studies in 22 personal cases. Two of these cases were particularly instructive. In one, the distal bowel contained a segment of gut which appeared to be the remnant of an intussusception. In the other, the blind ends were separated by tissue resembling necrotic bowel which had undergone torsion. Louw considered these cases as providing evidence of two different mechanisms which might be responsible for interference with the blood-supply to a portion of the bowel.

The 1955 *Lancet* article also cited earlier turn of the century work and publications of continental workers, especially that of Spriggs[16] (1912), concerning hypothetical "strangulation of the fetal gut". They published examples which by appearances suggested gut strangulation by various in utero mechanisms including volvulus, intussusception, snaring at the umbilical ring, kinks and bands.

The 1955 article also cites the very important and pertinent work of Harold Laufman and associates[17] of Chicago and Northwestern University which was published in 1949 in *Archives of Surgery* (59:550-564). They demonstrated that isolated, devascularized and "sterilized" loops of bowel when left in the dogs peritoneal cavity in this condition become converted into sterile bands or disappear entirely. Louw and Barnard, in their 1955 article, speculated that strangulated fetal bowel may end in disappearance of the infarcted portion with, at most, a complicating meconium peritonitis.

The authors of the 1955 *Lancet* publication[15] were encouraged by these observations and went to the laboratory to try to reproduce the atresia anomaly by interruption of the blood-supply to a segment of fetal gut. The operations were carried out by C.N. (Christiaan) Barnard, then as well as later, a particularly determined as well as skilled surgeon. Despite many disappointments, success ultimately was achieved in two animals born at two and 12 days following gut blood-supply deprivation by ligation of mesenteric vessels supplying a short segment of intestine. Intestinal obstruction was produced in both with necrosis predominating in the five day postligation pup and the classical form of atresia with separated blind ends and a mesenteric gap in the 12-day postligation pup.

I shared an office at the Medical College of Virginia in Richmond for three months in the Autumn of 1968 with Christiaan Barnard and was engaged with him in a number of surgical efforts of considerable difficulty in a number of experimental animals ranging in size from the rat to the baboon and can testify, with feeling, as to the extraordinary skill, drive and determination of this C.N. Barnard of the 1955 *Lancet* publication.

Subsequent studies by Louw and Barnard, as well as others, have confirmed and extended these experimental findings in other animals (rabbits and sheep) as well as in dogs.

At the end of the 1955 publication, the authors made the point that there was a practical application of their clinical and laboratory observations and findings. This applications was based on the assumption that the blood supply of bowel immediately adjacent to the atresia blind ends likely is defective and should be resected prior to an anastomosis.

It is of particular interest that also in 1955 two reports appeared concerning the involvement of in utero intussusception in postnatal ileal atresia[18] and in meconium peritonitis.[19] An additional case of antenatal intussusception-induced ileal perforation and meconium peritonitis appeared in 1956.[20]

The frequency of this cause of antenatal intestinal necrosis, perforation and atresia was indicated by an important 1958 publication in *Surgery* by Parkkulainen[21] from the Children's Hospital of the University of Helsinki in Finland. He described three cases of intrauterine intussusception induced intestinal atresia seen during a recent three year period. The atresia and intussusception in all three were in the ileum. Two of the three survived resection and anastomosis. One boy also had marked scrotal swelling at birth and meconium peritonitis with fluid and deposits of calcium in the atresia area at operation indicating meconium peritonitis as well as ileal atresias and causative antenatal ileoileal intussusception.

I have had personal experience with two cases of antenatal ileo-ileal intussusception as a cause of ileal atresia in the newborn in the past two years.[14] One patient had a divided ends and mesenteric gap type of atresia (Type III) with no gross evidence of meconium peritonitis and a clearly palpable intussusceptum in the distal segment. Both ends were enlarged with rather massive enlargement in the proximal end. In the other case, meconium peritonitis intraabdominal calcification was identified at birth by X-ray as well as marked pneumoperitonium. At operation, this patient was found to have a closed distal atresia end which contained the intussusceptum. Proximal to a mesenteric gap was an open proximal end of ileum with considerable meconium staining and marked local calcium deposits. Both patients were managed successfully by resection and primary end-to-end anastomosis. This experience as well as the prior cited report of Parkkulainen[21] strongly suggest that antenatal intussusception is a more frequent cause of ileal atresia than generally recognized. All reported cases of antenatal intussusception causing atresia are small bowel into small bowel.

With the notable exception of a remarkable 1967 report of 33 cases of small bowel atresia and stenosis with 31 survivors (94%) by Professor Jan Louw[22] of Cape Town, South Africa, the mortality elsewhere remained high in cases of midgut atresia until the dawn of the age of "hyperalimentation"/total parenteral nutrition (TPN).

In 1969, deLorimer et al[23] reported in *Surgery* the collective experiences of members of the Surgical Section of the American Academy of Pediatrics with 619 cases of jejunal and ileal atresia seen over a 10 year period (1957 to 1967) at 65 different institutions. Thirty-six percent of the atresias were found in the distal ileum, 33% in the central area and 31% in the proximal jejunum. Multiple atresias were identified in 38 patients (6%) and evidence of fetal bowel infarction was found in association with the atresia in 42% of 449 patients in which this information was available. Stenosis was encountered in only 25 of the 619 cases (4%). The mortality for ileal atresia was 28% and that for jejunal atresia was 41.7%.

The dramatic turn-around in the management results of surgery for midgut atresia and stenosis in the age of TPN is best presented in the 1985 report in *Surgery* by Rescorla and Grosfeld[24] from Indianapolis and the Indiana University Medical Center James Whitcomb Riley Hospital for Children. Their report concerned 52 cases of jejunoileal atresia and stenosis (49 atresias and 3 stenoses) and 12 cases of colonic atresia or stenosis (atresia in 11 and stenosis in one). Their survival rate was 87% for jejunoileal cases and 100% for colonic cases. These outstanding results were achieved despite six infants with cystic fibrosis and nine with gastroschisis. Sepsis and TPN-related choleostasis related progressive liver failure were the major causes of death in the jejunoileal cases.

One of the most severe forms of midgut atresia is the "apple peel" type with a proximal jejunal dilated blind-ending stump and a distal collapsed ileum wound around a persisting marginal blood supply with massive associated loss of gut and mesentery. This form was characterized as "apple peel" by Santulli[25] in a major publication on midgut atresia published in *Annals of Surgery* (154:939-948) in 1961. Other descriptive terms applied to this rather unusual and somewhat frightening conformation have been "Christmas tree" by Weitzman[126] in 1966 and "maypole" by Nixon and Tawes[27] in 1971. Other terms include "corkscrew" and "helical" by Zerella and Martin.[28] Both the frequency and severity of this type of atresia are shown by the 1970 report of Dickson[29] of 15 cases from a London (U.K.) experience with a mortality of 80% (12 of 15 cases).

This type of atresia is the next most severe and qualifies for classification as Type IV and next only to Type V, midgut amputation, deletion or "extinction" of the type described by me in 1986[8] (Fig. 5.1). In this type the midgut has been "guillotined" and very proximal beginning jejunum and mid-transverse colon end blindly in a cord structure and are adjacent to one another supported by a common "meso" (mesentery/mesocolon) supporting structure.

Colonic atresia may accompany small bowel atresia in multiple atresia cases. When it occurs alone as a single atresia, closed-loop difficulties may produce ischemic and necrotic complications after birth. Such a case was reported by me in 1978.[7]

Three types of midgut atresia should be considered separately from the common type considered above. Two share the in utero ischemia/necrosis etiology but have additional complicating factors. These are atresias and necrosis accompanying gastroschisis (considered in detail in chapter 4) and atresias with gut perforation and pseudocyst formation encountered in patients with cystic fibrosis and meconium ileus. The cystic fibrosis/meconium ileus problem is a genetic, as well as a surgical, problem. The recent cloning of the cystic fibrosis gene opens exciting prospects for genetic engineering.

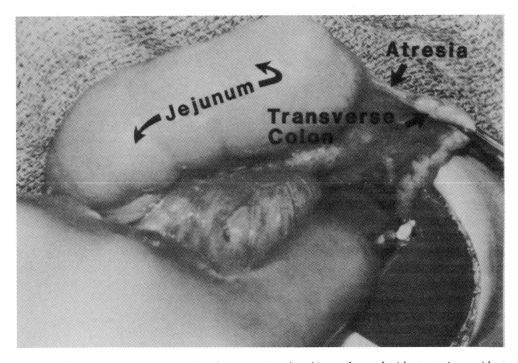

Fig. 5.1. Photograph taken at operation demonstrating the ultimate form of midgut atresia as midgut deletion/amputation with a small and dilated proximal jejunum just distal to the ligament of Treitz connected by a short fibrous cord to the patent distal transverse colon and with a common mesentery/ mesocolon. Reprinted with permisison from Moore TC. High jejunal atresia with midgut deletion. J Pediatr Surg 1986; 21:951-952. ©W.B. Saunders Company.

A third type which may extend beyond the midgut in both directions is the "hereditary" type reported from Ireland (Dublin)[30] and Canada (Montreal).[31] This type may be associated with pyloric and antral atresia, epidermolysis bullosa and may be so extensive and involved as to be incurable.

Although meconium peritonitis is an integral part of the midgut atresia picture, two infrequent complications of meconium peritonitis deserve mention. These are the occurrence of giant cystic meconium peritonitis[5] and the occurrence of intestinal obstruction later on in infancy which may produce a complete but delayed mechanical intestinal obstruction.[6] I have encountered and published experiences with both of these complications of meconium peritonitis.[5,6] In giant cystic meconium peritonitis, a great enlargement of the peritoneal cavity at birth is produced by a huge thick-walled and calcified meconium-filled cyst into which the proximal and open end of small bowel empties. This may be diagnosed antenatally by detection of calcium deposits.[4] The remaining midgut is collapsed and plastered against the posterior part of the obliterated former abdominal cavity. In the acquired, adhesion and calcification-induced mechanical small bowel obstruction, intestinal continuity had been reestablished in utero by auto-anastomosis and no obstruction existed at birth. Both of these patients were managed successfully by surgical intervention. The later-in-infancy adhesion-obstruction case was managed by simple operative lysis of the adhesions. The giant cystic meconium peritonitis case management was more complicated with two operations first for cyst emptying and midgut mobilization by decortication of the posterior abdominal wall and later by decortication of the extrahepatic biliary tract to relieve a persisting and intractable obstructive jaundice. Intestinal continuity was reestablished by use of the

Mikulicz double enterostomy and spur crushing technique.

The in utero auto-anastomosis phenomenon is of particular interest in terms of the "lessons of nature" and applicability to the necrotizing enterocolitis use of "patch, drain and wait" to be developed in more detail in the next chapter. Because of this, a major ischemic/necrotic vascular catastrophe may occur in utero with no obstructive or other symptoms at birth. In the male, only a swollen scrotum with X-ray demonstrated calcification may occur.

CHALLENGES

1. The most important and intriguing challenge in the area of this chapter is to use detailed studies of in utero midgut vascular ischemia/necrosis catastrophes as "experiments of nature" to design maximum gut salvage scenarios for use in necrotizing enterocolitis and midgut volvulus. This will be discussed in the next two chapters.

The combination of placental nutrition ("hyperalimentation"/TPN) and a sterile intra-uterine environment and their influence on the consequences of massive, catastrophic ischemia/necrosis in utero are worthy of study and constructive planning. The phenomenon of in utero auto-anastomosis to restore gut continuity after massive gut necrosis is of particular interest.

2. The problem of the greatly enlarged proximal jejunal blind end, often with extensive distal gut loss, presents a major challenge of a technical nature with respect to restoration of intestinal continuity with normal peristalsis and with maintenance of maximal mucosal absorptive surface.

The initial published approach to this problem appeared in an article in *Surgery, Gynecology and Obstetrics* in 1969 by Colin Thomas[32] of the University of North Carolina (Chapel Hill). He suggested and illustrated a jejunoplasty undertaking. This was an important beginning to this difficult problem. The most rational and mucosal saving approach was published in 1983 in the *Journal of Pediatric Surgery* by Alfred

deLorimer and Michael Harrison[33] of San Francisco. Their approach was an imbrication operation which achieved the best of both worlds with jejunum narrowing for appropriate anastomosis sizing and satisfactory peristalsis achievement and for maximal mucosal surface maintenance.

CONCLUSION

This is the first of three chapters to deal with the major challenges deriving from catastrophic and extensive ischemic midgut necrosis and gangrene in the antenatal and early postnatal periods and with their consequences of perforation, meconium peritonitis, gut and mesentery absorption, atresia/stenosis, fistula formation and the phenomenon of auto-anastomosis in both periods. This chapter is concerned with these happenings before birth in utero in a sterile environment where the observations may serve as "experiments of nature" wherein observations may contribute to a practical and effective scenario or scenarios for the management of those happenings occurring after birth in a nonsterile environment in the form of the dreadful acquired post-natal disorders of necrotizing enterocolitis and midgut volvulus with extensive ischemia and gangrene. These topics will comprise the next two chapters.

REFERENCES

1. Moore TC, Stokes GE. Congenital stenosis and atresia of the small intestine. Surg Gynec Obstet 1953; 97:719-730.
2. Moore TC. Congenital intrinsic duodenal obstruction: Report of 32 cases. Ann Surg 1956; 144:159-164.
3. Moore TC. Annular pancreas. Surgery 1953; 33:138-148.
4. Speck CR, Moore TC, Stout FE. Antenatal diagnosis of meconium peritonitis. Am J Roentgenol 1962; 88:566-570.
5. Moore TC. Giant cystic meconium peritonitis. Ann Surg 1963; 157:566-572.
6. Moore TC. Internal hernia with high jejunal obstruction in infants due to adhesions from antenatal meconium peritonitis. J Pediatr Surg 1973; 8:971-972.
7. Moore TC. Atresia of the colon at the splenic

flexure with absence of the distal colon and ischemic destruction of the proximal colon. J Pediatr Surg 1978; 13:89-90.

8. Moore TC. Jejunal atresia with midgut deletion. J Pediatr Surg 1986; 21:951-952.

9. Moore TC, Stokes GE. Gastroschisis: Report of two cases treated by a modification of the Gross operation for omphalocele. Surgery 1953; 33:112-120.

10. Moore TC. Gastroschisis and omphalocele: Clinical differences. Surgery 1977; 82: 561-568.

11. Moore TC, Nur K. An international survey of gastroschisis and omphalocele (490 cases): I. Nature and distribution of additional malformations. Pediatr Surg Int 1986; 1:46-50.

12. Moore TC. Management of midgut volvulus with extensive necrosis by "patch, drain and wait" in early infancy and childhood: Report of three cases. Pediatr Surg Int 1991; 6:313-317.

13. Moore TC. The role of labor in gastroschisis bowel thickening and prevention by elective preterm and prelabor cesarian section. Pediatr Surg Int 1992; 7:256-259.

14. Lai E, Cunningham TC, Moore TC. In utero intussusception producing ileal atresia and meconium peritonitis with and without free air. Pediatr Surg Int. (Submitted for publication).

15. Louw, JH, Barnard CN. Congenital intestinal atresia: Observations on its origin. Lancet 1955; 2:1065-1067.

16. Spriggs NI. Guy's Hospital Reports 1912; 66:143.

17. Laufman H, Martin WB, Method H et al. Observations in strangulation obstruction: II. The fate of sterile devascularized intestine in the peritoneal cavity. Arch Surg 1948; 59:550-564.

18. Rachelson MH, Jernigan JP, Jackson WF. Intussusception in the newborn infant with spontaneous expulsion of the intussusceptum; A case report and review of the literature. J Pediatrics 1955; 47:87-94.

19. Lannin BG, Leven NL, Tongen LA. Congenital obstruction of the small intestine and colon. Arch Surg 1955; 70:808-817.

20. Shnitka TK, Sherbaniuk RW. Congenital intussesception complicated by meconium peritonitis; Report of a case. Obstet Gynecol 1956; 7:293-298.

21. Parkkulainen KV. Intrauterine intussusception as a cause of intestinal atresia. Surgery 1958; 44:1106-1111.

22. Louw JH. Resection and end-to-end anastomosis in the management of atresia and stenosis of the small bowel. Surgery 1967; 62:940-950.

23. deLorimer AA, Fonkalsrud EW, Hays DM. Congenital atresia and stenosis of the jejunum and ileum. Surgery 1969; 65: 819-827.

24. Rescorla FJ, Grosfeld JL. Intestinal atresia and stenosis:Analysis of survival in 120 cases. Surgery 1985; 98:668-675.

25. Santulli TV, Blanc WA. Congenital atresia of the intestine: Pathogenesis and treatment. Ann Surg 1961; 154:939-948.

26. Weitzman JJ, Vanderhoof RS. Jejunal atresia with agenesis of the dorsal mesentery; with "Christmas tree" deformity of the small intestine. Am J Surg 1966; 111:443-449.

27. Nixon HH, Tawes R. Etiology and treatment of small intestinal atresia: Analysis of a series of 127 jejunoileal atresias and comparison with 62 duodenal atresias. Surgery 1971; 69:41-51.

28. Zerella JT, Martin LW. Jejunal atresia with absent mesentery and a helical ileum. Surgery 1976; 86:550-553.

29. Dickson JAS. Apple peel small bowel: An uncommon variant of duodenal and jejunal atresia. J Pediatr Surg 1970; 5:596-600.

30. Puri P, Fugimoto T. New observations on the pathogenesis of multiple intestinal atresias. J Pediatr Surg 1988; 23:221-225.

31. Guttman FM, Braun P, Gavance PH et al. Multiple atresias and a new syndrome of hereditary multiple atresias involving the gastrointestinal tract from stomach to rectum. J Pediatr Surg 1973; 8:633-640.

32. Thomas CG. Jejunoplasty for the correction of jejunal atresia. Surg Gynec Obstet 1969; 129:545-546.

33. deLorimer AA, Harrison MR. Intestinal plication in the treatment of atresia. J Pediatr Surg 1983; 18:734-737.

INVITED COMMENTARY

J. Eugene Lewis, Jr., M.D.
Professor Emeritus of Pediatric Surgery
St. Louis University

The midgut, supplied by the superior mesenteric artery, is the most frequent target of catastrophic intestinal necrosis and gangrene in utero. However, in utero the catastrophes occur in a sterile environment and nutrition is provided by the mother and her placental circulation. The literature documents the in utero interference with the midgut blood supply including intussusception. The term "lessons of nature" seems particularly pertinent.

Despite improved surgical management the mortality remained high. However, we all experienced the dramatic improvement in surgical management of midgut atresia with the addition of TPN. Further progress has been documented with the addition of imbrication of the dilated proximal bowel.

The "lessons of nature" gave us improved salvage with the addition of nutritional support. The lessons prepared us for further progress in the management of the extensive necrotic lesions.

REFERENCES

1. Boix-Ochoa J. Meconium Peritonitis. J Pediatr Surg 1968; 3:715-722.
2. Lorimer WS, Ellis DA. Meconium Peritonitis. Surgery 1966; 60:470-475.

H. Biemann Othersen, Jr., M.D.
Professor of Surgery and Pediatrics
Chief of Pediatric Surgery and Medical Director
The Children's Hospital
Medical University of South Carolina, Charleston

The author has reviewed here the experimental evidence which supports the pathogenesis of intestinal atresias and meconium peritonitis. That evidence indicates that intrauterine gangrene will lead to gut resorption and eventual atresia but occasionally auto-anastomosis. Dr. Moore has challenged us to use these intrauterine events as a model for treatment of the intestinal loss which occurs from necrotizing enterocolitis and malrotation with midgut volvulus. Just as plastic surgeons have become enthralled by fetal wound healing and are investigating that phenomenon, pediatric surgeons should study the intrauterine environment which allows resorption of gangrenous tissue. The concept is intriguing and certainly challenging and will be discussed further in the ensuing two chapters (6 and 7).

Raymond A. Amoury
Katherine Berry Richardon Professor of Pediatric Surgery
University of Missouri, Kansas City
Surgeon-in-Chief, Children's Mercy Hospital, Kansas City, MO
President, American Pediatric Surgical Association 1993-1994

Dr. Moore has nicely outlined the natural history of intra-uterine mesenteric vascular accidents causing intestinal necrosis. I would like to specifically address five areas.

1. The first is the clinical presentation of newborns with intra-uterine volvulus who present at birth with a pseudocyst consisting of necrotic and as yet, unresorbed intestine. As Dr. Moore has noted, there is a fibrous sheath overlying the remaining viable intestine which the operator must "pick through" until the underlying intact intestine, with two viable ends, is encountered. As Dr. Moore has suggested, if this process is intercepted postnatally later in its evolution, a conventional atresia with only two blind, atretic ends will be seen as the intervening necrotic intestine will have been resorbed by the fetus.

2. The second point concerns the need to screen patients with intestinal atresia for cystic fibrosis (CF). A significant number of neonates with ileal atresia will have cystic fibrosis as an underlying etiology. In these cases the thick, viscid meconium (characteristically found in newborns with meconium ileus due to cystic fibrosis) probably serves as a torque mechanism in producing a segmental rather than a midgut volvulus.

3. The third point concerns examining boys for inguinal hernias. If an enlarged, firm scrotum is encountered, it should not be assumed that this is a testicular tumor. A plain film or an ultrasound examination of the scrotum should be done. If calcificaiton is seen, this indicates an unusual presentation of a pre-existing, intra-uterine, intestinal perforation leading to meconium peritonitis with calcificaiton. In such a case, meconium has been discharged into the peritoneal cavity through a perforation. The spilled meconium then tracks its way down through the patent processus vaginalis, into the tunica vaginalis testis which surrounds the testicle and makes it appear enlarged and hard on inspection and palpation. These patients may have had a diagnosis of cystic fibrosis documented previously—if not, they should be screened for CF by a sweat test.

4. The fourth point that deserves emphasis is duodenojejunal atresia and the "apple-peel" anomaly.[1] Patients who have undergone successful resection of the atretic ends and primary anastomosis are very likely at increased risk to develop postoperative necrotizing enterocolitis (NEC). This is discussed in chapter 6. In our initial report on postoperative NEC[2] there were two infants with "apple-peel" anomaly who developed this complication. Both succumbed.

5. Finally, I would like to comment briefly on a hereditary form of multiple intestinal atresias. The atresias can occur from the gastric antrum to the distal colon. Patients with, what we have termed the "string of pearls" anomaly,[3] show a characteristic roentgen appearance of multiple, dense calcifications which appear centrally (intraperitoneally) rather than in the retroperitoneum. This is essentially an uncorrectable condition. Once the diagnosis is made, further attempts to salvage the infant by conventional means should be discontinued. The possible role of intestinal transplantation in these infants is very uncertain at the present time.

REFERENCES

1. Leonidas JC, Amoury RA, Ashcraft KW et al. Duodenojejunal atresia with "apple peel" small bowel. A distinct form of intestinal atresia. Radiology 1976; 118:661-665.
2. Amoury RA, Goodwin CD, McGill CW et al. Necrotizing enterocolitis following operation in the neonatal period. J Pediatr Surg 1980; 15:1-8.
3. Martin CD, Leonidas JC, Amoury RA. Multiple gastrointestinal atresias with intraluminal calcifications and cystic dilatation of bile ducts:A newly recognized entity resembline "a string of pearls". Pediatrics 1976; 57:268-271.

Robert J. Touloukian, M.D.
Professor of Surgery and Pediatrics
Yale University
Chief of Pediatric Surgery, Yale-New Haven Hospital

The emphasis in this chapter is on the pathogenesis of midgut atresia and meconium peritonitis with ample discussion given to the early pathology and experimental work from which we derive our current understanding of etiology.

The outstanding survival, reaching 90%, cited by current authors is a reflection of the importance of early detection, avoiding respiratory and metabolic complications, as well as meticulous surgical technique in reconstructing the GI tract. Prenatal diagnosis is available more often than not, particularly by 28 to 30 week gestation, when hydramnios is present. The importance of referral to a maternal high risk unit cannot be overemphasized, and early operation is facilitated by prompt transfer to a tertiary care pediatric surgery center.

The first operation for a baby with atresia will often determine outcome. The author has mentioned the importance of tapering the megaduodenum and jejunum to avoid the complications of a stagnant, nonperistaltic proximal limb. As important, are to sacrifice the large, bulbous segment and doing a spatulated primary anastomosis that avoids the blind loop syndrome. Saline or mineral oil should be milked into the colon in search of a membranous distal obstruction. Preserving even 2 or 3 cm of terminal ileum may be vital in preventing the short gut syndrome and severe TPN cholestasis.

David Tapper, M.D.
Professor of Surgery and Pediatrics
Vice Chairman of the Department of Surgery
University of Washington
Surgeon-in-Chief
Children's Hospital and Medical Center, Seattle

Review of the mechanisms of atresias, and presentation is accurate and descriptive. The majority of children with these abnormalities present early. Disasters occur when distended proximal atretic portions of intestine perforate. Polyhydramnios may be the initial clue and prenatal ultrasound can confirm intestinl pathology. Aspiration of greater than 30 cc of gastric fluid from newborns' stomach in the delivery room is indicative of some type of intestinal obstruction. This reviewer believes that this maneuver should always be done.

In our experience Type IV atresia (apple peel or Christmas tree) has shown improved survival recently. Our results have improved we believe related to minimal handling of intestine, surgically tapering a proximally dilated jejunum and hyperalimentation. Survival with hyperalimentation has improved dramatically although the length of hospitalization often exceeds 6 weeks.

This reviewer feels compelled to comment on the author's concept of the mechanisms of atresia and the creation of an in utero sterile environment. Without question, the mechanism that the author describes has been proven based on previous publications and multiple observations. The extension of this experiment-in-nature to the treatment of necrotizing enterocolitis and midgut volvulus is a greater step than this reviewer is willing to accept.

David L. Collins, M.D.
Pediatric Surgeon, Medical Group of San Diego
Clinical Professor of Surgery
University of California, San Diego

I agree with Dr. Moore that the contribution by Jan Louw concerning the dysfunction of the blind end of the atretic intestine, was most significant.

However, I believe his advice that the dilated blind end must be excised, while effective, will lead to unnecessary and, in some cases, significant loss of functional intestine. This intestine can be made to function quite effectively by simply plicating it, which will narrow the diameter down to the point that the peristaltic wave produces coaption, and, thus, effective propulsion of bowel contents. Failure of coaption is the reason that the dilated bowel, even though quite viable, will not adequately propel its contents.

The reason that plication, although proposed by Harrison and others, has not found favor, is that the stitches tend to pull out, and obstructive symptoms recur. At a second operation, the bowel is found in its original state.

I have found that this can be completely prevented using the technique of Teflon felt plication. One millimeter thick strips of Teflon felt about 3 millimeters wide, are placed along the sides of the bowel at points 180 degrees opposite from each other. They are an equal distance from the mesenteric attachment. The bowel is then folded together, and horizontal mattress sutures of nonabsorbable material are placed through the felt, the bowel, a third strip of felt which is placed in the middle of the plication, bowel again, felt again, and then back to be tied. This technique can be used at any level of the bowel, including ileum, jejunum or duodenum.

It would probably also work in the colon, although I have tended simply to do an end colostomy for colonic atresia with subsequent secondary closure.

CHAPTER 6

NECROTIZING ENTEROCOLITIS

INTRODUCTION

Isolated case reports of gastrointestinal perforation in the newborn and early neonatal period have dotted the pediatric and surgical literature from time immemorial. This low-key and somewhat sleepy area was jolted suddenly and dramatically in the mid-1960s by the thunderbolt of an epidemic of the highly lethal occurrence and the increasing frequency of necrotizing enterocolitis. The onset of this dreadful plague occurred during the onset of the increasing use of neonatal intensive care units and the increasing salvage of increasingly premature and increasingly fragile and low birth weight newborns. The onset of this new and frightening disorder was chronicled beautifully by a trio of major and classic publications between November 1964 and October 1967 from the Departments of Radiology, Pediatrics, Pathology and Pediatric Surgery of the Columbia University College of Physicians and Surgeons and the Columbia Presbyterian Medical Center and Babies Hospital of New York City.[1-3]

The 1964 paper in *Radiology* (83:879-887) by Berdon et al[1] reported 21 patients and three of their four survivors were treated surgically by resection of necrotic bowel. This experience clearly indicated the surgical nature of this fulminant new disease and its high overall mortality (81%). Their report also detailed the dramatic increase in the frequency of this disorder. Although their report spanned the period of 1954 to 1964, seven of their 21 patients (one third) were seen in a brief period of six months in 1963.

The 1967 report by Touloukian, Berdon, Amoury and Santilli[3] in the October issue of the *Journal of Pediatric Surgery* is one of the great classics of the pediatric surgery literature. In the quarter of a century (26 years) since the publication of this classic, little has been added to our understanding of the spectrum of this disease, nor its cause and cure—and its lethality and morbidity remain frighteningly high.

This 1967 report was concerned with 25 cases of necrotizing enterocolitis in the newborn. Their incidence of prematurity was high as only seven of their 25 patients (28%) weighed over 2500 g at birth. Following an early and rather limited latent period, the pattern of disease progression was rather consistent and reproducible involving fast abdominal distention and prolonged gastric emptying and vomiting which often contained bile. The initially normal stools became blood streaked and occasionally diarrheal as well. Increasing lethargy and pallor were followed by septic shock and death. Although both operative and nonoperative treatment were utilized, four of the six survivors were among the 15 patients operated upon and only two were in the 10 patients in the nonoperative group.

Roentgen findings were major factors involved in both patient monitoring and in treatment decisions and results analysis. Intestinal distention in the form of multiple loops of dilated small bowel was the most common roentgen finding and was encountered in 23 of the 25 patients (92%). It was the only X-ray finding in five patients and four died (80%). Intramural air (pneumatosis intestinalis) was an important but subtle and difficult-to-demonstrate finding. It appeared as small linear and bubbly extraluminal and subserosal collections of air and was demonstrated in eight patients, seven of whom died (88%). Pneumatosis peritoneum (free peritoneal air) as a clear indication of intestinal perforation and a clear indication for operation was found in four patients all of whom were operated upon with two deaths (50% mortality). The last and most ominous roentgen sign was "portal vein gas" (actually air dissecting along and outside the portal vein rather than within its lumen as air emboli). This finding was encountered in four patients all of whom died (100% mortality).

The discussion of the gross findings at operation or autopsy in the 1967 report by Touloukian et al[3] was particularly valuable and lucid. The diseased intestine was described as dilated and hemorrhagic, gray or necrotic (or all three) depending upon the extent of involvement. They made the important observation that grossly involved areas and the seemingly normal adjacent portions of intestine showed considerable friability. This suggested more extensive involvement than visually detectable. They emphasized that the most extensively involved gut area was the submucosa where

superficial ulcerations and submucosal hemorrhage were encountered along with the necrotic process. They pointed out that in many areas the denuded mucosa was covered by a slimy grayish coat of agglutinated inflammatory cells, fibrin and necrotic epithelium which formed a pseudomembrane. Impending perforation was identified as "ballooned-out" zones which were quite common with intact serosa alone preventing the breakthrough. Perforations occurred in 13 of their 25 cases (52%) and were located in the ileum in six cases, in the colon in five cases in the jejunum in two cases. They found perforation generally to be associated with necrosis of considerable length of intestine. Nonetheless, in two cases (ileum) it was localized. In addition to the perforation and pseudomembrane formation, they found gross and microscopic evidence of intramural gas (pneumatosis intestinalis) in the form of strips and bubbles involving both the submucosa and subserosa. It was of particular interest and importance that little cellular organization (or evidence of "healing") was encountered at the margins of these gas containing spaces.

Their appreciation of the surgical pitfalls of this awesome condition was both readily assessed and incisive. It was soon apparent that the pneumatosis intestinalis frequently was a premonitory sign of perforation. It was their quite reasonable hope that early operation based on the radiological finding of pneumatosis intestinalis alone might improve the dismal results of waiting for perforation. This was in line with a long surgical tradition of "operate before it ruptures". To their surprise and dismay the outcome in five cases so managed was uniformly fatal.

Because they considered small bowel distention alone too nonspecific to indicate or mandate operation, they established a policy of repeated roentgenograms over four hours to detect more readily the more specific roentgen findings of pneumatosis and/or pneumoperitoneum. Their conclusion has stood the test of time (26 years) and bears direct quotation:

The decision to limit surgery to patients who have actual perforation is a difficult one, but is deemed necessary in view of our inability to define adequately the extent of disease or to assess properly the site of involvement in the operating room when roentgenograms have shown only multiple distended loops of intestine or pneumatosis. Four of the six survivors were in babies where perforation had occurred and prompt radiographic identification was followed by resection which included the site of perforation.

Very little of significance has been added to these major and critical and most perceptive observations in the 30 years which have passed since the first of this trio of publications in 1963. The occurrence of necrotizing enterocolitis in association with exchange transfusions and umbilical vein catheterizations[4-6] and umbilical artery catheterization[7,8] have been added to the principal prematurity precursor since 1963.

Both the mortality and the morbidity have remained high. Attempts to replace resection and enterostomy with resection and primary anastomosis have not fared well.[9]

A 1969 report by Wilson and Woolley[10] from the Children's Hospital of Los Angeles in *Archives of Surgery* described 16 cases of necrotizing enterocolitis with nine operations and six deaths (67% mortality). In 1970 a 57% mortality of operation (7 cases) was reported from Oxford University (U.K.).[6] In 1973, Dudgeon et al[11] from Los Angeles Children's Hospital recorded a surgical mortality of 74% (14 of 19 patients).

Also in 1973, Ann Kosloske and Lester Martin[12] of the University of Cincinnati and the Cincinnati Children's Hospital made an important presentation before the Central Surgical Association describing not only the mortality of necrotizing enterocolitis but also its morbidity and complications. Surgical complications occurred in 10 of their 22 necrotizing enterocolitis patients and required 17 operations and

was associated with a 30% mortality. Many of their infants who survived the acute disease suffered serious late complications which included stricture of both colon and small bowel, enteric fistula, abscess formation, malabsorption and sepsis. In a discussion of this important paper William Sieber[13] of the Pittsburgh Children's Hospital stated that only one of eight premature infants operated upon for necrotizing enterocolitis at his institution had survived (an 88% mortality).

The stricture problem has been particularly troublesome with the incidence in major reported series ranging from 25% to 38%.[14-16] Strictures also have been reported with enterocyst formation and internal fistulas.[17]

The reported nonuniversity/community hospital experience with necrotizing enterocolitis was no better. In 1977, Roty et al[18] reported from the Bronson Medical Center of Kalamazoo, Michigan an experience with 61 cases of necrotizing enterocolitis. Twenty-six of these patients were treated medically/nonsurgically with 14 deaths and 12 survivors (54% mortality). Thirty-five of these patients were operated upon with 24 deaths and 11 survivors for a 69% mortality.

In 1981, Lester Martin and Wallace Noblett[18] of Cincinnati lamented in a *Journal of Pediatric Surgery* publication that the increased mortality with perforation in necrotizing enterocolitis and the frequent finding of massive intestinal necrosis have hampered efforts to improve survival. They express the dilemma quite well:

Operative indications for NEC vary widely. Numerous criteria have been used in an effort to coordinate timing of operation with demarcation of gangrenous intestine to avoid unnecessary resection of salvageable bowel. At operation, the viability of borderline intestine has been difficult to establish despite various methods to assess intestinal blood flow.

In 1986, Thomas Weber and Gene Lewis[19] from St. Louis (Cardinal Glennon

Children's Hospital) recorded an interesting experience with "second look" laparotomy in necrotizing enterocolitis. The most critically ill 14 (of 32) newborns with NEC and perforation underwent a planned second-look laparotomy at 24 to 36 hours after the initial operation to assess questionable viable bowel and resect if necessary, to irrigate out purulent material and to search for further perforations. Culture positive pus was found in all 14 cases, additional necrotic bowel in six and additional perforation was encountered in two. The survival in this group was 71% (10 of 14). Survival in the less ill group of 18 not receiving the second-look operation was 66% (12 of 18). This experience clearly demonstrates the relentless progression of the necrotic process despite operative attempts at cure by resection and stoma.

A very major publication in 1986 by Grosfeld, West and associates[20] of Indianapolis clearly and vividly delineates the spectrum of agony and disappointment in morbidity as well as mortality in the surgical care of necrotizing enterocolitis. Of 125 infants who underwent surgery for necrotizing enterocolitis (1972-1984) only 63 survived short-term (more than 30 days) for a mortality of 50%. In addition, there were 15 additional long-term (late) deaths for a total 62% mortality. Twenty-four of the survivors (38%) had the short bowel syndrome. Additional medical problems included cholestasis (17 cases), TPN induced cirrhosis of the liver (3 cases), meningitis (3 cases), seizures (8 cases) and nutritional rickets (6 cases). Furthermore, significant additional developmental and intellectual delays were encountered. Twenty-three of 48 long-term survivors (48%) were less than the fifth percentile for weight and/or height for their age. Only seven of the entire surviving group of 48 (14.5%) were greater than the 50th percentile.

Jackman et al[21] of London, U.K. (Queen Elizabeth Hospital for Children) in 1990 reported in the *British Journal of Surgery* a recent six year experience with 74 neonates with necrotizing enterocolitis of whom 40 (54%) were operated upon. The early post-operative mortality was 23% and there was one late death. The long-term results were rather disheartening. Of the 30 survivors, two had short bowel syndrome, two have chronic respiratory disease, two are partially sighted and five have experienced severe developmental delay. Only 50% of the survivors (15) enjoy good health.

In 1977, Sigmund Ein, Donald Marshall and David Girvan[22] of Toronto reported an experience with 5 cases of peritoneal drainage under local anesthesia for perforations from necrotizing enterocolitis. This procedure had first been carried out by one of the authors, Donald Marshall.[23] It was intended to be a temporizing rather than a definitive therapeutic undertaking and the mortality was 40%. A later, 1980, report from the same institution (Hospital for Sick Children, Toronto) by Janik and Ein[24] described 15 additional cases with 8 deaths and a mortality of 53%. The weights of these infants ranged from 600 to 3040 g.

The definitive answer to this approach of Ein and associates was provided in a 1988 article from Pittsburgh (Children's Hospital) by Cheu, Skarochana and Lloyd.[25] In their reported experience with 169 patients with established NEC, 92 (55%) underwent operation. Primary laparotomy was carried out in 41 of the 92 (45%) and 51 patients (55%) underwent primary peritoneal drainage (one third of those had a subsequent laparotomy within seven days). The mortality for the primary laparotomy group was 17% and that for the primary peritoneal drainage group was 47%—considerably higher. The authors concluded that primary peritoneal drainage is not an alternative to laparotomy.

A 1990 report by Ein et al[26] extended the local anesthesia drainage experience to 37 infants. It was still recommended as a temporizing procedure. Nonetheless, the mortality remained high at 44% and the morbidity was not addressed. Excluding the 12 infants who responded to drainage only and who presumably had minimal disease, the mortality in the other 25 infants was 64% (16 of 25).

In 1989, I[27] published in *Pediatric Surgery International* an entirely new definitive surgical approach to the management of necrotizing enterocolitis which was triggered by a sad and disastrous experience with the old approach of operation, resection of necrotic bowel and enterostomy.

This sad experience had its beginning in October of 1982 when I was asked to see a newborn infant who was quite ill with necrotizing enterocolitis with gut perforation and a large amount of free air in the peritoneal cavity on X-ray. At operation, extensive necrosis of the ileum and distal jejunum was encountered with multiple perforations. The necrotic and perforated small intestine was resected and a distal jejunal stoma was brought out through a stab wound to the right of the upper midline linea alba incision. A Stamm gastrostomy was carried out followed by placement of small Penrose drains loosely from the undersurface of both diaphragms to exit sites through stab wounds at the lowest parts of both lower quadrants with extra loops placed in the pelvic area. The peritoneal cavity was irrigated with warm salt solution to clear out remaining fecal contents and other debris. The patient was markedly improved the next day. The jejunostomy stoma which early on appeared pink and healthy grew steadily more dusky and then cyanotic and necrotic with progressive dry gangrene prior to its slough and disappearance in about five days following operation. Shortly thereafter, liquid intestinal contents appeared at both dependent drainage sites and were collected in standard enterostomy bags both for measurement and to prevent skin erosion and damage. The infant's general condition remained unchanged during these happenings. As this enteric volume did not diminish, a TPN Broviac catheter was placed in the external jugular vein. The patient tolerated all of this remarkably well and continued to improve and gain weight for the next eight weeks. As the drainage site enteric fluid output continued, it was concluded that this was time for a reexploration to restore intestinal continuity.

At operation, the stunning finding was that all of the small intestine had disappeared with at most one or two centimeters of jejunum at the ligament of Treitz. This clearly was incompatible with life and the patient died shortly thereafter. I then firmly resolved *never again* to do either a bowel resection or an enterostomy in a case of necrotizing enterocolitis.

An important observation from this experience was that internal intestinal fistulation could be "captured" by extensive peritoneal cavity drainage by Penrose drains creating "de facto" and quite adequate enterostomies. Gastrostomy and Broviac TPN, not always employed in early cases, soon became standard and routine.

The basic principle of this approach was to achieve maximum salvage of all salvageable intestine, large and small, and to simulate as nearly as possible the in utero "lesson of nature" in which maximum gut salvage occurred with only a limited atretic segment or segments despite catastrophic in utero ischemia and gangrene (see chapter 5 for more details on this fascinating matter).

Broviac TPN simulated the maternal placental circulation for nutrition and the sterile fetal peritoneal cavity was simulated by drainage exit of fecal contents and prompt adhesion elimination of the peritoneal cavity (hence no place for peritonitis to occur).

The extensive peritoneal cavity drainage by Penrose drains came easily to the me because I had relied extensively on them to keep me out of trouble for some 30 years. In a 14 year period (1952-1966) early in my surgical career when my private practice was largely (95%) adult, Penrose drains were employed in all cholecystectomies, all gastric resections in which a closed duodenal stump was left behind, in all ruptured appendices and in all sigmoid colon resections for cancer and diverticulitis (usually supplemented by an Argyle chest tube passed by anorectum beyond the primary anastomosis for venting and stenting in lieu of colostomy).

Interestingly, the last case of necrotizing enterocolitis operated upon by me had extensive necrosis and loss of the distal transverse and descending colon and sigmoid and was managed by intraluminal gut chest tube venting and stenting beyond the most proximal perforation, supplementing suture "patching" of multiple large necrotic perforations. This infant survived and did not develop Penrose drain sites enteric fistula discharge.

This approach of "patch, drain and wait" also has been employed successfully in the management of midgut volvulus with extensive necrosis and gangrene[28] and will be considered in greater detail in the Challenges section.

CHALLENGES

1. The overwhelmingly most important challenge in the management of necrotizing enterocolitis is how to achieve maximum salvage of both functioning baby and functioning gut.

The disastrous results over many, many years and despite improved facilities, TPN, antibiotics, etc. with resection and either enterostomy or primary anastomosis clearly demand a new approach. Both resection and enterostomy or primary anastomosis in the face of continuing and on-going necrosis and gangrene end up being largely gut losing and gut destructive processes.

The basic and foremost principle of the "patch, drain and wait" approach is to lose no gut by resection or stoma creation trauma.

The in utero environment for maximum salvage of extensive ischemic and necrotic gut is simulated by TPN for maternal placental nutrition and extensive peritoneal cavity drainage, fistula capturing and peritoneal cavity obliteration (no chance for peritonitis in nonexisting peritoneal cavity) simulate a "de facto" "sterile" (or at least an infection-free or infection-controlled) peritoneal cavity. Inflammation-induced neovascularization doubtless makes a major contribution to the salvage of bowel of borderline viability. This neovascularization may be rather exuberant early on and may pose a serious hazard if attempts to reoperate to reestablish intesti-

nal continuity are made too soon after the initial operation. One infant, quite early in this experience died of excessive and uncontrollable bleeding during a second and too early operation.

The development of the "patch, drain and wait" approach was evolutionary rather than revolutionary. As indicated in the Introduction section, its inception germinated from a disastrous failure of the old resect and stoma approach and important observations during this sad experience.

At the time of the 1989 publication, a seven year experience had accumulated and a definitive management protocol was well established. Its essence was and is as follows:

1. First of all, a Broviac catheter for fluid and electrolyte administration and for TPN is inserted via the external or internal jugular vein into the central venous area. This is done and secured, isolated and sterile, prior to laparotomy and the spread or potential spread of hazardous bacteria, etc. across the torso from the peritoneal cavity.

2. The peritoneal cavity is entered quickly by a supra-umbilical mid-line lineal alba vertical incision which provides both speed and an essentially bloodless field (electrocautery dissection) which, with comparatively heavy interrupted sutures, provides a very strong wound closure as well. It also may readily be extended downward if needed (seldom is).

3. On entering the peritoneal cavity, the level(s) and degree of necrotic and perforated damage are assessed after careful and atraumatic suction and irrigation of accumulated fecal matter, necrotic fragments and other debris. The entire gastrointestinal tract is carefully inspected from the diaphragm to the pelvic floor with a very minimum of intestinal "handling".

4. If extensive or total intestinal necrosis and fragmenting are encountered, no "patching" is attempted as there is nothing to patch. The operator then pro-

ceeds with extensive bilateral Penrose drain draining, gastrostomy and wound closure. Discrete perforations or necrotic thin "veil" covered impending perforations in other cases are approximated loosely by fore and aft interrupted 6-0 silk sutures with no attempt at water-tight closure or traditional "anastomosis"-type of closure.

5. A Stamm gastrostomy then is carried out and secured to the anterior abdominal wall with interrupted sutures.

6. Small Penrose drains are inserted into the peritoneal cavity bilaterally through stab wounds in the most dependent portions of both lower quadrants. Long segments of Penrose drain are loosely brought from the undersurface of the domes of both diaphragms to the exit sites in both lower quadrants with additional loops into the pelvis and flanks and are secured with heavy (2-0) silk sutures at the exit sites.

7. The linea alba incision is firmly and securely closed with interrupted heavy sutures with a small rubber wick drain in the lower part of the incision subcutaneous tissue with staples for quick skin closure.

The 1989 report included details of five representative and illustrative cases all of whom survived despite near total intestinal necrosis and fragmentation (intestine in shreds) in two. It also described briefly a then recent 11 month experience with eight additional infants with necrotizing enterocolitis and birth weights ranging from 800 to 1800 g with perforation which had been managed successfully by the "patch, drain and wait" approach. The captured "de facto" enterostomies closed spontaneously in six of these infants and in two operative closure was required—all successfully. The 1991 report in *Pediatric Surgery International*[28] increased the number of cases without mortality, stricture or short bowel syndrome to 14 consecutive cases. In the author's most recent 18 consecutive cases of necrotizing enterocolitis with perforation there has been no mortality, no short bowel syndrome and no stricture formation.

It is estimated from these experiences that the captured enteric fistula "de facto" enterostomies will close spontaneously in from two thirds to three fourths of the cases. It is presumed that this spontaneous reestablishment of intestinal continuity is similar to the in utero auto-anastomosis phenomenon observed in meconium peritonitis cases without intestinal obstruction at birth.

The absence of intestinal diversion may have contributed to the absence of stricture formation. This issue was addressed beautifully by Irving Enquist and Bernard Levowitz[29] of Brooklyn (N.Y.) and the Medical School of the State University of New York in their brilliant experimental study of stricture formation in defunctionalized segments of colon in dogs and published in the December 1956 issue of *Surgery* (40:1085-1093).

CONCLUSION

Necrotizing enterocolitis is a 30-year old epidemic of catastrophic intestinal ischemia, necrosis and perforation of still unknown cause which occurs largely in premature newborn infants with an unabating mortality and an awesome and debilitating morbidity for which the long-time standard surgical approaches of resection and stoma formation or primary anastomosis have been disappointing failures despite all the important advances in the care of premature infants which have taken place in the past 30 years.

I have proposed an entirely new approach which I term "patch, drain and wait". Neither resection nor enterostomy is a part of this approach, which emphasizes maximum salvage of compromised intestine. Major features of this method are prolonged total parenteral nutrition/TPN, gastrostomy, minimal bowel handling, loose transverse approximation ("patching") of the upper and lower margins of a limited number of major perforations and extensive and prolonged drainage of the peritoneal cavity by Penrose drains placed from both diaphragms to exit sites in the inferior aspects of both lower quadrants.

Marked improvement in the infant's condition occurs within hours. Enteric fistulas develop in the majority of cases and are "captured" by one or both of the Penrose drains with disappearing peritonitis and the formation of "de facto" enterostomies at one of the drainage sites (generally the left side). The approximately 25% of the "de facto" enterostomies which do not close spontaneously may be closed operatively. The last 18 cases of necrotizing enterocolitis with perforation managed by this approach by me have been managed with no mortality, no short bowel syndrome and no stricture formation. These results are infinitely better than those with any other approach reported to date.

This "patch, drain and wait" approach is modeled on the experiment of nature in which extensive gut necrosis from a vascular catastrophe in utero may result in only a limited atresia or may eventuate only in a meconium peritonitis with telltale calcification and no intestinal obstruction. Broviac hyperalimentation/TPN functions as the placenta for nutrition and the Penrose drains simulate a sterile in utero peritoneal cavity as "de facto" enterostomies are established and as adhesion obliteration of the peritoneal cavity and inflammation-induced angiogenesis, with adequate antibiotics on board, lead to maximum gut preservation, large and small, in a comparatively aseptic environment.

This approach has also been used by me with success in the management of midgut volvulus with extensive necrosis as the next chapter will consider in more detail and as reported in 1991 in *Pediatric Surgery International*.[28]

The late 1940s experimental studies of Laufman et al[30] and Davis et al[31] provide some interesting observations pertaining to the "patch, drain and wait" central concept of salvage of severely damaged ischemic gut by revascularization. The citation of the important studies of Laufman et al[30] by Louw and Barnard[32] is discussed at length in chapter 5 on midgut atresias and meco-

nium peritonitis as experimental evidence in support of their proposal of in utero intestinal ischemia as the cause of intestinal atresia. Laufman et al of Chicago reported in 1949 in *Archives of Surgery* that intestinal ischemia-induced autolysis of small intestine in the peritoneal cavity of dogs in the relative absence of bacteria resulted in a residual fibrous cord or complete absence of the ischemic devascularized segment of gut. Another important observation of this Laufman et al report is as follows:

> Another feature of these preliminary experiments was the striking observation that whenever the blood supply to one of these closed loops was severed and the loop placed back into the peritoneal cavity, it soon acquired a new blood supply through omental and serosal adhesions.

Laufman et al cited similar results obtained by Davis et al[31] of Los Angeles using rabbits in which a new blood supply of surviving devascularized small intestine was formed from omental and serosal adhesions as well as from revascularization from the mesentery and speculated that "the bowel in these experiments (of Davis et al[31]) apparently never reached the stage of irreversible autolysis but, being almost sterile, was able to survive until a new blood supply was formed."

In their 1948 report in *Surgery, Gynecology and Obstetrics*, Davis et al[31] stated that

> examination of the devascularized loops of surviving animals showed that the blood supply to the devascularized area came from five sources: adherent loops of intestine, growth of mesenteric vessels, the omentum which was frequently found adherent to the damaged loop, vascularized adhesions from the parietal peritoneum and the devascularized loop of bowel and collateral circulation through the intramural blood vessels.

REFERENCES

1. Berdon WE, Grossman H, Baker DH et al. Necrotizing enterocolitis in the premature infant. Radiology 1964; 83:879-887.

2. Mizrahi A, Barlow O, Berdon W et al. Necrotizing enterocolitis in premature infants. J Pediatr 1965; 66:697-703.

3. Touloukian RJ, Berdon WE, Amoury RA et al. Surgical experience with necrotizing enterocolitis in the infant. J Pediatr Surg 1967; 2:389-401.

4. Orme RL, Edes SM. Perforation of the bowel in the newborn as a complication of exchange transfusion. Br Med J 1968; 4:349-351.

5. Caralps-Riera JM, Cohn BD. Bowel perforation after exchange transfusion in the neonate: Review of the literature and report of a case. Surgery 1970; 68:895-898.

6. deSa DJ, Mucklow ES, Gough MH. Neonatal gut infarction. J Pediatr Surg 1970; 5:454-459.

7. Marchildon MB, Buck BE, Abdenour G. Necrotizing enterocolitis in the unfed infant. J Pediatr Surg 1982; 17:620-624.

8. Roty AR, Kilway JB, Brown AL. Acute necrotizing enterocolitis in neonates. Am Surg 1977; 43:392- 394.

9. Cooper A, Ross AJ, O'Neill JA et al. Resection with primary anastomosis for necrotizing enterocolitis. J Pediatr Surg 1988; 23:64-68.

10. Wilson SE, Woolley MM. Primary necrotizing enterocolitis in infants. Arch Surg 1969; 99:563-566.

11. Dudgeon DL, Coran AG, Lauppe FA et al. Surgical management of necrotizing enterocolitis in infancy. J Pediatr Surg 1973; 8:607-614.

12. Kosloske AM, Martin LW. Surgical complication of neonatal necrotizing enterocolitis. Arch Surg 1973; 107:223-228.

13. Sieber WK. Discussion of paper by Kosloske AM, Martin LW. Arch Surg 1973; 107:228.

14. Schwartz MZ, Richardson J, Hayden CK et al. Intestinal stenosis following successful medical management of necrotizing enterocolitis. J Pediatr Surg 1986; 15:890-897.

15. Born M, Holgersen LO, Shahrivar F et al. Routine contrast enemas for diagnosing and managing strictures following nonoperative treatment for necrotizing enterocolitis. J Pediatr Surg 1985; 20:461-463.

16. Ross MN, Wayne ER, Janik JS et al. A standard of comparison for acute surgical necrotizing enterocolitis. J Pediatr Surg 1989; 24:998-1002.

17. Lloyd DA, Cwyes S. Intestinal stenosis and enterocyst formation as late complications of neonatal necrotizing enterocolitis. J Pediatr Surg 1973; 8:479-486.

18. Martin LW, Noblett WW. Early operation with intestinal diversion for necrotizing enterocolitis. J Pediatr Surg 1981; 16: 252-255.

19. Weber TR, Lewis JE. Role of second-look laporotomy in necrotizing enterocolitis. J Pediatr Surg 1986; 21:323-325.

20. Cikrit D, West KW, Schreiner R et al. Long-term follow-up after surgical management of necrotizing enterocolitis: Sixty-three cases. J Pediatr Surg 1986; 21:533-535.

21. Jackman S, Breveton RJ, Wright VM. Result of surgical treatment of neonatal necrotizing enterocolitis. Br J Surg 1990; 77:146-148.

22. Ein SH, Marshall DG, Girvan D. Peritoneal drainage under local anesthesia for necrotizing enterocolitis. J Pediatr Surg 1977; 12:963-967.

23. Marshall DG. Peritoneal drainage under local anesthesia for necrotizing enterocolitis. Presented at meeting of Canadian Association of Pediatric Surgeons, Winnipeg, Manitoba, January 1975.

24. Janik JS, Ein SH. Peritoneal drainage under local anesthesia for necrotizing enterocolitis perforation: A second look. J Pediatr Surg 1980; 15:565-568.

25. Cheu HW, Sukarochana K, Lloyd DA. Peritoneal drainage for necrotizing enterocolitis. J Pediatr Surg 1988; 23:557-561.

26. Ein SH, Shandling B, Wesson D et al. A 13 year experience with peritoneal drainage under local anesthesia for necrotizing enterocolitis perforation. J Pediatr Surg 1990; 25:1034-1037.

27. Moore TC. The management of necrotizing enterocolitis by "patch, drain and wait". Pediatr Surg Int 1989; 4:110-113.

28. Moore TC. Management of midgut volvulus with extensive necrosis by "patch, drain and

wait" in early infancy and childhood. Pediatr Surg Int 1991; 6:313-317.

29. Enquist IF, Levowitz BS. The development of anastomotic strictures in defunctionalized bowel. Surgery 1956; 40:1085-1093.

30. Laufman H, Martin WB, Method H et al. Observations in strangulation obstruction: II. The fate of sterile devascularized intestine in the peritoneal cavity. Arch Surg

1949; 59:550-564.

31. Davis HA, Gaster J, Marsh RL et al. The effect of streptomycin in experimental strangulation of the bowel. Surg Gynec Obstet 1948; 87:63-67.

32. Louw JH, Barnard CN. Congenital intestinal atresia. Observations on its origin. Lancet 1955; 2:1065- 1067.

INVITED COMMENTARY

J. Eugene Lewis, Jr., M.D.
Professor Emeritus of Pediatric Surgery
St. Louis University

Necrotizing enterocolitis has been a catastrophic event in my surgical career. Beginning as an occasional phenomenon, the incidence rapidly increased with the improved salvage of premature infants. The devastating intestinal ischemia, necrosis and perforation occurring largely in premature infants have produced an unabating mortality and awesome expensive morbidity. Standard surgical approaches of resection, primary anastomosis and stoma formation have been disappointing failures.

This chapter documents these failures despite the important advances in the care of premature infants. The second look operation offers very little improvement in results.

The author proposes an approach which he describes as "patch, drain, and wait". Neither resection or enterostomy is part of the approach. Maximum salvage of compromised intestine is the goal with total parenteral nutrition, gastrostomy, loose closure (patching) of major perforations and extensive and prolonged drainage of the peritoneal cavity from both diaphragms to exit sites in the abdomen. The results have been most impressive. The treatment has been modeled on the results of in utero vascular catastrophes.

I have no experience with this approach as definitive treatment. However, the surgical approach seems to have great merit. The author emphasizes the factors in success as the use TPN functioning as the placenta for nutrition; the penrose drains simulating a sterile in utero peritoneal cavity as "de facto" enterostomies are established; and adhesion obliteration of the peritoneal cavity and inflammation-induced angiogenesis, with antibiotics, leading to a maximum gut preservation in a comparatively aseptic environment. The author's results and the experimental studies of Enquist and Levowitz justify further use of this approach.

H. Biemann Othersen, Jr., M.D.
Professor of Surgery and Pediatrics
Chief of Pediatric Surgery and Medical Director
The Children's Hospital
Medical University of South Carolina, Charleston

Dr. Moore again has challenged physicians to consider the in utero events which allow correction of the abdominal catastrophe of mesenteric vascular occlusion by resorption of gangrenous gut and healing of the adjacent intestine. It is the author's contention that a central catheter furnishing total parenteral nutrition may substitute for the placenta and peritoneal drainage might mimic the sterile intrauterine environment. I can see the rationale of the first proposition but when the gut is colonized soon after birth, a sterile intestinal content is difficult to obtain. Adequate drainage of the peritoneal cavity may prevent accumulation of pus and produce fistulas rather than abscesses.

This concept is an interesting one worthy of serious consideration. However, one must remember that sometimes intrauterine accidents result in near total loss of intestines with multiple atresias or a very short bowel. All intrauterine vascular events are not completely corrected by the time of birth. Even so, the concept is worth exploring in very premature infants whose survival by conventional approaches has been poor.

Raymond A. Amoury, M.D.
Katherine Berry Richardson Professor of Pediatric Surgery
University of Missouri, Kansas City
Surgeon-in-Chief, Children's Mercy Hospital, Kansas City, MO
President, American Pediatric Surgical Association 1993-1994

Doctor Moore has nicely outlined the historical aspects of necrotizing enterocolitis (NEC) from its recognition as a distinct entity, through the various methods used in the medical and surgical management of these critically ill infants.

I would like to emphasize again the appearance of NEC in postoperative patients. In 1980 NEC following operation in the neonatal period was described for the first time from The Children's Mercy Hospital. Necrotizing enterocolitis appeared in the less familiar postoperative setting in nine infants.[1] All showed the clinical findings of NEC, as well as the characteristic roentgen finding of pneumatosis intestinalis. Three had portal vein gas. A search of the literature at that time showed a paucity of information regarding NEC as a complication following operations at any age, but especially in the newborn period. Of the nine patients described in this original report one had esophageal atresia with a distal TEF, one tetralogy of Fallot, two had duodenojejunal atresia with the "apple peel" anomaly, three had gastroschisis, one had supralevator anorectal atresia with a rectosigmoid fistula, and one had multiple small intestinal atresias. I have commented on the occurrence of NEC in infants who have undergone repair of gastroschisis in chapter 3 "Gastroschisis". The two infants in our original report with the "apple peel" anomaly were progressing satisfactorily following resection of the atretic ends of the intestine and primary anastomosis, when they developed signs and symptoms of NEC. Both patients succumbed rapidly. As Dr. Moore has indicated, (chapter 5) it is important to note that the intestinal circulation in the "apple-peel" anomaly is precarious, based as it is on retrograde flow from the superior mesenteric artery via the right colic artery. In addition, the intestine is unfixed and its "apple-peel" configuration puts it more at risk for ischemia. Any shift in circulatory pattern, for example, from dehydration, could result in a low flow state in the intestinal microcirculation and necrosis. Aggressive feeding programs, especially with hyperosmolar feedings, probably served to initiate a cascade of NEC in this setting which proved lethal in our two patients. In summary, gastroschisis and the "apple-peel" anomaly should be regarded as risk factors for NEC.

I would like to add another possible risk factor, namely, cocaine exposure to the fetus. A review of our experience at The Children's Mercy Hospital and the Truman Medical Center, University of Missouri-Kansas City School of Medicine by Downing, Horner, and Kilbride[2] strongly suggested a cause and effect relationship. Cocaine is an amino-alcohol with vasoconstrictive properties. Several possible mechanisms, both prenatally and postnatally, could predispose to the onset of NEC. These include reduced uterine blood flow resulting in fetal hypoxemia, tachycardia, hypertension, and chronic placental insufficiency which may also result in intrauterine growth retardation and altered blood flow to the gastrointestinal tract. Diminished splanchnic circulation may also occur secondary to cocaine-induced low cardiac output in the newborn.

Czyrko et al[3] reported on their experience in ten infants born to cocaine abusers. These neonates showed a 2.38-fold increase in risk of developing NEC compared with controls matched for race, sex, and birthweight. A greater percentage of the cocaine-positive infants with NEC required operation (70% versus 42% of controls) and their mortality was significantly higher (50% versus 23%).

We have had a somewhat different experience at The Children's Mercy Hospital. During a two year period 5,937 live births occurred at the Truman Medical Center, University of Missouri-Kansas City School of Medicine, with 794 of these babies admitted to our neonatal intensive care unit. Of these admitted 69 (8.6%) tested positive for cocaine metabolites. The overall incidence of NEC was 3.2% (26/794). Of the infants with NEC, 38% (10/26) had documentation of maternal cocaine exposure. Their gestational ages were greater, and the onset of disease was earlier than in noncocaine infants developing NEC. Two of these NEC patients were term infants with no known risk factors for NEC. Three additional infants were not fed prior to the onset of NEC. Some reports from large urban centers have shown no increase in the incidence of NEC in cocaine-positive babies, whereas others have shown a significant increase in very low birth weight (VLBW-under 800 grams) infants exposed to cocaine.

The possible role of reperfusion injury, toxic oxygen radicals, and toxic radical scavengers in the pathogenesis of NEC has been briefly reviewed.[4] Clark and colleagues have examined the contribution of oxygen-derived free radicals in experimental NEC[5] and the protective effects of the scavenger enzyme superoxide dismutase (SOD).[6] Finally, Clark et al[7] have focused on the role of specific nutrients and intraluminal biochemical events in the pathogenesis of NEC and the reparative effects of nitric oxide (NO) on chemically injured gut.[8]

REFERENCES

1. Amoury RA, Goodwin CD, McGill CW et al. Necrotizing enterocolitis following operation in the neonatal period. J Pediatr Surg 1980; 15:1-8.
2. Downing GJ, Horner SR, Kilbride HW. Characteristic of perinatal cocaine-exposed infants with necrotizing enterocolitis. Am J Dis Child 1991; 145:26-27.
3. Czyrko C, Del Pin C, O'Neill JA Jr. et al. Maternal cocaine abuse in necrotizing enterocolitis: Outcome and survival. J Pediatr Surg 1991; 26:414-421.
4. Amoury RA. Necrotizing enterocolitis. In: Ashcraft KW, Holder TM. eds. Pediatric Surgery, 2nd. ed. Philadelphia: W.B. Saunder Company, 1993, p. 341-357.
5. Clark DA, Fornabaio DM, McNeill H et al. Contribution of oxygen-derived free radicals to experimental necrotizing enterocolitis. Am J Pathol 1988; 130:537-542.
6. Miller MJS, McNeill H, Mullane KM et al. SOD prevents damage and attenuates eicosanoid release in a rabbit model of necrotizing enterocolitis. Am J Physiol 1988; 255:G556-G565.
7. Clark DA, Thompson JE, Weiner LB et al. Necrotizing enterocolitis: Intraluminal biochemistry and bacteria and an animal model. Pediatr Res 1985; 19:919-921.
8. Miller MJS, Zhang XJ, Sadowska-Krowicka H et al. Nitric oxide release in response to gut injury. Scand J Gastroenterol 1993; 28:149-154.

John G. Raffensperger, M.D.
Professor of Surgery, Northwestern University
Surgeon-in-Chief, Children's Memorial Hospital, Chicago
Editor, *Swenson's Pediatric Surgery*

Regarding atresias, meconium peritonitis, necrotizing enterocolitis or midgut volvulus, it seems to me that you have covered these very well. I disagree with you completely, however, on the management of necrotizing enterocolitis. We treat a large number of these babies in one of two ways. In the very small infants, we simply make a right lower quadrant incision and insert a drain under local anesthesia. It is amazing how well this works. As you say, there is something mysterious going on because, in many cases, when there has been an obvious perforation with free air, the intestine heals itself. On the other hand, if the infant is unstable, weighs over 1,000 grams, has signs of peritonitis and a dropping platelet count, we always operate, resect the most involved bowel and create a double stoma. If there is total gut necrosis, we simply close and advise the parents that nothing should be done.

Arnold M. Salzberg, M.D.
Professor of Surgery and Pediatrics
Division of Pediatric Surgery
Medical College of Virginia, Richmond

In spite of the "patch, drain and wait" approach, there are a number of newborns with NEC who benefit from bowel resection and stomal construction in the presence of a fore-shortened mesentery, tenuous bowel and diminished mesenteric blood flow. With the usual end enterostomy, the mesenteric side of the bowel is tethered and cannot be comfortably exteriorized without tension even with division of mesentery, which then jeopardizes viability. Revisions may sacrifice precious bowel.

To avoid this problem, a short terminal loop enterostomy is formed over a rod. The bowel end is closed and a short loop of adjacent intestine is brought through an ample opening in the abdominal wall and sutured to fascia and peritoneum. A 1 cm anti-mesenteric longitudinal enterostomy is matured. Conservation of intestinal mesentery assures bidirectional stomal blood flow without tension. Later, stomal closure is performed with minimal loss of bowel length.

This technical supplement of terminal anti-mesenteric short loop enterostomy has proven useful in constructing stomas in newborns with NEC, in whom the traditional end enterostomy seemed precarious because of tension or viability.

REFERENCE

1. Alaish SM, Pendurthi TM, Michna Ba, Drucker DEM, Krummel TM, Bousamra M, Salzberg AM. Terminal short loop enterostomy in necrotizing enterocolitis. (To be published)

David Tapper, M.D.
Professor of Surgery and Pediatrics
Vice Chairman of the Department of Surgery
University of Washington
Surgeon-in-Chief
Children's Hospital and Medical Center, Seattle

This is an extensive review of necrotizing enterocolitis. The author clearly states that as a result of his personal experiences with resection and anastomoses, he has evolved a technique of "patch, drain and wait". This technique is based on the assumption mentioned in chapter 5 related to intestinal atresias in the sterile abdominal cavity (the so-called experiment-in-nature). Although the author's results are excellent and clearly better than other reported series, I have difficulty accepting the in utero atresia model as an explanation for the success of the treatment. The fetal intestine has no air within the bowel lumen to cause increased pressure and displacement of bacteria into capillaries and portal circulation. If the abdominal cavity becomes obliterated by the inflammatory reaction, what is the morbidity and mortality of later operation to establish intestinal continuity. In addition, I do not believe that any formulation of total parenteral nutrition approximates the nutrition in the amniotic cavity.

One group of patients not mentioned is the larger neonate who develops signs and symptoms of necrotizing enterocolitis. I believe the pathophysiology is different in these children and the disease may present more quickly and be more virulent. Prompt and early intervention, prior to perforation, has a greater chance of salvaging these infants. When compared to the 600-900 gram neonate on a ventilator, this larger infant tolerates surgery better and should be treated when signs of worsening peritonitis occur. Primary excision with anastomoses can often be performed.

David L. Collins, M.D.
Pediatric Surgeon, Medical Group of San Diego
Clinical Professor of Surgery
University of California, San Diego

I have nothing to add, but agree completely with the principles Dr. Moore espouses. I have not yet had a case of extensive patchy necrosis, which would be suitable one on which to try the "patch, drain and wait" technique of Dr. Moore. However, I am planning to use it at my next opportunity.

CHAPTER 7

MIDGUT VOLVULUS

INTRODUCTION

Midgut volvulus with extensive midgut ischemia, necrosis and gangrene is one of the most awesome, frightening, disabling and lethal acquired conditions to occur in childhood, or any other, years. It was quite aptly labeled "The Deadly Vomit" by Millar et al[1] in a 1987 publication of 137 cases seen in a 28 year experience. The high and unrelenting mortality has been unchanged over the years as cited in numerous publications and as clearly documented in a 1992 publication of 182 cases of malrotation and its complications by Messineo et al[2] of the Hospital for Sick Children of Toronto.

The frequent occurrence of symptomatic malrotation of the intestine in the early neonatal period due to duodenal obstruction from Ladd's bands or midgut volvulus with early bilious vomiting ("the deadly vomit") and occasional blood in the stools and the high mortality of midgut volvulus with midgut ischemia, necrosis and gangrene were addressed well in early publications dealing with this illusive topic.[3-5]

Snyder and Chaffin[3] of Los Angeles provided clear illustrations of the fixation (normal or non and short) of the dorsal mesentery and of the comparative ease of torsion of the nonfixed dorsal mesentery bowel and the resulting catastrophe of midgut volvulus and torsion-triggered acute interruption of the blood supply to the volvulus involved midgut. Bill and associates[4] made important observations concerning Ladd's bands and their management.

Stewart et al,[5] in 1976, reported a 15 year experience (1951-1966) with 164 patients with symptomatic malrotation of the bowel from the Children's Hospital of Boston. Five of their patients died of midgut volvulus before surgical treatment could be rendered. Midgut volvulus was present in 77 of the 159 patients operated upon (48%). Twelve of the 77 patients with midgut volvulus required resection (15%). The mortality of these 77 and 12 patients is not specifically identified.

Important publications appeared in 1970 and 1972 from New York regarding the roentgen diagnosis of midgut malrotation and volvulus by Berdon, Santulli and associates[6] of Columbia University and Babies Hospital and by Simpson, Becker, Schneider and associates[7] of the Mount Sinai Hospital and Medical School. These two reports were particularly thorough and well illustrated and agreed that the most important initial contrast X-rays should be upper gastrointestinal.

In 1976, an important report from Mt. Sinai Hospital and Medical School by Krasna, Becker, Schneider and associates reported the combined use of antithrombotic low molecular weight dextran and a second-look operation 36 to 48 hours after the initial operation for ischemic midgut volvulus in five cases. Symptoms of abdominal distention and bile stained vomiting had appeared early after birth in all five (at 12, 28, 30, 33 and 48 hours). Remarkable recovery of seemingly destroyed bowel at the first operation had occurred in all five cases and four of the five survived. The one death resulted from septic thrombosis of the superior vena cava. Each case is well and clearly presented. The authors express well and feelingly the dilemma of this problem:

> Unfortunately, however, the appearance of the involved bowel at the time of derotation and Ladd procedure is not a reliable enough way to determine viability or nonviability. The early appearance of infarcted bowel is closely mimicked by that of still viable, hemorrhagic, congested, bluish and pulseless bowel that has just been derotated in a child in shock. At this time, a surgical decision on the extent of resection required, is very likely to result in the removal of very long segments of bowel.

In 1981, the simultaneous occurrence of malrotation with intussusception[9,10] and with Hirschsprung's disease[10] was reported from the USA and from Britain. The report by Filston and Kirks of Duke University was titled "Malrotation—The Ubiquitous Anomaly" and was concerned with 34 gut rotational anomalies seen at Duke during a four year period (1976-1980). Twenty-one of these cases (62%) were associated with significant congenital anomalies other than abdominal wall defects or diaphragmatic hernias. Twenty-two of their patients presented with symptoms of obstruction related to malrotation and four of their patients had signs of intestinal

ischemia prior to operation. Midgut volvulus was found in 17 of the 22 patients operated upon for obstruction (77%) and four required extensive resection because of necrosis. One infant died of unrecognized malrotation and volvulus at operation for obstruction thought to be due to Hirschsprung's disease.

An important 1982 publication from the Children's Hospital of Philadelphia by Howell et al[11] drew attention to the role and importance of patient nutrition in the malrotation and ischemic bowel picture. They reviewed a five year experience with 50 cases of anomalies of midgut rotation and fixation. Forty-four of these children were operated upon. Two additional infants died rapidly of profound shock before operation could be attempted and intestinal gangrene was confirmed at autopsy. Nine of 15 children coming to operation in the first week of life had an associated midgut volvulus (60%) and two of the nine were found to have intestinal gangrene (22%). Four of 10 infants operated upon between the first week and first year of life also had midgut volvulus (40%) but no gangrene. Six of the 14 late presenting children (over 1 year of age with two over 7 years of age) also had midgut volvulus (43%) and one of the six (17%) had gangrene. They reported that 90% of the patients with volvulus had malnutrition as compared with only 58% without volvulus. One of their patients also had intussusception associated with a midgut volvulus.

The 1987 Millar et al[1] "deadly vomit" publication in *Pediatric Surgery International* reviewed their 28 year experience with 137 cases of malrotation and midgut volvulus to study and emphasize the patterns of clinical presentation. Twenty percent of their patients were over one year of age, while 62% were neonates. Vomiting was the paramount symptom (97%), but was not initially bile stained in 20% of their cases. It was of interest that diarrhea was a major symptom in 16% of their cases. Abdominal pain was a major symptom in 96% of their patients who were over one year of age. Two of their important findings were particularly disturbing. They found that clinical signs were not apparent in most cases until gut infarction had occurred. They also observed that radiographic examination of the abdomen was considered "normal" in more than 20% of their cases. They reported that barium meal was the contrast examination with most accuracy and that it should be diagnostic— if interpreted accurately. The found sadly that the significant mortality (19%) in all age groups was invariably related to delay in presentation and diagnosis.

The most important and perceptive and thorough publication concerning malrotation and midgut volvulus of the past 40 years was published in 1989 in the *Journal of Pediatric Surgery* (24:777-780) by Powell, Othersen and Smith[12] of the Medical University of South Carolina in Charleston. They reviewed the charts of 70 consecutive children with midgut volvulus as a consequence of malrotation. They reviewed the full spectrum of this serious and potentially catastrophic complication of gangrenous midgut volvulus and did not concentrate on any limited age group. The ages of their 70 patients ranged from one day to 78 years and their oldest fatality was at 68 years with ischemic gangrene of the entire midgut.

Although 39% of their patients (27 cases) had presenting symptoms in the first 10 days of life, one half of their patients (35 cases) were older than two months of age at the onset of symptoms. The authors made and recorded the important observation that the older children often had a longer course of vague and indistinctive antecedent symptoms which included intermittent, nonbilious vomiting and chronic abdominal pain among others. Bilious and nonbilious vomiting occurred with equal frequency in children over two years of age. Of equal importance was their observation that volvulus, intestinal gangrene and mortality occurred regardless of age or chronicity of symptoms. The majority of the morbidities and all seven fatalities were encountered in patients with volvulus and intestinal necrosis.

They also encountered a remarkable number of additional associated congenital anomalies. A total of 56 anomalies were found in 32 of the 70 patients (46%). It was of particular interest in this regard that laparotomy for one of these associated anomalies provided the opportunity for the definitive diagnosis in 14 patients.

Upper gastrointestinal series was diagnostic in 29 patients (41%) with no false negative studies. In comparison with these clear-cut results, five of 29 patients undergoing contrast enemas had inconclusive results and required subsequent upper gastrointestinal contrast studies to verify the diagnosis. It was of particular interest that nine patients were found to have malrotations while undergoing laparotomy for conditions unrelated to malrotation such as appendicitis, peptic ulcer disease, etc. In a similar vein, contrast roentgen studies discovered malrotation as an unexpected ("serendipitous") finding in six additional patients being investigated for such remote conditions as sleep apnea, failure to thrive, occult blood in stool and fissure-in-ano. Four of these six patients had symptoms whose chronicity exceeded two months.

Sixty-two of their patients underwent Ladd's procedure (lysis of Ladd's bands), including appendectomy. At the time of laparotomy or postmortem examination, midgut volvulus was demonstrated in 31 of 70 patients (44%). The age breakdown of this finding was: 15 of 31 in children under two months of age (43%) and 16 of 31 in children older than two months (46%). A particularly chilling statistic was that 15 of the 31 with associated midgut volvulus (48% of those with volvulus and 21% overall of the total of 70 patients) required resection on average of 50 cm of intestine for gangrene. Seven of these patients required TPN for an average of 86 days (3 months).

In addition to the need for prolonged TPN, of the 15 patients requiring intestinal resection for necrosis, nine suffered serious morbidity (catheter sepsis in seven, pneumonia in five, wound infection in three, renal failure in three, urinary tract infection in two and hepatic failure in two). The seven deaths (10% overall morbidity) all occurred in the group of patients with volvulus and intestinal gangrene (a mortality of 47% for this group). Three of the deaths involved children less than two months of age and four involved the older than two months of age group.

The authors make the important point that malrotation is neither "harmless" nor completely "asymptomatic" and they document these points quite well with their own experience. They report that all of their serendipitously discovered patients were managed by Ladd's procedure without complication and furthermore and quite importantly with *resolution of symptoms.*

Their conclusions and recommendations are unequivocal and sound and are as follows: "Given the broad spectrum of symptoms and signs, we question the labeling of patients as having 'asymptomatic' or 'incidental' malrotation. Because the initial manifestations might be unpredictable and the possibility of catastrophic complications exist regardless of the age, chronicity of symptoms, or manner of presentation, we recommend prompt elective Ladd's procedure in all patients found to have abnormalities of intestinal rotation and fixation, even if the diagnosis is a serendipitous discovery."

I am vividly aware of the hazard of midgut volvulus beyond childhood years and the perplexing chronicity of symptoms.[13] An 18-year-old woman in the fourth month of her first pregnancy was seen because of progressive nausea and vomiting of two weeks duration. She had experienced recurrent episodes of crampy abdominal pain with nausea and vomiting since childhood. Despite hospital admissions at 11 and 12 years of age, the cause of her symptoms had remained elusive. Upper gastrointestinal barium studies revealed a marked narrowing of the third portion of the duodenum. At operation she was found to have a midgut volvulus with no fixation of the dorsal mesentery. Numerous ancient adhesions bound the midgut and mesentery together but there was

no ischemia at this time, rather the upward pressure of a rapidly expanding uterus had converted a near complete duodenal obstruction into a complete one with the twisted superior mesenteric vessels providing the obstruction. Partial derotation of the volvulus was followed by a bypassing duodenojejunostomy. The postoperative course and remaining pregnancy were normal as was childbirth and child. The patient on long-term follow-up remained completely free of the symptoms which had plagued her so frequently and for so many years.

The 1992 Messineo et al[2] publication from Toronto, cited earlier in the introduction, was concerned with symptomatic malrotation of the intestines in 182 children seen between 1964 and 1989 (25 years). One hundred and eleven of the patients (61%) had midgut volvulus. Of these, 79 had no necrosis and experienced only one fatality. For the 32 patients with necrosis, the mortality was 47% (15 cases). They observed then the probability of dying was at least 65% when more than 75% of the bowel is necrotic.

My 1989 report[14] on the use of the "patch, drain and wait" approach to necrotizing enterocolitis suggested the usefulness of this approach and principle as well in cases of midgut volvulus with extensive gut ischemia and necrosis. Its use in three cases was published in 1991[15] and will be dealt with more completely in the Challenges section of this chapter.

CHALLENGES

1. As with necrotizing enterocolitis, the overwhelmingly most important challenge in the management of midgut volvulus with extensive ischemia, necrosis and gangrene is how to achieve maximum salvage of both functioning baby and functioning gut.

As with necrotizing enterocolitis, the awesome morbidity with midgut volvulus and extensive ischemia, necrosis and gangrene is almost as bad as its mortality, with greatly prolonged hospitalization, short gut problems, prolonged TPN and TPN problems, etc., etc.

The lessons of nature to be derived from in utero intestinal vascular catastrophes with resultant midgut atresias and meconium peritonitis with and without intestinal obstruction are as pertinent and as applicable to midgut volvulus and necrosis as to necrotizing enterocolitis. Total parenteral nutrition substitutes for placental circulation for meeting nutritional and growth needs. Extensive bilateral Penrose drain drainage of the peritoneal cavity simulates a "sterile" peritoneal cavity as "de facto" enterostomies are established and adhesions obliterate the peritoneal cavity (hence no further chance for peritonitis). With antibiotic coverage, exuberant neovascularization of adhesions and parietal and visceral peritoneum provide maximum opportunity and support for maximum gut salvage over a period of time (weeks).

In the author's 1991 report of the use of "patch, drain and wait" (details of method in chapter 6) in three cases of extensive midgut necrosis associated with volvulus, all of the major features and consequences of in utero vascular intestinal catastrophe were found in long-term results of "patch, drain and wait" usage. Extensive gut necrosis (40%) disappeared leaving only two nearby short classical atretic segments. In another case, global midgut ischemia evolved into considerable gut loss but also a surprising amount of gut salvage where none at all was expected. The ultimate appearance was of multiple atresias with both open and closed gut ends of the persisting and salvaged gut segments.

The second and third look approaches may save some visually questionable gut, but miss out on the longer-term healing and restorative features of the "patch, drain and wait" approach and principle and fail in the end to take advantage of the associated gut preservation aspects of "resect no gut" and "do no enterostomies".

2. The second major challenge comes on the catastrophe prevention front and involves the Othersen group's recommendation of doing the Ladd's procedure in all identified cases of malrotation whether or not "symptomatic".

To me, the reasoning of the Othersen group is sound, their documentation impressive and convincing and their advice good.

3. A somewhat lesser yet real challenge relates to what to do after the Ladd's procedure with respect to tacking down the dorsal mesentery as suggested by Bill and Grauman[16] in 1966 as a measure to prevent volvulus recurrence.

Stewart et al[5] in their report of the extensive experience of the Children's Hospital of Boston with intestinal malrotation did not encounter recurrence of midgut volvulus and recommended against this approach. The experience of the Othersen group[12] was similarly free of volvulus recurrence and they reported uniformly excellent results with the Ladd's procedure alone. Snyder and Chaffin[3] in their scholarly 1954 report before the American Surgical Association, which was published in the *Annals of Surgery*, provide a beautiful and instructive drawing (their Fig. 13) illustrating the duodenojejunal segment which has been freed from its attachment to the mesentery of the small intestine and placed against the psoas muscle in the right gutter. They emphasize this step in the correction of malrotation to be important for stabilization of the mesentery of the small intestine to prevent recurrence of volvulus.

CONCLUSION

Midgut volvulus with extensive ischemia, necrosis and gangrene is not only a challenge but a blood curdling and nerve shattering experience for the surgeon as well. Prevention when possible must be accorded high priority.

While second and third "looks" may avoid resection of some visually borderline gut at the first operation, maximum salvage as afforded in theory and in limited practice by the "patch, drain and wait" approach and principle is missed.

While the use of "patch, drain and wait" for midgut volvulus with extensive ischemia, necrosis and gangrene is, as yet, limited, it is sufficiently encouraging for wider use and more careful study. The alternatives certainly are anything but attractive.

REFERENCES

1. Millar AJW, Rode H, Brown RA et al. The deadly vomit: Malrotation and midgut volvulus. Pediatr Surg Int 1987; 2:172-176.
2. Messineo A, MacMillan JH, Palder SB et al. Clinical factors affecting mortality in children with malrotation of the intestine. J Pediatr Surg 1992; 27:1343-1345.
3. Snyder WH, Chaffin L. Embryology and pathology of the intestinal tract: Presentation of 40 cases of malrotation. Ann Surg 1954; 140:368-380.
4. Schultz LR, Lasher EP, Bill AH. Abnormalities of rotation of the bowel. Am J Surg 1976; 101:128-133.
5. Stewart DR, Colodny AL, Daggett WC. Malrotation of the bowel in infants and children: A fifteen year review. Surgery 1976; 79:716-720.
6. Berdon WE, Baker DH, Bull S et al. Midgut malrotation and volvulus (which films are the most helpful? Radiology 1970; 96:375-383.
7. Simpson AJ, Leonidas JC, Krasna IH et al. Roentgen diagnosis of midgut malrotation: Value of upper gastrointestinal radiographic study. J Pediatr Surg 1972; 7:243-252.
9. Ornstein MH, Land RJ. Simultaneous occurrence of malrotation and intussusception in an infant. Br J Surg 1981; 68:440-441.
10. Filston H, Kirks DR. Malrotation—The ubiquitous anomaly. J Pediatr Surg 1981; 16:614-620.
11. Howell CG, Vozza F, Shaw S et al. Malrotation, malnutrition, and ischemic bowel disease. J Pediatr Surg 1982; 17:469-473.
12. Powell DM, Othersen HB, Smith CD. Malrotation of the intestines in children: The effect of age on presentation and therapy. J Pediatr Surg 1989; 24:777-780.
13. Moore TC. Vomiting during pregnancy due to midgut volvulus with duodenal obstruction. Am J Obstet Gynec 1957; 74:1356-1360.
14. Moore TC. Management of necrotizing enterocolitis by "patch, drain and wait". Pediatr Surg Int 1989; 4:110-113.
15. Moore TC. Management of midgut volvulus with extensive necrosis by "patch, drain and wait" in early infancy and childhood. Pediatr Surg Int 1991; 6:315-317.
16. Bill AH, Grauman D. Rationale and technique for stabilization of the mesentery in cases of malrotation of the midgut. J Pediatr Surg 1966; 1:127.

INVITED COMMENTARY

J. Eugene Lewis, Jr., M.D.
Professor Emeritus of Pediatric Surgery
St. Louis University

The tragic results of midgut volvulus and resulting midgut ischemia are well documented. Early diagnosis and prompt surgical intervention are essential to the salvage of the infant or older child.

Midgut volvulus is the end result of malfixation of the right colon and the duodenojejunal limb. In 1936 William E. Ladd presented his classic paper describing 21 cases of malrotation and midgut volvulus. The thin bands crossing the duodenum were divided and henceforth referred to as "Ladd's bands". These bands are the attachment of the colon to the right parietal peritoneum. They do not obstruct the duodenum.

The bands enclosing the duodenum and the cecum produce the obstruction and must be divided. The duodenojejunal limb is now free and moved to the right. The cecum and colon are moved to the left with the mesentery spread out across the posterior peritoneal cavity. The problem is one of malfixation rather than malrotation. The malfixation creates the potential for tragic volvulus. The correction leaves a malrotation.

I believe with Othersen that all malfixations should be corrected when diagnosed. Tragic results can be avoided in the older child or adult. I do not favor fixing the bowel to its new location. This would seem to offer little value and a potential for harm.

Second look operations have been used and seem a reasonable approach when the viability of the bowel seems questionable. If extensive necrosis is present, the use of "patch and drain" technique may offer an improvement in salvage. Certainly the results of extensive resection have been tragic.

If intestinal grafting becomes a safe predictable alternative, many lives can be saved and returned to constructive endeavor.

REFERENCES

1. Ladd WE. Surgical diseases of the alimentary tract in infants. New Eng J Med 1936; 215:705.
2. Lewis JE. Partial duodenal obstruction with incomplete duodenal rotation. J Pediatr Surg 1966; 1:47.

H. Biemann Othersen, Jr., M.D.
Professor of Surgery and Pediatrics
Chief of Pediatric Surgery and Medical Director
The Children's Hospital
Medical University of South Carolina, Charleston

Again Dr. Moore has challenged us to think without constraint from accepted dogma. In malrotation the basic problem is mechanical twisting of the mesentery as opposed to necrotizing enterocolitis where the exact pathogenesis is unknown. In midgut volvulus, mesenteric venous obstruction progresses to arterial insufficiency and gangrene of the involved intestine. Many surgeons have found that exploratory laparotomy often is insufficient to distinguish the gut which is severely congested from that which is infarcted. Perhaps the technique suggested by Dr. Moore of "patch, drain and wait" may be successful when there is a considerable amount of congested bowel with only minimal gangrene. However, there are many tragic cases where the entire gut is obviously gangrenous and thin-walled and incapable of surviving with no blood flow. When the infarcted bowel is resected, immediate recovery can be expected. However, long-term morbidity and eventual mortality are the substitute when there is not enough small bowel remaining for nutrient absorption. With early successes in small bowel transplantation, there may be hope for these unfortunate children.

Raymond A. Amoury, M.D.
Katherine Berry Richardson Professor of Pediatric Surgery
University of Missouri, Kansas City
Surgeon-in-Chief, Children's Mercy Hospital, Kansas City, MO
President, American Pediatric Surgical Association 1993-1994

Dr. Moore has thoroughly outlined the lethal threat of incomplete rotation and incomplete mesenteric fixation of the intestine. The lethal component of this anomaly is the potential for volvulus of the midgut, which is suspended on a primitive, unfixed dorsal mesentery continuing the superior mesenteric artery and vein.

In newborns presenting with bile-stained vomitus their primary diagnostic consideration should be intestinal obstruction. Dr. Moore has emphasized the need for conservatism in resection when dealing with apparently gangrenous intestine. Interstitial hemorrhage can look like intestinal gangrene and "second look" and even "third look" laparotomies are reasonable procedures and conservative. I have not had experience with Dr. Moore's "patch, drain and wait" procedure. The concept has the advantage of avoiding resection of questionably gangrenous intestine. It is always tempting to want to eliminate "necrotic" intestine, however, an inaccurate assessment may be made, especially where there is a significant amount of intramural intestinal hemorrhage.

I would like to emphasize that the baby vomiting bile mandates that the diagnosis of malrotation and volvulus be ruled out (usually by an upper gastrointestinal study) or, that the patient be operated upon promptly. If the possibility of a rotational anomaly with volvulus is eliminated, the patient can be approached more deliberately with any metabolic or other abnormalities corrected. If, however, the diagnosis is in question, the patient should undergo prompt operation to avoid the tragic consequences of midgut gangrene.

I feel that consideration of volvulus, or the documentation of a volvulus, constitutes the most important emergency in the newborn period requiring laparotomy.

I have carried out unnecessary emergency laparotomies in two patients. I felt it critical to operate on both of these infants who presented with bile-stained vomiting and equivocal contrast studies. I have had a converse and tragic experience in an infant who presented at one week of age with a severe anemia and only moderate abdominal distention and dilatation of intestinal loops on roentgenograms. In this infant extensive interstitial hemorrhages had occurred secondary to volvulus and obstruction of the baby's mesenteric venous and lymphatic drainage while maintaining an arterial pressure which allowed arterial inflow. This resulted in disruption of mesenteric capillaries and lymphatics and intramural hemorrhage and anemia.

Neonates with volvulus may appear to show a scaphoid abdomen early in the course of volvulus as the small bowel may empty itself and the stomach may decompress itself by vomiting. When intestinal dilatation is clinically manifest by abdominal distention, and plain x-rays show dilated intestinal loops in a baby with volvulus, the baby's course is already advanced.

In short, malrotation with the possibility of a midgut volvulus should be in the differential diagnosis of infants who present with bile-stained vomiting. It is the most pressing anomaly requiring emergency operation. If exploratory laparotomy is not to be carried out promptly, then the diagnosis of midgut volvulus should be eliminated by a contrast study.

Arnold M. Salzberg, M.D.
Professor of Surgery and Pediatrics
Division of Pediatric Surgery
Medical College of Virginia, Richmond

Laparotomy in a six-day-old newborn with a 14 hours history of vomiting demonstrated a 720° volvulus, with black midgut thought to be gangrenous. Detorsion and gastrostomy, without resection, warm compresses and periarterial Lidocaine concluded the procedure without improvement in the bowel.

Three hours later, a superior mesenteric arteriogram under general anesthesia demonstrated occlusion of the SMA (superior mesenteric artery), three centimeters distal to its origin. Because of the possibility of spasm, Papaverine was given into the SMA by injection and infusion. Repeat arteriogram showed increased flow in the SMA and its branches. Papaverine was continued for 12 hours and a second look operation showed some viable and black bowel. No resection was done. Papaverine was continued with heparin and 24 hours later at the third operation necrotic bowel was resected and four stomas constructed, leaving 78 centimeters of viable small intestine plus the ileo-cecal valve and the entire colon. Papaverine was discontinued 6 hours following operation. Ostomies were of good color and functional. Renal failure, hypernatremia, acidosis and pulmonary edema occurred with death at 36 hours postoperatively.

The arterial inflow from the SMA is compromised by volvulus, edematous bowel loops and spasm. The latter may be seminal in the bowel ischemia. Papaverine intra-arterially, while not affecting organic occlusion, may obviate the ischemia secondary to spasm and lead to less bowel compromise, more viable bowel and improved outcome.

REFERENCES

1. Williamson SL, Tisnado J, Cook DE, Barnhardt G, Salzberg AM. Intra-arterial infusion of Papaverine to relieve superior mesenteric artery vasoconstriction in a neonate with midgut volvulus. Vasc Surg 1986; 4:236-239.

David Tapper, M.D.
Professor of Surgery and Pediatrics
Vice Chairman Department of Surgery
University of Washington
Surgeon-in-Chief
Children's Hospital and Medical Center, Seattle

The author's extensive review of Powell's et al, paper highlights this chapter. From the author's standpoint "patch, drain and wait" is the procedure of choice for midgut volvulus with extensive necrosis. Once again, the "resect no gut" philosophy relies on the in utero atresia experience.

Regarding Dr. Bill's suggestion to fix the dorsal mesentery after Ladd's procedure, Bill has subsequently recanted this suggestion. Bill reviewed his extensive experience and concluded that fixation does not decrease the incidence of recurrent volvulus.

David L. Collins, M.D.
Pediatric Surgeon, Medical Group of San Diego
Clinical Professor of Surgery
University of California, San Diego

Second Challenge:

I agree that the asymptomatic patient who has a more or less incidental nonrotation diagnosed, should be operated on because of the definite likelihood of volvulus with gangrene taking place.

Third Challenge:

Although I have routinely performed a simple Ladd procedure with division of bands and separation of the cecum and the jejunum, I have had two patients in which secondary volvulus has taken place. I have then done the fixation procedure as suggested by Bill. I do not yet do this in all cases, however, because I am concerned about the possibility of internal hernias taking place around the cecum, which is pexed to the abdominal wall in the left upper quadrant.

=== CHAPTER 8 ===

BILIARY ATRESIA
AND RELATED CONDITIONS

INTRODUCTION

Few challenges in pediatric surgery have been more formidable and resistant to clear resolution than biliary atresia and related conditions. I can look back on a good 40 years of struggle in this arena of pitfalls[1-10] starting with three major publications in 1953 which included original publications in the February issue of *Surgery, Gynecology and Obstetrics*[1] and the July issue of *Annals of Surgery*[2] and an invited editorial in *The American Surgeon*[3] titled "Early Operation for Atresia of the Bile Ducts". The 1953 *Surgery, Gynecology and Obstetrics* article contained the first published suggestion of a Roux-Y "hepatojejunostomy" at the hilum of the liver for extrahepatic biliary atresia even though those bile ducts "at the hilum of the liver may not be large enough for a single enteric anastomosis."[1]

The dramatic and brilliant work of Professor Morio Kasai[11-14] of Sendai, Japan (Tohoku University School of Medicine) in the late 1950s (first operation for "noncorrectable" biliary atresia in March 1957)[12] and subsequently has brought the above hope and dream into striking reality and has changed the outlook of biliary atresia infants from near universal disaster and hopelessness into the radiant and promising realm of effective surgical therapy. Professor Kasai's first publication relating to his new operation appeared in Japanese in *Shujutsu* (*Operation*) in 1959 (13:733-739) with S. Suzuki as a co-author.[11] The author of this book was gratified to see his 1953 *Surgery, Gynecology and Obstetrics* article cited in this classic and breakthrough publication of Professor Kasai.

Although the etiology of biliary atresia and related conditions remains unknown, there appears to be a continuum between these conditions which include neonatal hepatitis, extrahepatic biliary atresia, spontaneous perforation of the extrahepatic bile ducts in infancy, cystic dilatations of the extrahepatic bile ducts (choledochus cysts) and cystic dilatations of the intrahepatic bile ducts (Caroli's disease).[7,8] At times these conditions may coexist in a single patient simultaneously or sequentially. The occurrence of biliary atresia as discordant in monozygotic/identical twins suggests an acquired rather than genetic etiology[6,7] and the tendency of some of these conditions, especially choledochus cyst and Caroli's disease, toward malignant degeneration and transformations suggests a viral and likely oncogenic viral etiology.

The gross and microscopic appearances resemble a combined destructive and obstructive cholangiopathy. The discussion in this chapter will be limited to those conditions which are surgical in nature, as well as surgically challenging.

EXTRAHEPATIC BILIARY ATRESIA

Atresia of the extrahepatic biliary tract has long been the most frequent as well as the most troubling and agonizing of these conditions.

The early literature divided extrahepatic biliary atresia cases into the rare "operable" category in which a patent extrahepatic segment communicated unobstructed with the intrahepatic biliary tract system and which could accordingly and theoretically, be anastomosed to some appropriate or adjacent segment of the alimentary tract. The great majority without this connection were classified as "inoperable" in type. As the surgeon did not know without "operating" whether the obstruction was "operable" or "inoperable", in my 1953 *Surgery, Gynecology and Obstetrics* publication I took the liberty of renaming these obstructions as "correctable" and "noncorrectable". These terms at the time seemed quite proper and "correct" in terms of semantic accuracy. Professor Kasai adopted and used these new terms in his classic 1959 publication[11] and subsequently[12] despite his clear and important demonstration the most "noncorrectable" extrahepatic atresias actually were "correctable" by his brilliant new operation. Nonetheless the classification battle[15,16] has raged quietly ever since, leaving me (an inadvertent terminology culprit) with a mild sense of suppressible "guilt". Confession, even 40 years delayed, may have some redeeming merit.

My three 1953 publications concerning biliary atresia resulted from the stimulus of a flurry of interesting cases of neonatal obstructive jaundice and biliary

atresia seen and operated upon by me during his year as chief resident in surgery at the Indiana University Medical Center in Indianapolis. The 1953 report in *Annals of Surgery* (138:111-114) described the first and youngest successful use of common bile duct exploration and drainage for obstructive neonatal jaundice due to two isolated areas of atresia in the distal common duct and proximal common hepatic duct. Two figures in that publication (a drawing and a cholangiogram) illustrate the unique method of common duct drainage employed and the successful result.

The 1953 *Surgery, Gynecology and Obstetrics* publication (96:215-225) represented a major effort to explore the spectrum, challenge and theoretical opportunities in extrahepatic biliary atresia through the clinical picture, treatment results and histological pathology of 31 proved cases of extrahepatic biliary atresia seen at the Indiana University Medical Center during a 17 year period (1935 to 1952).

As cited above, I discarded the terms of "operable" and "inoperable", then in use, as both meaningless and confusing since operation was required to determine correctability by the standards of that time. Hence, the substitution of the then more meaningful terms of "correctability" and "noncorrectability". Although eight of the 31 patients (26%) were "correctable", only one survived surgical attempts at correction. The tragic statistic was that five of the eight "correctable" patients were in excess of $5^1/_2$ months of age when first seen. In the Discussion section of this publication, the author made the strong statement and recommendation as follow: *"Neonatal jaundice should, in effect, be regarded as an emergency. The work-up should be prompt and thorough and operation should be carried out without delay when there is a reasonable suspicion of biliary atresia."* (italics added)—this some 40 years ago!

A particularly important part of this overall study was the review of the histological finding of sections of liver available in 19 of the 31 cases. Round cell infiltration and portal fibrosis were found to progress rapidly in the first four weeks of life and were well established and of formidable presence and appearance by six and eight weeks of life. This clearly narrowed the "window of opportunity" for successful surgical correction before irreparable fibrotic and cirrhotic damage was done to these fragile newborn livers.

Of equal importance was the finding that intrahepatic bile ducts were present in 18 of the 19 cases. This clearly indicated the potential for operative intrahepatic biliary tract communication and decompression into the alimentary tract. The concept of "cholangioenterostomy" was mentioned and it was stated that the situation of the majority of patients with "noncorrectable" biliary atresias "might be improved if some effective method could be devised for draining off the accumulating bile into the intestinal tract before the onset of portal fibrosis." It was further stated that "this decompression might be achieved by the anastomosis of a Roux-Y limb of jejunum to a cut surface of the liver"—a Roux-Y "hepatojejunostomy". In the last item in the Summary of this publication, I stated:

> It is urged that renewed efforts be made to bring within the realm of effective surgical management that unfortunate majority of patients whose extrahepatic biliary atresia is of the type considered noncorrectable by contemporary standards. The use of a Roux-Y hepatojejunostomy, supplemented by cholagogues and antibiotics, is perhaps worthy of further consideration and investigation.

These strong suggestions and recommendations, as above, in the author's February 1953 Surgery, Gynecology and Obstetrics publication triggered an invitation from the editors of The American Surgeon to me to write an editorial on the topic of "Early Operation for Congenital Atresia of the Bile Ducts". It was done and published later in 1953.[3] The conclusion of the next-to-last paragraph is as follows:

Since associated intrahepatic biliary atresia is encountered in only a very small percentage of these patients, the possibility exists that some means of achieving hepatic biliary decompression ultimately may be shown to be practicable. The use of an anastomosis of a Roux-Y limb of jejunum to a cut surface of liver has been suggested. However, a number of problems remain to be solved. If it can be shown that there is hope for some of the infants with *noncorrectable* atresia, the importance of early operation will be even greater in these patients than in those of the correctable type.

Five years before this 1953 report (1948), Professor William P. Longmire Jr.,[17] then at Johns Hopkins, reported in Surgery (24:264-276, 1948) a description of a new operation for biliary obstruction presented at the annual meeting of the Society of University Surgeons in 1948 (New Orleans). His new operation for treating extensive obstructions of the common duct or common hepatic duct involved anastomosis of one of the intrahepatic ducts to the jejunum following partial resection of the left lobe of the liver. He employed a loop of jejunum with an enteroenterostomy below the hepatic anastomosis. He reported one successful case in an adult with recurrent common hepatic duct obstruction and three unsuccessful cases of its use for congenital biliary atresia. All three of the biliary atresia patients had been operated upon unsuccessfully before the Longmire procedure was carried out. Their ages at the time of the Longmire operation were not given but it is likely that they were well beyond the four week cut-off period and had extensive and likely intractable biliary atresia generated liver fibrosis and cirrhosis. Further successful experience with this operation in adults was reported before the American Surgical Association in 1949 and published in Annals of Surgery (130:455-460).[18] A Roux-Y segment of defunctionalized jejunum was used in later cases rather than the jejunal loop described in the original operation and report. In discussions of this important paper and approach, the Longmire operation was hailed an "ingenious" approach by such distinguished biliary tract surgeons as Richard B. Cattell, Warren Cole, Frank H. Lahey and Waltman Walters.

Few operations in pediatric surgery have generated more excitement, attempts to equal or improve results or more publications of all sorts than Kasai's. As few operations, in or outside of pediatric surgery, are more demanding of exquisite technical surgical skill and extreme care in management judgment, many authors had difficulty equaling Professor Kasai's results and some even questioned them, as well as the fact that his first publication had appeared in his own native Japanese language.[11,12] An occasional person even recommended abandonment of the operation.[19] It is to Professor Kasai's credit that he persisted with patience and determination which resulted in a steady improvement of his results over the years.

In addition to Professor Kasai,[20] other Japanese surgeons were working vigorously and resourcefully toward resolution of the biliary atresia and related problems. Professors Suruga[21,22] and Sawaguchi[23,24] deserve special mention.

In 1967, Professor Keijiro Suruga et al[21] of Tokyo reported an experience with 50 infants with congenital biliary atresia. On the theoretical basis that in cases of congenital biliary tract obstruction that the thoracic duct might act as a compensatory channel for the excretion of bile, he and his associates carried out and reported 15 cases in which the thoracic duct was transplanted into the sublingual part of the oral cavity. Five of their 15 infants survived the operation more than two years. They made the important observation that in all cases where the infant was less than two months of age at the time of operation, the jaundice diminished but never disappeared completely. They considered this operation not as curative but as protection against progressive cirrhosis. In a 1972 report, Suruga et al[22] had expanded their experience with biliary atresia to 101 cases. By

this time, the thoracic duct drainage procedure which had been designed in 1962 was largely abandoned except in cases of no intrahepatic ducts. The Suruga I operation was described and illustrated (their Fig. 1). Their new approach involved a cutaneous enterostomy for the isolated jejunal conduit to the porta hepatis and dissecting out the porta hepatis. With these innovations, they reported that bile flow had been achieved in 20 of 25 cases (80%) operated upon since 1968.

Sawaguchi et al[23,24] made important contributions toward diminishing the frequent and highly destructive ascending cholangitis problem by staging the operation and employing a porta hepatis conduit detached from the functioning intestinal tract stream of contents. Their 1968 publication[23] described the use of the staged operation.

A 1976 report in *Surgery* by Suruga et al[25] described the use of microsurgery as an important advance in the surgical treatment of biliary atresia. An important 1981 report by Suruga et al[26] described the improved results from both microsurgery and the introduction of a major new innovation and improvement on the Suruga I operation termed the Suruga II. This anatomic improvement is illustrated well in Figure 4 of their publication in the *Journal of Pediatric Surgery* (16:621-626, 1981).[26] Adjacent stomal contamination of the isolated porta hepatis conduit is eliminated by use of a Witzel enterostomy tube access to the Roux-Y limb between the skin and peritoneum—an ingenious contribution. In their 1981 report, Suruga et al[26] reported that 25 of 29 biliary atresia patients (86.2%) between 1972 and 1979 by their new approach were alive with bile excretion and in a satisfactory general condition. I have used the Suruga II operation by preference since first reading of it in 1982.[10]

In the past 10 years, steady if slow progress has been made in refinements of technique and management. In 1982, Suruga et al[27] advocated and reported experiences with reoperation and porta hepatic curvetage for reestablishment of bile flow when it had stopped. Since 1977, all seven of their cases who underwent rehepatic-portoenterostomy with porta hepatis cuvetage showed bile excretion and three of these seven were relieved of their jaundice. Also in 1982, Kosloske and associates[28] of Albuquerque described successful endoscopic recanalization (via conduit stoma) of a portoenterostomy with bile flow reestablished and maintained during one year of follow-up. This option for reestablishment of bile flow without an anesthetic or a major operation is a further major plus for a cutaneous stoma of an isolated jejunal conduit to the porta hepatis. There are others including avoidance of ascending cholangitis, measurement of bile output and bile content of bilirubin, etc.

Professor John Lilly and associates[29,30] of Denver have made and published important observations concerning bilirubin output and prognosis of biliary atresia. In their 1989 report[30] they studied bile bilirubin during the first month after the Kasai operation in 67 patients. Thirty-nine of the 67 patients died (58%) of these 38 (97.4%) excreted less than six mg of bilirubin per day during the first postoperative month. Nine additional patients of the 67 (13.4%) also excreted less than 6 mg of bilirubin per day. While these patients were still alive at the time of this report, all were either jaundiced or awaiting transplantation. Of the 19 of the 67 patients who excreted 6 mg or more per day of bilirubin (28.3%) all were alive with normal or near normal liver function. Their 1979 report[29] considered two other important survival determinants in addition to concentration of bile bilirubin, age of patient and large bile ducts. They found bile bilirubin concentration greater than 8.8 mg/100 ml to be a favorable determinant as well as large bile ducts. With respect to age of patient at time of operation, they found an age below 10.5 weeks of age to be important. With the three important survival determinants all in the "favorable" category and using actuarial analysis, the expected four-year survival of biliary atresia

patients following the Kasai-type of operation was determined to be 89%. In their 1990 publication in *Pediatric Surgery International* (5:87-90),[31] they again address the patient age at operation component of long-term survival. In their Denver series of 131 infants with biliary atresia, long-term survival was found to be 46% in patients operated upon in the first $2^1/_2$ months and *only* 24% in patients operated upon after $2^1/_2$ months of age. The importance of early age at operation also was stressed by Lilly et al in their important 1989 presentation before the American Surgical Association (*Annals of Surgery* 210:289-294, 1989).[32] The age at operation is repeated throughout the literature relating to biliary atresia. In Professor Kasai's[33] first major publication in English (*J Pediatr Surg* 3:665-675, 1968), he lamented toward the end of the Comment section of his paper that "not a few cases with 'incorrectable' biliary atresia, namely cases of Type 3, might be curable, if hepatic portoenterostomy could be carried out before 4 months of age, preferable within 3 months after birth."

The continuing productivity and improving approaches and survival statistics by the Kasai group of Sendai have been major factors in achieving world-wide acceptance of this important approach to biliary atresia of the largely "noncorrectable" type. In a 1978 report in the *World Journal of Surgery* (2:571-580), Kasai et al[34] described their experience with 174 patients with proved biliary atresia of whom 172 underwent "curative" operation (portoenterostomy or portocholecystostomy). Twenty-seven of the 172 patients, 15.7% had what they termed Type 1 atresia (involving common bile duct). Fourteen of these 27 patients (52%) had experienced bile flow and disappearance of jaundice. Thirty of the 172 patients (17.4%) had Type II atresia (common hepatic duct). Five of these 30 patients (16.7%) had bile flow and disappearance of jaundice. One hundred and fifteen of the 172 patients (67%) had Type III atresia (porta hepatis, "noncorrectable"). Of this group of 115 with "noncorrectable"/porta hepatis atresia, 33 (28.7%) had bile flow and disappearance of jaundice. Since 1972, when they went to a double Roux-Y portoenterostomy to prevent postoperative cholangitis, their cure rate increased to 55.4% in 65 patients. In this group, 10 of 11 infants less than 60 days of age had active bile flow achieved (91%). This 1978 report indicated Professor Kasai, at that time, had 47 patients living without jaundice with 22 surviving longer than five years and nine more than 10 years. The longest survivor then was 23 years of age. They attribute these fine and improving results to early operation, appropriate operative technique and the prevention of postoperative cholangitis.

A 1985 report by the Kasai group[35] addressed the reoperation problem. They reported that excellent bile drainage was obtained after reoperation in 13 of 15 patients with good bile flow after the first operation (87%) but that, on the contrary, good bile flow was obtained by reoperation in only 4 of 12 cases (33%) without active bile flow after the initial operation. A 1989 publication by Kasai et al[36] addresses the need and desirability of liver transplantation in an age of increasing success of the Kasai-type of hepatic portoenterostomy. Here again the age of the patient loomed large as they concluded that liver transplantation should be considered as the primary treatment for biliary atresia *only* for patients over 120 days of age (4 months) with enlarged and hard livers.

The crucial importance of early operation and of age of the patient at the time of operation has become increasingly clear over the years as one plows through an avalanche of case and series reports. The findings of two groups particularly stand out, those of the Kasai/Sendai group[37] of Japan and those of the Canty and Collins group of San Diego.[38,39]

The 1990 Sendai/Ohi/Kasai group's report[37] was of major interest regarding age at operation and long-term survival. They reported the 10-year survival of patients treated before the age of 60 days (8.6 weeks) to be *73% while* the 10-year survival of patients treated after 91 days (8 of 71) was *13%*.

Of the 25 patients operated upon in the Canty/San Diego experience[39] (1974 to 1985), 18 were operated upon in the first 10 weeks of life and 17 of the 18 (94%) were alive and jaundice free between one and 13 years postoperative as compared with only 2 of 7 over 10 weeks (28.6%) and the two alive with their own livers functioning were 11 weeks of age at operation. The Sawaguchi modification was used in all with stoma closures from 4 to 10 months after the original procedures and with short conduits and continuity reestablishment near the ligament of Treitz. In the under 10 weeks of age at operation group, 5 of the 18 (28%) were under four weeks of age at operation, 12 were under 6 weeks of age at operation (67%) and 16 of the 18 (89%) were under eight weeks of age. With these young ages at operation and the Sawaguchi approach, it was of particular interest that the incidence of cholangitis in the under 10 weeks of age operation was only one of 18 (5.5%) and that for the over 10 weeks of age (with 2 of the 7 at 11 weeks of age) was 1 of 7 (14.3%).

A particularly important paper appeared in 1990 by Vacanti et al[40] of Boston and the Children's Hospital (Harvard). The paper presented a balanced approach to biliary atresia by a group of talented pediatric surgeons doing both traditional pediatric surgery (including biliary atresia) and liver transplantation. The title of their paper in the *Journal of Pediatric Surgery* (25:149-152) was "The Therapy of Biliary Atresia Combining the Kasai Portoenterostomy with Liver Transplantation: A Single Center Experience". Their study involved 28 infants born between 1981 and 1988 who underwent Kasai's operation as a primary surgical treatment. Sixteen of these patients (57.1%) achieved total biliary drainage, while 5 of 28 (17.9%) achieved partial biliary drainage and 7 of 28 (25%) achieved no drainage. Nine of 28 (32.1%) have undergone liver transplantation and 25 of the 28 (89.3%) were alive at the time of this report. Twenty of the 25 (80%) living were jaundice free. Sixty-five percent of these living and jaundice free patients had the Kasai operation only. These are important results. It is unfortunate that the age of each patient at Kasai operation, and correlation with results, is not given. They do state that the mean age at Kasai operation was 8.5 weeks with a range from 3 to 15 weeks.

Two major events of the past 25 years have served to seriously hinder the development of sound and logical approaches to biliary atresia in North America. The first was the tragic Gellis "pronouncement" which bore the authority of "holy writ" to pediatricians. This "dictum" was presented in four back-to-back publications in the September 1968 issue of the *American Journal of Diseases of Children*.[41-44] These studies from Boston were based on a retrospective study of data (charts, slides, etc.) from a distant and foreign city (Toronto).

The first two reports[41,42] stated that infants with neonatal hepatitis surgically explored in the first four months of life developed cirrhosis three times as often as infants not operated upon and blamed surgical and anesthetic "trauma" for these "results". The third report[43] starts as follows: "Successful repair of bile ducts continues to be a rare occurrence. On the other hand, abdominal surgery increases the mortality and morbidity of neonatal hepatitis, and appears to be an adverse factor in long-term prognosis." They concluded this report with a Summary statement that "these findings reveal that factors other than age play a role in the development of cirrhosis in biliary atresia." This despite my published observations 15 years earlier quite to the contrary. (I did not make the references list of this publication which had a *grand* total of six citations.) The fourth of these appalling publications[44] concludes with the following statement:

> As far as the diagnostic management of infants with neonatal hepatitis is concerned, a wait of up to 4 months of age is

suggested before exploratory laparotomy is undertaken. This approach carries the least danger for infants with neonatal hepatitis, without jeopardizing the possibility of complete recovery in the rare salvageable case of biliary atresia.

This monstrous misstatement had a devastating effect on pediatric surgeons attempting to improve the results in cases of biliary atresia by early operation including the Kasai operation (first reported some nine years earlier) and in the same year of its first appearance in the English literature. Referring pediatricians took this nonsense to be holy gospel and biliary atresia referrals shrank to nothing. I, as a chief of pediatric surgery at a University teaching hospital did not see a non"terminal" case of biliary atresia for many, many years despite most vigorous protests including the passing around of copies of 1953 publications, etc.

The second major harmful event was the arrival of liver transplantation as a "competing" modality of surgical treatment of biliary atresia. Thanks to cyclosporine and to an inordinate amount of media "hype", transplantation became the only way to go in the treatment of biliary atresia. "Transplant" surgeons who knew little or nothing of pediatric surgery and little of transplantation immunobiology beyond the dose of cyclosporine became television "celebrities" and began slapping livers in all over the place.

The absurdity of this is quite evident in Professor Lilly's 1989 report before the American Surgical Association which reads as follows:

> For some time surgery of the biliary atresia has been one of the most controversial areas in pediatric surgery. The doyen of clinical pediatricians, Dr. Sidney Gellis,[45] wrote recently that treatment will be confined to liver transplantation. Dr. Thomas Starzl[46] publicly stated that the Kasai operation was of only 'historic' significance.

SPONTANEOUS PERFORATION OF EXTRAHEPATIC BILE DUCTS

Spontaneous perforation of the extrahepatic bile ducts in early infancy is a comparatively rare and infrequently reported occurrence of unknown etiology. It is a biliary atresia related inflammatory destructive and obstructive phenomenon and may be found in association with biliary atresia distal to the site of perforation which occurs most frequently at or near the junction of the cystic, common hepatic and common ducts. While the onset is insidious in most cases, it may be acute in approximately 25% of the cases. The major symptoms and findings are abdominal distention and jaundice. The younger the patient at onset the more likely is jaundice to be found and the onset acute.

Important review articles relating to this problem were published in 1970 by Prevot and Babut[47] and in 1974 by Lilly et al.[48] The classic 1974 article published by Lilly et al[48] in *Surgery*, stimulated the me to have a diagnosis and handle to publish a case of my own seen many years before of dramatic nature but no clear and established diagnostic classification.[5] This patient had been seen in 1962 at four weeks of age with a massive and rapidly progressing bile peritonitis. At operation most of the infant's extrahepatic biliary tract had sloughed away in a necrotic reaction which left only a small remnant of common hepatic duct and very distal atresia near the duodenal segment of the common bile duct. This difficult and challenging problem was managed successfully by anastomosis of a Roux-Y limb of jejunum to the tiny common hepatic duct remnant. He remained anicteric for 21 years. At 21 years of age, he suddenly became sharply and acutely icteric without pain. A transhepatic cholangiogram revealed complete obstruction near the junction of the right and left hepatic ducts. As those perforations in infancy with their frequently associated "sacs" which resemble prepseudocysts may predispose to the ultimate development of pseudocysts of the

extrahepatic bile ducts with an established potential for malignant degeneration, I, still this patient's surgeon, was quite concerned that the present acute obstruction or some future one might be malignancy generated. At operation in April 1983, a tense but benign stricture was found and opened with a T-tube left in place and brought out of the Roux-Y limb in the manner of a Witzel enterostomy. A T-tube cholangiogram three years postoperatively demonstrated a patent anastomosis with normal intrehepatic bile ducts. The T-tube was removed at that time and the patient has remained jaundice-free in the seven years since T-tube removal.

As 25 additional cases of spontaneous perforation of the extrahepatic bile ducts in infancy had been reported since the classic Lilly et al report of 1974, I, together with Cameron[8] undertook an updating of the published literature supplemented by a questionnaire to the author's of published reports of cases with emphasis on long-term follow-up and possible long-term malignancy. A 1978-report in *Gastroenterology* by Kagawa et al[49] reviewed 48 reported cases of carcinoma arising in choldochal cysts. They found that one half of the patients were 30 years of age of younger with five of them being teenagers. A recent, 1990, report by Iwai et al[50] of Kyoto (Japan) described the finding of an adenocarcinoma arising in a choledochal cyst in a 12-year old girl. They indicated that this was the youngest patient reported up to that time with adenocarcinoma in a choldochus cyst.

My 1986 report with Cameron[8] in *Pediatric Surgery International* included 77 reported cases of spontaneous extrahepatic biliary tract perforations managed operatively up to that time. There was a slight preponderance of females (56 to 44%). Birth weights generally within normal limits and malformations beyond the biliary tract were rare. Two patients were dizygotic twins with the other twin not involved. The most frequent clinical findings were abdominal distention (82%) and jaundice (70%). Other important clinical features were nausea and vomiting and the presence of ascites and abdominal hernias. Jaundice was found to be more frequent in cases where symptoms began in the early weeks of life.

The age of the patients at the onset of symptoms ranged from birth to four years of age. The onset of symptoms was in the first two weeks in 39% of the cases, in the first month of life in 61% and in the first $3^1/_2$ months of life in 79%.

The interval in weeks from the onset of symptoms to operation was of particular interest. Eighteen of the patients (25%) were operated upon within one week and their clinical course may be regarded as acute. In 30 patients (42%) the interval ranged from two to four weeks and their clinical picture may be regarded as subacute. In 24 cases (33%), the clinical course was more chronic or indolent with the interval from the onset of symptoms to operation ranging from five to 16 weeks.

The site of perforation found at operation most often involved the common bile duct near its junction with the cystic and common hepatic ducts. Occasionally the perforation involved the gallbladder or the cystic duct. In many cases, an edematous mass was found in the subhepatic or portahepatic areas which variously was described as a sac, a pseudocyst or a pseudopseudocyst. In 12 cases obstruction of the common duct was found between the site of common duct perforation and the duodenum. An anomalous junction of the pancreatic and biliary ductal systems was described in six cases.

Eighty-two operations were carried out on the 77 patients. Five required a second operation. Seventy-one percent of the first operations were of simple drainage, suture, cholecystostomy or cholecystectomy type. All five reoperations occurred in this group. Anastomosis/bypass operations were utilized in 27% of the first operations and four of the five reoperations. Ten of the 77 operatively managed patients died (13%) with seven of the 10 deaths (70%) in the drainage group of cases. Since 1971, the anastomosis/bypass approach has pre-vailed over the drainage-type operations by a 60:40 ratio. There have been no reported deaths since 1974.

A sobering observation may be found in the first case of Prevot et al.[51] At the first operation, a perforation of the common hepatic duct near its junction with the cystic duct was found and managed by a drainage procedure. Intraoperative cholangiography demonstrated a patent but narrowed biliary tract down to the duodenal junction. Large amounts of bile drainage continued after operation, even following removal of the drainage tube on the 13th postoperative day. The persistent biliary fistula necessitated reexploration 32 days following the initial operation. Cholangiography at this operation showed obliteration of the biliary tract beyond the site of the former perforation. This was managed successfully by hepaticojejunostomy. This experience clearly indicated a continuing and on-going of extrahepatic biliary tract inflammation and obliteration. A recent, 1992, report by Megison and Vottler[52] in *Surgery* described a similar operative finding with distal common bile duct obstruction and proximal perforation. Their patient was managed by drainage and cholecystostomy. The common bile duct obstruction persisted for five weeks following operation. At this time the obstruction disappeared as cholangiography through the cholecystostomy demonstrated free flow of contrast media into the duodenum through a normal appearing common duct. This finding suggests that an obstructed common bile duct may "recanalize" and did. The frequency of this is unavailable from current data but from the above cited experience, it is unlikely to be the expected outcome. An important feature of this case report was that nuclear DISIDA scan was of value in demonstrating bile extravasation from the common bile duct. Both scans with DISIDA and cholecystostomy cholangiograms may be of value in following these cases regardless of the operative approach elected.

The determination of the incidence of malignancy in these cases long-term and their involvement in choledochal cyst formation will await the careful long-term study and evaluation of a much larger number of cases—perhaps a "registry".

CHOLEDOCHUS CYST (DILATATION OF EXTRAHEPATIC BILE DUCTS)

A considerable controversy concerning the management of choledochus cyst occurred in the late 1960s with most American surgeons preferring anastomosis of the cyst to an adjacent portion of the intestinal tract, usually the duodenum and Japanese surgeons and some European ones preferring excision of the cyst and restoration of intestinal tract continuity. Most American surgeons were influenced by the R.E. Gross 1933 publication[53] on this topic which suggested that resection carried too high a mortality. This was a review of the literature (52 cases) and a report of two cases.

In 1968, Alois Schärli and Marcel Bettex[54] reported from Berne, Switzerland in the *Journal of Pediatric Surgery* the successful resection of a large choledochal cyst with biliary tract reconstruction by anastomosis between the common hepatic duct and the distal remnant of the common bile duct. They cited the morbidity of unresected choledochal cysts from both stones (reported 15 times) and malignant degeneration of the cyst which had been recorded four times.[55]

Two particularly important publications from major Japanese centers, Sendai and Tokyo, appeared in the November issues of *Annals of Surgery* and *Surgery* by Kasai et al[56] and Ishida et al.[57]

The Kasai et al[56] report was of 21 patients with choledochal cysts. Eight of their patients had complete atretic obstruction of the distal choledochus with symptoms (jaundice) from birth (38%). An abdominal mass was palpable in only three of these eight patients and pain and fever were not components of their presentation. The onset of symptoms in these 13 patients without distal common bile duct atresia was from three months to seven months of age. Eight of their patients were managed by internal drainage procedures and 13 by cyst resection and restoration of continuity by Roux-Y anastomosis. The only deaths (5) occurred in the distal atresia group. They cited the Schärli-Bettex experience but observed that some of their distal atresia patients also had hepatic duct hypoplasia which would have made the Schärli-Bettex approach impossible in these cases. They also cited the high incidence of carcinoma occurring in choledochal cyst walls, at least 14 cases up to that time. Of these 14, 10 were 35 years of age of younger and two were 18 years old. They concluded that the choice of surgical operation for choledochus cyst should be resection of the cyst followed by reconstruction by hepaticojejunostomy in Roux-Y fashion.

Ishida et al[57] reported 31 cases of choledochal cysts seen at the University of Tokyo during a 16 year period (1953 to 1969). Nineteen of their patients were treated by cyst excision and Roux-Y reconstruction of the biliary tract with excellent results in 14 (74%) and only transient postoperative difficulties in two more patients (10.5%). There were three deaths in this cyst excision group (16%), one early (shock) and two late (anastomosis stricture and irreversible liver cirrhosis in one case each). Of the nine Roux-Y cystjejunostomy cases, three died of cholangitis and one developed carcinoma in the retained choledochal cyst. They recommended primary excision of the choledochal cyst as the operation of choice—and for good reason.

In 1971, a report of 11 cases of choledochus cyst was published in *The American Surgeon* by O'Neill and Clatworthy.[58] Ten of the 11 were managed by drainage of the cyst into the duodenum and one by a Roux-Y drainage. On X-ray barium contrast studies, reflux into the biliary tree occurred in all duodenal drainage cases and not in the Roux-Y drainage case. Five of their 10 duodenal drainage cases had recurrent cholangitis with frequent symptoms. Also in 1971, Peter Jones, Durham Smith and associates[59] reported five consecutive successful cases of choledochal cyst excision in a two year period from Melbourne in Australia.

In 1979, Professor J.R. Lilly[60] of Denver presented an important report to the American Pediatric Surgical Association which was published with discussions in the *Journal of Pediatric Surgery* (14:643-646). This report concerned other biliary tract malformations coexisting with choledochal cyst and their surgical management. Additional malformations occurred in five of 13 cases of choledochal cyst and included main hepatic duct cysts in five, common hepatic duct stenosis in one, left hepatic duct stenosis in one and Caroli's[61] disease (intrahepatic bile duct cystic dilatations) in one. The coexistence of choledochal cyst with Caroli's disease had been reported earlier by Engle and Salmon[62] (1964) and Gots and Zuidema[63] (1970) and these reports have helped to establish the important interrelations of these disorders within the broad spectrum of "biliary atresia and related disorders". In his discussion of this important paper, R. Ohi[64] of Sendai (Japan) emphasized malformations which may occur distal to the cyst. These included anomalous pancreatic duct-common bile duct junctions of the type initially reported by Babbitt[65] in 1969 and Babbitt et al[66] in 1973. Ohi[64] cited an experience in Sendai involving total excision of a choledochal cyst in 26 consecutive patients in the latter half of which experience a deliberate effort was made by ERCP or operative cholangiography to ascertain the precise location of the pancreatic duct-common bile duct location. In all instances in which these efforts were successful, the common bile duct-pancreatic duct junction was found to be abnormal. In one instance, the pancreatic duct separately opened into the cyst. This opening had to be excised separately as a part of the cyst and anastomosed to the duodenum in order to preserve satisfactory pancreatic drainage.

Also in 1979, Arima and Akita[67] from Kagoshima University (Japan) reported in the *Journal of Pediatric Surgery* the identification of an anomalous junction of the pancreaticobiliary ductal system in six of 28 children with congenital dilatation of the bile ducts (21.4%), in three of 57 children with congenital biliary atresia (5.3%) and in two of 17 children with infantile hepatitis (11.8%). These important observations raise interesting questions regarding these anomalous connections and their etiology—acquired as inflammatory sequelae or congenital and causes of biliary tract inflammation.

The use of antenatal ultrasound to detect and follow the development of choledochal cysts and antenatal ultrasound and CT scanning may also contribute to the accumulation of important data toward a better understanding of choledochal cysts, including causes, progression, management, etc. A 1980 report by Araki et al[68] indicated the value of CT in both diagnosing choledochal cysts in conjunction with ultrasound but can also be useful when ultrasonography fails to provide useful information. Three of their 15 patients were found to have cholangiocarcinomas arising from their choledochal cysts. In 1983, Howell et al[69] from the Children's Hospital of Philadelphia described an interesting and important experience with ultrasound antenatal diagnosis of choledochal cyst which demonstrated the choledochal cyst in the fourth ultrasound and at 31.5 weeks of gestation. Progressive changes in the cyst in the first 10 days of life led to prompt excision of the cyst. No abnormal junction of the pancreatic and common bile duct was identified in this case. The cyst in this case not only enlarged steadily over the initial 10 postnatal days but also was found to have a striking increase in the amount of sludge within the cyst. With the exception of the 1968 Schärli-Bettex case,[54] this was one of the earliest postnatal successful resections of a choledochal cyst.

An especially important and very major publication concerning congenital bile duct dilatation appeared in 1985 from Sendai, Japan by Ohi, Kasai and associates.[70] In a group of 47 patients suffering from congenital dilatation of the extrahepatic bile ducts whose intrahepatic bile ducts could clearly be demonstrated by operative cholangiogram or preoperative ERCP, 39 patients (83%) had dilatation of the intrahepatic bile ducts. Extended (1 to 11 years) follow-up revealed no morbidity which could be attributed to the dilatation of the intrahepatic bile ducts following the standard excision and bile drainage by hepatico-enterostomy in all cases. Postoperative studies in 21 patients showed marked decreases in the sizes of the intrahepatic bile ducts in all but two patients with huge cystic dilatations of the intrahepatic bile ducts. The form of dilatation of the intrahepatic bile ducts was cystic in 14 cases and fusiform in 25. Of 22 patients with cystic dilatation of the extrahepatic bile ducts, the intrahepatic bile duct dilatation was cystic in 10 cases and fusiform in 12. In all cases of extrahepatic fusiform dilatation the intrahepatic dilatation was fusiform as well. Cancer was not encountered in any of the 47 choledochal cyst patients in this series managed by choledochal cyst resection.

Not all news on the choledochal cyst excision front is good however. A 1986 report in *Gastroenterology* by Yoshikawa et al[71] is of ominous import throughout this field with particularly troublesome questions which may be raised on the liver transplantation for biliary atresia field. In this publication a 27-year-old woman who had had excision of a choledochal cyst at 14 years of age was found to have developed an adenocarcinoma which seemed to arise from the intrapancreatic terminal choledochus connecting with the remnant cyst. This is the fourth patient to be reported with a biliary carcinoma developing after primary resection of a choledochal cyst. In one case, the carcinoma appeared at the anastomosis and in two it appeared in the intrahepatic bile ducts. The case recorded here was the first to appear in the terminal intrapancreatic choledochus.

In another 1986 report from Japan (University of Tokushima) by Komi et al,[72] 5 of 23 adult patients with choledochal cysts managed by cyst excision (21.7%) were found to have adenocarcinoma in their cyst walls.

A 1990 follow-up of the Sendai experience by Ohi et al[37] includes 100 cases of congenital dilatation of the bile ducts. There were no deaths nor malignancy in their late complication analysis. Ninety-one of the 100 patients had undergone their standard operation of total excision of the extrahepatic bile ducts and reconstruction by Roux-Y hepaticojejunostomy. Intrahepatic bile duct dilatation is best managed by completely free bile drainage from the dilated intrahepatic biliary system which should be achieved by careful and adequate anastomotic hook-up at the initial radical cyst resection operation.

DILATATION OF THE INTRAHEPATIC BILE DUCTS (CAROLI'S DISEASE)

From the above sections of this Introduction, it is clear that intrahepatic dilatation of the bile ducts is a frequent occurrence in association with choledochus cyst (extrahepatic dilatation of the bile ducts) and is best managed by cyst excision and good drainage. Malignant degeneration also remains a continuing hazard in Caroli's disease.

CHALLENGES

1. The most important single challenge in the management of biliary atresia and biliary atresia related conditions which also may coexist with extrahepatic biliary atresia and may include neonatal hepatitis is to get these infants to the operating room for definitive relief of obstructive jaundice and the hazard of obstruction induced serious and progressive liver damage (cirrhosis) at the earliest hint of obstructive jaundice with targeting toward the first week of life.

Work-up, including rapid ruling out alpha 1-antitrypsin deficiency, should proceed at lightning speed, rather than at the snail's pace of the past. Nuclear scans can rapidly be carried out as can ultrasonography studies. Antenatal findings may also be alerting and greatly hasten and direct the rapid work-up. As neonatal hepatitis is a part of this "package" of conditions and may coexist with the extrahepatic and other ongoing processes, its presence or absence, should not delay the rapid undertaking of direct visualization of the extrahepatic biliary tract and rapid relief of obstruction by incisional or laparoscopic operation. With the wretched alternative of liver transplantation with its awesome morbidity and a lifetime of disabling and mutilating immunosuppression with its own set of serious problems including cancer induction, absolutely every effort should be made to preserve the infant's own God-given autogenous liver and to make every effort to protect it from short or long-term trauma particularly ascending cholangitis.

2. The early (hours/days) laparoscopic option with bile duct and hepatic hiliar dissection and resection accompanied by Penrose drain placement, through a stab wound at the hilar area to permit rapid and early bile escape and measurement (stoma-type bag at drain exit site) and convenient tissue rim formation around hilar drainage to permit later (7-10 days) intestinal conduit anastomotic hook-up.

Laparoscopy surgery, long a staple for adult biliary tract disease, is particularly appealing as a very early and minimally invasive assault on biliary atresia-types of neonatal obstructive/destructive jaundice disorders. The use of hiliar resection followed by Penrose drain drainage of hilar bile only has been employed successfully by me and was cited in my published discussion[10] of Professor J.R. Lilly's paper before the American Surgical Association in 1989. This approach might diminish hilar obstructive scar formation by not adding immediately an intestinal anastomosis wound healing challenge to the resection of fragile hilar area of indeterminate number of ducts and early bile outpouring potential.

3. The importance of a public (parent and pediatrician) awareness of the importance of early referral and definitive operation to relieve obstructive jaundice in biliary atresia and related conditions to save the infant's own and best-ever liver is of the highest priority.

The superlative efforts at early referral and early operation for biliary atresia of Tim Canty and Dave Collins[38,39] in San Diego represent a "role model" pattern for this important part of patient care of an early warning and preventative nature. Their outstanding efforts at early operation, as well as their own excellence in technical surgical skills and judgment, have made important contributions to their 94% jaundice free survival at one to 13 years following operation for biliary atresia done before 10 weeks of age. The outstanding long-term results of the pioneering Sendai/Kasai group37 with a 73% 10 year survival of infants operated upon before 60 days (8.6 weeks) in comparison with a survival at 10 years of only 13% in those operated upon after 91 days of age, should reinforce parent and pediatrician confidence and hopeful outlook regarding the Kasai-type portoenterostomy for biliary atresia when carried out early and before irreparable liver damage results from tragic delay in operation.

The competing "siren song" of the now 25 year old Gellis pronouncements[41-44] that surgery before four months of age for biliary atresia leads to fatal neonatal hepatitis related cirrhosis can hardly have died out completely. Add to this residual of Gellis-generated pediatrician concern, the new media "siren song" blitz by the liver transplantation "lobby" and the job of the pediatric surgeon in securing the best and safest management of biliary atresia patients is anything but easy and peace-of-mind generating. An informed public and profession is a *major challenge*, but it is also the only recourse!

4. What is the role of liver transplantation in the management of biliary atresia and related conditions in infancy?

I[73-77] have a long and in-depth personal involvement in clinical and experimental tissue and organ transplantation, including liver, and is fully aware not only of the many advantages of organ transplantation but also of its pitfalls and hazards.

Lethal delay in referral for porto-enterostomy well beyond four months with a rock hard liver probably would justify liver transplantation as the primary surgery because of the greatly diminished likelihood of a successful portoenterostomy at this very, very late date endstage of disease. A clearly failed portoenterostomy also would clearly be an indication for liver transplantation.

A recent (1993) abstract from a major organ transplantation center[78] recommends liver transplantation for biliary atresia on the basis of their experience with 62 liver transplants into 45 patients (1.4 liver transplants per patient). Six patients required two transplants, four patients required three transplants and one patient required four transplants. Thirty-six percent of their patients required at least one reoperation (excluding retransplantation). Thirty-six of the 45 patients (80%) required 158 hospital readmissions (4.3 per patient) and 53.7% experienced 45 rejection episodes (2.0 per patient). A total of 175 infections were recorded (3.9 per patient) and there were five deaths (11.1%).

In comparing this awesome infant and childhood transplantation-induced trauma with the excellent long-term results of Canty/Collins and the Kasai group of actual (not "actuarial") patient jaundice free survival for 1-13 years of 94% and the Kasai group 10 year survival with early operation of 73%, the superiority of portoenterostomy and one's own liver (despite media "hype") is quite clear.

Not only is portoenterostomy much less traumatic in both morbidity and mortality than liver transplantation, it preserves the infant's and child's own autogenous God-given liver and without need of the plague-for-life of life-time immunosuppression with all of its known and yet to be discovered hazards. As biliary atresia and related and often coexisting conditions are likely of viral and oncogenic viral etiology and with an established clinical tendency toward malignant transformation without immunosuppression, an organ transplant (here liver) with life-time immunosuppression imposes a totally unacceptable risk unless there is absolutely no other choice.

The last paragraph of the author of this book's discussion[9] of Tim Canty's superlative report[39] to the 1987 meeting of the Pacific Coast Surgical Association addresses the issue and is as follows:

With respect to the question of hepato-portoenterostomy versus liver transplantation as primary therapy for biliary atresia, it must be recalled that biliary atresia is almost certainly an acquired disorder (having been observed in only one of two identical twins[6,7]) and likely of viral and oncogenic viral cause. Biliary atresia appears to be a part of a complex that includes neonatal hepatitis, spontaneous rupture of the extrahepatic bile ducts, choledochal cyst and Caroli's disease, which may coexist and have an established potential of malignancy over time. This complex may be regarded as falling within a general classification of acquired destructive neonatal cholangiopathy, perforating and dilating as well as obstructing. With a likely oncogenic viral cause and a known potential for the development of malignancy in this complex, transplantation and long-term immunosuppression may have an additional risk factor of immunosuppression-fostered malignancy in biliary tract remnants and other involved host tissues.

5. Is it desirable to have a stoma at the first operation or the second operation if the laparoscopy initiative is pursued and how long should it remain open (Suruga II-type operation)?

The isolated porta hepatis-to-skin conduit has been a major factor in cholangitis avoidance, in monitoring assays of volume and concentration of bile and bilirubin output and as an access for endoscopic follow-up of bile flow and for curettage in case of sudden stoppage of bile flow.

I strongly agree with the need for this stoma and the Suruga II subcutaneous Roux-Y catheter access for returning collected bile free of the contaminating potential of an adjacent open second stoma. This involves little specialized care and is associated with few complications. Canty[39] has observed similar ease of stoma management. Eighteen months of conduit stoma use before reanastomosis to the subcutaneous nearby Roux-Y jejunal limb is recommended.

6. Should the management of spontaneous perforation of the extrahepatic bile ducts involve simple drainage with a cholecystostomy for monitoring and follow-up or resection and Roux-Y hepaticojejunostomy?

As essentially all of the reports are of single cases, it is quite difficult to gain the sort of clinical "feel" for treatment as affecting outcome. An international or national collective study as done with childhood cancers with prospective randomized studies with safety-net provisions might help resolve these problems. It is my current feeling that if extensive necrosis and disappearance of the extrahepatic bile ducts is found, Roux-Y hepaticojejunostomy is the best immediate approach. If, however, a localized perforation is found, Penrose drain drainage and cholecystostomy for ductal drain and subsequent cholangiographic monitoring to determine ultimate opening or persistence of refractory distal (terminal/duodenal area) obstruction would be acceptable for a limited period of time. Here again a collective/cooperative approach with protocols and registry for data information distribution might be desirable.

7. A major, long-time and perhaps receding challenge is how to manage choledochal cysts, by resection or internal drainage into the duodenum (original efforts) or into a Roux-Y limb of jejunum (later favorite of internal drainers).

From the Introduction section data regarding choledochal cyst, this issue would appear to have been rather decisively determined in favor of resection on three major issues: 1) safety, 2) avoidance of reflux and cholangitis, 3) occurrence of cancer in unresected cysts. The World Pediatric Surgery community owes an immense debt to the determination, technical skill and wise judgment of multiple talented and resourceful Japanese surgeons who rendered this former "controversy" no longer "controversial".

8. The determination of the etiology or etiologies and agent or agents: genetic or nongenetic, viral or nonviral and onco- genic or nononcogenic for biliary atresia and related conditions is a challenge of immense importance.

From the limited available data of significance or conviction in this area, a major collaborative prospective effort would appear to be very much in order and in need. Antenatal imaging detection of these conditions as well as improved techniques of isotope and CT scanning, viral study and tissue histo- and immunohistochemical investigation, including in situ hybridization, etc. will greatly expand the potentials for critical information gathering in this area.

CONCLUSION

The past 40 years have been a period of near miraculous progress in the surgical management of biliary atresia and related conditions. Disorders which, 40 years ago, were almost universally regarded as quite hopeless (particularly "noncorrectable" extrahepatic biliary atresia) are now quite within the realm of excellent short and long-term survival results in experienced, knowledgeable and skillful hands. A giant share of the credit for this remarkable turnaround must be given to teams of brilliant, determined, hard-working, skilled and resourceful Japanese surgeons, particularly to Professor Morio Kasai and associates at the Tohoku University School of Medicine in Sendai, Japan.

The twin North American blights *initially* of the highly publicized and widely believed (by pediatricians) Gellis edict[41-44] that surgery for biliary atresia before four months of age produced fatal liver cirrhosis and that repair of biliary atresia could quite safely wait beyond four months of age and *more recently* the second major blight produced by the transplantation "lobby" (media and pediatrician) promotion of liver transplantation as the primary surgical approach to biliary atresia have been great, sad and tragic "crosses" for the Pediatric Surgeons community of North America to bear. These daggers of misinformation have deflected and disturbed patient care and have contributed to excessively long "work-ups" and loss of important and critical early repair advantages. The rather wide-spread abandonment of conduit stomas would appear to be another inappropriate "concession" to liver transplant surgeon wishes for a soft and cushy transplant. We are fortunate that the Japanese pediatric surgeons have largely turned "deaf" ears to this North American-induced nonsense.

My three 1953 publications identifying patent intrahepatic bile ducts in the vast majority of cases of extrahepatic biliary atresia, their presence as multiple small ducts rather than a large single channel at the hilum of the liver and the rapid cirrhotic/fibrotic obliteration of these intrahepatic ducts within days and one to three weeks after birth led me to strongly advise and recommend early definitive repair operation,[1,3] to actually do this successfully in May of 1951 at 6 weeks of age in an infant with multiple extrahepatic bile duct atresias and a collapsed and nondistended extrahepatic biliary tract of the "noncorrectable" type *(Annals of Surgery* 138:111-114, 1953)[2] and to suggest the use of a Roux-Y "hepatojejunostomy" at the hilum of the liver with no attempt at individual bile duct anastomosis in cases of "noncorrectable" biliary atresia *(Surgery, Gynecology and Obstetrics* 96:215-225, 1953)[1] where early operation was considered of the greatest importance (as compared with the "correctable" type[3]). It is gratifying to me that at least one perceptive Japanese surgeon was familiar with at least one of these 1953 publications which he cited[1] in his classic landmark and breakthrough publication of 1959.[11]

The immediate post-obstructive jaundice appearance use of laparoscopy within hours of birth for extrahepatic biliary atresia diagnosis, tissue removal for viral, bacterial, histochemical and other study and resection of the biliary tract at porta hepatis followed by Penrose drain placement at the porta hepatis cited earlier in the Challenges section is quite exciting. This approach is based on reported experiences of the author[10] with Penrose drain stimulation both of increasing bile drainage within days (6 to 8) and of formation of an accompanying fibrotic ring of sub-

stance around the periphery of the dissected and exposed porta hepatis which will permit easy and secure interrupted porta hepatis rim suture to an isolated jejunal conduit.

REFERENCES

1. Moore TC. Congenital atresia of the extrahepatic bile ducts: Report of 31 proved cases. Surg Gynec Obstet 1953; 96:215-225.
2. Moore TC. Common duct exploration and drainage for obstructive neonatal jaundice. Ann Surg 1953; 138:111-114.
3. Moore TC. Early operation for congenital atresia of the bile ducts:An Editorial. Am Surgeon 1953; 19:1012-1013.
4. Moore TC, Hurley AG. Congenital duplication of the gall bladder; Review of the literature and report of an unusual symptomatic case. Surgery 1954; 35:283-289.
5. Moore TC. Massive bile peritonitis in infancy due to spontaneous bile duct perforation with portal vein occlusion. J Pediatr Surg 1975; 10:537.
6. Moore TC, Hyman PE. Extrahepatic biliary atresia in one human leukocyte identical twin. Pediatrics 1986; 78:182.
7. Moore TC. Pathogenesis of biliary atresia. Pediatrics 1986; 78:182.
8. Moore TC, Cameron RB. Spontaneous perforation of the extrahepatic biliary tract in infancy and childhood: Review of 77 operatively managed cases. Pediatr Surg Int 1986; 1:206-209.
9. Moore TC. Discussion of paper by Canty TG. Am J Surg 1987; 154:25-26.
10. Moore TC. Discussion of paper by Lilly JR et al. Ann Surg 1989; 210:294.
11. Kasai M, Suzaki S. A new operation for "noncorrectable" biliary atresia: Hepatic portoenterostomy. Shujutsu (Operation) 1959; 13:733-739 (in Japanese).
12. Kasai M, Watanabe I, Ohi R. Follow-up studies of long-term survivors after hepatic portoenterostomy for "noncorrectable" biliary atresia. J Pediatr Surg 1975; 10: 173-182.
13. Kasai M, Ohi R, Chiba T et al. A patient with biliary atresia who died 28 years after hepatic portojejunostomy. J Pediatr Surg 1988; 23:430-431.

14. Kasai M, Mochizuki I, Ohkohchi N et al. Surgical limitation for biliary atresia: Indications for liver transplantation. J Pediatr Surg 1989; 24:851-854.

15. Gans SL. Editorial: Correctable or non-correctable: Biliary atresia. J Pediatr Surg 1983; 18:107-108.

16. Lilly JR. Editorial: Choledochal cyst and "correctable" biliary atresia. J Pediatr Surg 1985; 20:299-301.

17. Longmire WP, Sanford MC. Intrahepatic cholangiojejunostomy with parital hepatectomy for biliary obstruction. Surgery 1948; 24:264-276.

18. Longmire WP, Sanford MC. Intrahepatic cholangiojejunostomy for biliary obstruction—Further studies. Ann Surg 1949; 130:455-460.

19. Arcari F. Discussion of paper by Altman RP et al. J Pediatr Surg 1975; 10:690.

20. Kasai M, Kimura S, Asakura Y et al. Surgical treatment of biliary atresia. J Pediatr 1968; 3:665-675.

21. Suruga K, Nagashima K, Hiral Y et al. A clinical and pathological study of congenital biliary atresia. J Pediatr Surg 1967; 2:558-564.

22. Suruga K, Nagashima K, Kohno S et al. A clinical and pathological study of congenital biliary atresia. J Pediatr Surg 1972; 7:655-659.

23. Sawaguchi S, Nakajo T, Hori T et al. Staged reconstruciton of the biliary tract for congenital biliary atresia. Presented before the 68th annual meeting of the Japanese Surgical Society, Kanazawa, 1968.

24. Sawaguchi S, Akigama H, Saeki M et al. The treatment of congenital biliary atresia, with special reference to hepatic portoentero anastomosis. Fifth annual meeting of the Pacific Association of Pediatric Surgeons. Tokyo, Japan. June 16, 1972.

25. Suruga K, Kono S, Miyano T et al. Treatment of biliary atresia: Microsurgery for hepatic portoenterostomy. Surgery 1976; 80:558-562.

26. Suruga K, Miyano T, Kitahara T et al. Treatment of biliary atresia: A study of our operative results. J Pediatr Surg 1981; 16:621-626.

27. Suruga K, Miyano T, Kimura K et al.

28. Graere AH, Volpicelli N, Kosloske AM. Endoscopic recanalization of a portoenterostomy. J Pediatr Surg 1982; 17:901.

29. Hitch DC, Shikes RH, Lilly JR. Determinants of survival after Kasai's operation for biliary atresia using actuarial analysis. J Pediatr Surg 1979; 14:310-314.

30. Vazquez-Esteres J, Stewart B, Shikes RH et al. Biliary atresia: Early determination of prognosis. J Pediatr Surg 1989; 24:48-51.

31. Stewart BA, Hall RJ, Karrer FM et al. Long-term survival after Kasai's operation for biliary atresia. Pediatr Surg Int 1990; 5:87-90.

32. Lilly JR, Karrer FM, Hall RJ et al. The surgery of biliary atresia. Ann Surg 1989; 210:289-294.

33. Kasai M, Kimura S, Asakura Y et al. Surgical treatment of biliary atresia. J Pediatr Surg 1968; 3:665-675.

34. Kasai M, Suzuki H, Ohahi E et al. Technique and results of operative management of biliary atresia. World J Surg 1978; 2:571-580.

35. Ohi R, Hanamatsu M, Mochizki I et al. Reoperation in patients with biliary atresia. J Pediatr Surg 1985; 20:256-259.

36. Kasai M, Mochizuki I, Ohkohchi N et al. Surgical limitaiton of biliary atresia: Indication for liver transplantation. J Pediatr Surg 1989; 24:851-854.

37. Ohi R, Nio M, Chiba T et al. Long-term follow-up after surgery for patients with biliary atresia. J Pediatr Surg 1990; 25:442-445.

38. Canty TG, Self TW, Collins DL et al. Recent experience with a modified Sawaguchi procedure for biliary atresia. J Pediatr Surg 1985; 20:211-215.

39. Canty TG. Encouraging results with a modified Sawaguchi hepato portoenterostomy for biliary atresia. Am J Surg 1987; 154:19-24.

40. Vacanti JP, Shamberger RC, Eraklis A et al. The therapy of biliary atresia combining the Kasai portoenterostomy with liver transplantation: A single center experience. J Pediatr Surg 1990; 25:149-152.

41. Thaler MM, Gellis SS. Studies in neonatal

Reoperation in the treatment of biliary atresia. J Pediatr Surg 1982; 17:1-6.

hepatitis and biliary atresia:I. Long-term prognosis of neonatal hepatitis. Am J Dis Child 1968; 116:257-261.

42. Thaler MM, Gellis SS. Studies in neonatal hepatitis and biliary atresia: II. The effect of diagnositic laparotomy on long-term prognosis of neonatal hepatitis. Am J Dis Child 1968; 116:262-270.

43. Thaler MM, Gellis SS. Studies in neonatal hepatitis and biliary atresia: III. Progressing and regression of cirrhosis in biliary atresia. Am J Dis Child 1968; 116:271-279.

44. Thaler MM, Gellis SS. Studies in neonatal hepatitis: IV. Diagnosis. Am J Dis Child 1968; 116:280- 284.

45. Gellis SS. Pediatric notes. The weekly Pediatric Commentary. 1984; 8:43.

46. Starzl TE. Guest presentation. 19th Annual Meeting. American Pediatric Surgical Association. Tucson, Arizona 1988.

47. Prevot J, Babut JM. Spontaneous perforation of the biliary tract in infancy. Prog Ped Surg 1970; 1:187- 208.

48. Lilly JR, Weintraub WH, Altman RP. Spontaneous perforation of the extrahepatic bile ducts and bile peritonitis in infancy. Surgery 1974; 75:664-673.

49. Kagawa Y, Kashihara S, Kuramoto S. Carcinoma arising in a congenitally dilated biliary tract. Gastroenterology 1978; 74:1286-1294.

50. Iwai N, Deguchi E, Yanagihara J et al. Cancer arising in a choledochal cyst in a 12-year old girl. J Pediatr Surg 1990; 25:1261-1263.

51. Prevot J, Vert P, Babut JM. Deux cas de perforation spontance des voies biliares chez le nourisson. Rev Pediatrie 1970; 6: 541-546.

52. Megison SM, Vottler TP. Management of common bile duct destruction associated with spontaneous perforation of the biliary tree. Surgery 1992; 111; 237-239.

53. Gross RE. Idiopathic dilatation of the common bile duct in children: Review of the literature and report of two cases. J Pediatr 1933; 3:730-755.

54. Schärli A, Bettex M. Congenital choledochal cyst: Reconstruction of the normal anatomy. J Pediatr Surg 1968; 3:604-607.

55. Alonso-Lei F, Rever WE, Pesagno DJ. Con- genital choledochal cyst, with a report of 2 and an analysis of 94 cases. Int Abstr Surg 1959; 108:1-30.

56. Kasai M, Asakura Y, Taira Y. Surgical treatment of choledochal cyst. Ann Surg 1970; 172:844-851.

57. Ishida M, Tsuchida Y, Saito S et al. Primary excision of choledochal cysts. Surgery 1970; 68:884-888.

58. O'Neill JA, Clatworthy HW. Management of choledochal cyst: A fourteen year followup. Am Surg 1974; 37:230-237.

59. Jones PG, Durham Smith E, Clarke AM et al. Choledochus cysts: Experience with radical excision. J Pediatr Surg 1971; 6: 112-120.

60. Lilly JR. Surgery of coexisting biliary malformations in choledochal cyst. J Pediatr Surg 1979; 14:643- 646.

61. Caroli J, Soupault R, Kossakowski J et al. La dilatation polykystique congenital des roies biliares intrahepatiques. Essai de classification. Sem Hop Paris 1958; 34:488-495.

62. Engle J, Salmon PA. Multiple choledochal cysts. Arch Surg 1964; 88:345-349.

63. Gots RE, Zuidema GD. Dilatation of the intrahepatic biliary ducts in a patient with a choledochal cyst. Am J Surg 1970; 119:726-728.

64. Ohi R. Discussion of paper by Lilly JR. J Pediatr Surg 1979; 14:647.

65. Babbittt DP. Congenital choledochal cysts: New etiological concept based on anomalous relationship of common bile duct and pancreatic bulb. Ann Radiol 1969; 12: 231-240.

66. Babbitt DP, Starshak RJ, Clemett AR. Choledochal cyst: A concept of etiology. Am J Roentgenol 1973; 119:57-62.

67. Arima E, Akita H. Congenital biliary tract dilatation and anomalous junction of the pancreatico-biliary ductal system. J Pediatr Surg 1979; 14:9-15.

68. Araki T, Itai Y, Tasaka A. CT of choledochal cysts. Am J Roentgenol 1980; 135:729-735.

69. Howell CG, Templeton JM, Weiner S et al. Antenatal diagnosis and early surgery for choledochal cyst. J Pediatr Surg 1983; 18:387-393.

70. Ohi R, Koike N, Matusumoto Y et al. Chances of intrahepatic bile duct dilatation

after surgery for congenital dilatation of the bile duct. J Pediatr Surg 1985; 20:138-142.

71. Yoshikawa K, Yoshida K, Shirai Y. et al. A case of carcinoma arising in the intra-pancreatic terminal choledochus 12 years after primary excision of a giant choledochus cyst. Gastroenterology 1986; 81:378-384.

72. Komi N, Tamura T, Tsuge S et al. Relation of patient age to premalignant alterations in choledochal cyst epithelium: Histological and immunochemical studies. J Pediatr Surg 1986; 21:430-433.

73. Moore TC, Hume DM. The period and nature of hazard in clinical renal transplantation: I. The hazard to patient survival. Ann Surg 1969; 170:1-11.

74. Moore TC, Hume DM. The period and nature of hazard in clinical renal transplantation: II. The hazard to transplant kidney

function. Ann Surg 1969; 170:12-24.

75. Moore TC, Hume DM. The period and nature of hazard in clnical renal transplantaiton: III. The hazard to transplant kidney survival. Ann Surg 1969; 170:25-29.

76. Ohtawa T, Moore TC. Effects of cyclosporin A dose reduction and antibiotics on hemorrhage and rejection in rat heart allografting. IRCS Med Sci 1979; 7:256-257.

77. Moore TC. Neurovascular Immunology: Vasoactive Neurotransmitters and Modulators in Cellular Immunity and Memory (456 pages). Boca Raton:CRC Press Inc, 1993.

78. Kalayoglu M, D'Allesandro AM, Knechtle SJ et al. Long-term results of liver transplantation for biliary atresia. Central Surgical Association, Fiftieth Annual Meeting program, page 40, 1993.

INVITED COMMENTARY

William P. Longmire Jr., M.D.
Professor of Surgery and Chairman of the Department, Emeritus
University of California, Los Angeles
VA Distinguished Physician, Emeritus
President, American Surgical Association 1967
President, American College of Surgeons 1972-1973

This chapter covers in interesting detail the historical development of currently recommended treatments of the most common bile duct anomalies either constrictive (atresia) or dilatative (choledochal cysts, Caroli's disease, etc.). The author's concept that biliary atresia, neonatal hepatitis, choledochal cysts and Caroli's disease are part of a complex related to an acquired destructive neonatal cholangiopathy possibly with a viral cause is interesting and one that might be further investigated as intrauterine diagnostic procedures are developed.

The role of transplantation in the treatment of life-threatening biliary abnormalities remains somewhat controversial, but the author's recommendations of transplantation for the four or more month old infant with advanced cirrhosis, or the clearly failed portoenterostomy following an early exploration, cannot be faulted.

It is always refreshing to read an author's opinions and recommendations so clearly and vigorously expressed. Dr. Moore's ideas and opinions are solidly based on 40 years of experience in the field and any disagreements will hopefully only serve to stimulate further pro or con investigation and substantiation of whatever point of view is taken.

Timothy G. Canty, Sr., M.D.
Surgeon-in-Chief, Children's Hospital of Louisville 1974-1977
Associate Professor of Surgery, Chief, Div. of Pediatric Surgery
University of Louisville 1974-1977
Surgeon-in-Chief, Children's Hospital of San Diego 1977-1983
Associate Professor of Surgery, Chief, Div. of Pediatric Surgery
University of California, San Diego 1977-1983
Senior Surgeon, Children's Hospital of San Diego 1983-present

The author presents a very important historic perspective on the diagnosis and treatment of obstructive disorders of the biliary tract in children, most especially biliary atresia. Though these disorders were well described over fifty years ago, more recent pioneering efforts by many American, Mexican, and especially our Japanese colleagues in pediatric surgery, have made these previously fatal conditions survivable in a large number of cases. Important emphasis is placed on the significance of timing: early recognition and correction is mandatory for successful treatment of this disease. Biliary atresia operatively treated after eight to ten weeks of age has a very poor prognosis. However, if diagnosed and treated expeditiously, the survival and perhaps "cure" has been significant in several large series.

The continuing controversy over the most appropriate primary treatment for biliary atresia, liver transplantation or hepatoportoenterostomy, is discussed forthrightly. The compelling evidence is in favor of early portoenterostomy, a procedure with negligible early morbidity and mortality. Transplantation, on the other hand, should be reserved as a salvage procedure in those who fail hepatoportoenterostomy. The failure rate of portoenterostomy in experienced hands should be less than 50%.

This reviewer certainly agrees with the views and conclusions presented by the author in this chapter and salutes him on a significant contribution to the pediatric surgical literature.

Keijiro Suruga, M.D.
Professor Emeritus (Pediatric Surgery)
Juntendo University
Head and Director, Katsunan Municipal Hospital
Tokyo, Japan

Biliary atresia and related conditions continue to be the subjects of various discussions specifically regarding operative results in the field of pediatric surgery.

I am very much impressed by reading this chapter, titled "Biliary Atresia and Related Conditions" written by Professor T.C. Moore who suggested a Roux-Y hepatojejunostomy at the hilum of the liver for extrahepatic biliary atresia in 1953 before Professor Kasai reported his original operation.

As the author strongly recommended in this chapter, it is extremely important for biliary atresia patients to undergo early portoenterostomy before they have serious and progressive liver damage.

According to our postoperative 10 years follow-up study on biliary atresia and a number of follow-up studies reported from Japan, the number of patients who are jaundice free and have no findings of progressive liver fibrosis including portal hypertension is gradually increasing and operative procedures of portoenterostomy and pre- and postoperative treatment are also improving.

As the author stated, the indication for liver transplantation will be justified for biliary atresia patients who clearly failed portoenterostomy or have already had severe liver cirrhosis due to lethal delay in referral for portoenterostomy.

In cases of choledochal cyst, at present, most pediatric surgeons in the world are in favor of resection of the cyst. However, according to our follow-up study on choledochal cyst patients who underwent total excision of the cyst, we are further facing many problems like stenosis or dilatation of intrahepatic bile ducts, stone formation both in the liver and pancreas, pancreatitis and malignant change in relation to the anomalous junction of the pancreaticobiliary ductal system.

Pathogenesis of biliary atresia is still unknown. Recently, we reported our study on the role of hepatic lymphatics which is related to the pathogenesis of biliary atresia. Further studies on pathogenesis besides diagnosis and treatment should be continued in order to improve the operative result of this lesion.

Morio Kasai, M.D.
Emeritus Professor, 2nd Department of Surgery
Tohoku University School of Medicine
Sendai, Japan
Director, Tohoku Teishin Hospital (Sendai)

It took ten years for the radical operation for biliary atresia, hepatic portoenterostomy, to be generally accepted in Japan and more than twenty years in other countries, since the operation was first published in a Japanese journal in 1959. The first article reporting results of hepatic portoenterostomy from the United States in 1974 raised serious questions regarding the efficacy of the procedure, and similar results were reported from the United Kingdom in the same year. Some other pediatric surgeons even recommended to abandon the operation. On the other hand, reports of successful results with the procedure from countries other than Japan were first presented by French and Australian surgeons before the fifth annual meeting of the Pacific Association of Pediatric Surgeons in Tokyo in 1972. The first success in hepatic portoenterostomy from the United States was reported in 1974. Since then, pediatric surgeons who had once experienced successful hepatic portoenterostomy actively contended against presentations denying the operation, at medical meetings or in articles.

I am convinced that more than 80% of patients with biliary atresia can be cured by the radical operation when requirements indispensable for a successful operation are fulfilled: early operation, accurate operative techniques and adequate postoperative care. The curability may rise to nearly 90% without liver transplantation. Endoscopic surgery will be available for the treatment of biliary atresia. However, the conventional laparotomy will be evaluated again in the future when operative stress is extremely reduced and healing of surgical wounds is promoted by major developments in both anesthesiology and perioperative treatment.

CHAPTER 9

CONGENITAL DIAPHRAGMATIC HERNIA

INTRODUCTION

The early published literature relating to congenital diaphragmatic hernia had a decidedly schizoid character.[1] Reports from children's hospitals and large surgical referral centers presented this condition as a comparatively rare one of relatively mild risk and largely good results from surgical repair. The anatomical nature and infrequency of this condition attracted a certain amount of media attention as these cases were described as cases of "upside down stomachs". Maternity hospital and units statistics were quite different.

In a 1935 report in the *Journal of Thoracic Surgery* Orr and Neff[2] of the University of Kansas Medical School in Kansas City, Kansas recorded experience with operation in 17 cases of congenital diaphragmatic hernia with a 53% survival (9 patients). Ladd and Gross[3,4] of the Children's Hospital of Boston in 1941 had a 63% survival of 19 patients operated upon of a total of 28 cases of congenital diaphragmatic hernia. In 1945, E.J. Donovan[5] of the Babies Hospital of New York reported in *Annals of Surgery* a 76.5% survival of 17 patients operated upon (13 of 17 patients). In 1952, C. Everett Koop and Julian Johnson[6] reported from the Children's Hospital of Philadelphia in *Annals of Surgery* an operative experience with transthoracic repair of diaphragmatic hernia in 15 infants with a survival of 80% (12 patients). Riker,[7] in 1954, reported the Children's Memorial Hospital of Chicago experience with congenital diaphragmatic hernia before the Central Surgical Association. Thirty-one of their patients were operated upon with 25 survivors (80.6%). Seventeen of their operations were by the abdominal approach and 14 were transthoracic.

An impressive personal operative experience with seven cases of congenital hernia of the diaphragm from the Children's Hospital of Boston was reported in the *American Journal of Diseases of Children* in 1946 by Robert E. Gross[8] with a 100% survival. In the opening paragraph of this report, Gross states: "Surgical attack on these malformations has now reached a stage where it is usually possible to correct the deformity, regardless of the small size of the subject."

A large referral center (Mayo Clinic) experience with congenital diaphragmatic hernia appeared in a major 1948 article in *Surgery, Gynecology and Obstetrics* (86: 735-755) by Stuart Harrington.[9] Twenty-one of his 430 cases of surgically treated diaphragmatic hernia of all types were of the congenital type (4.9%) and 16 of these 21 survived (76%).

The literature from obstetrical hospitals and units has revealed strikingly different findings both with respect to the frequency and to the gravity of congenital diaphragmatic hernia. A major presentation in this area came from the Departments of Obstetrics and Surgery of the Evanston Hospital of Evanston, Illinois in an article in the September 1955 issue of *Obstetrics and Gynecology* by Bowers, McElin and Dorsey.[10] Their series consisted of 13 cases of congenital diaphragmatic hernia seen in the newborn at the Evanston Hospital between January 1944 and January 1954. During this period there were 5,556 deliveries giving living newborn infants with congenital diaphragmatic hernia quite a relatively frequent incidence of one in each 1,196 births (approximately twice as frequent as pyloric stenosis and much more frequent than any other major surgical birth malformation in the newborn).

The mortality for this Evanston Hospital obstetrical unit experience was 92.3%. Only two infants survived as long as 24 hours. Nine of the 13 babies (69%) expired within two hours of birth and were diagnosed at autopsy. Antemortem diagnosis was made in only four of the 13 (31%) and all were operated upon, with only one survival. This infant was operated upon at 11 hours after birth. The defect in this successful infant was left-sided, without a sac and was closed successfully with release from the hospital on the eleventh postoperative day.

These Evanston/Northwestern University authors cited the University of Chicago Lying-In Hospital experience where only one infant born at that obstetrical hospital with congenital diaphragmatic hernia had lived more than six hours and with a high in-stitutional incidence of pulmonary hypoplasia as cited in Edith Potter's[11] classic publication from that institution, *Pathology of the Fetus and Newborn*. Ten babies with congenital diaphragmatic hernia were born at the Chicago Lying-In Hospital during a period when there were 21,000 deliveries. As the autopsy rate for dead babies at this time was 95%, the incidence of diaphragmatic hernia during that period may be assumed to be no more than one in each 2,100 births—again a rather frequent occurrence, as well as a very high lethality.[11,12]

The 1955 publication in *Annals of Surgery* by Campanale and Rowland[13] from obstetrical and surgical units of the Ramey Air Force Base in Puerto Rico was of major importance in calling attention in the surgical literature to the importance of hypoplastic lung in association with congenital diaphragmatic hernia. In this nonreferral military base hospital with a large and active obstetrical unit five cases of congenital diaphragmatic hernia were seen within a short period of 18 months and with a mortality of 100%. Two of the newborn babies died without operation at 45 minutes and $3^1/_2$ hours of age. Three infants were diagnosed and operated upon at 45 minutes, two hours and $21^1/_2$ hours of age and died two hours, 45 minutes and nine hours postoperatively. Severe hypoplasia was encountered in all five babies. The hernia was on the right side in one case an on the left in four. The infant with a right-sided hernia died without operation at $3^1/_2$ hours of age. The right lung weighed 6 g and the left lung 18 g. The infant with a left sided hernia who died without operation at 45 minutes of age had a left lung which weighed 2.5 g while the right lung weighed 15 g. The three infants who were operated upon unsuccessfully all had left-sided diaphragmatic hernias and at autopsies their left lungs weighed 5.0, 5.5 and 5.5 g while their right lungs weighed 25, 11.5 and 15.5 g. This paper is beautifully illustrated with X-rays, gross pathology photographs and photomicrographs which document extensively the severe degrees of pulmonary hypoplasia seen in all five of these infants. The authors obtained personal communications from several other authors. With respect to their personal communication with R.E. Gross of the Children's Hospital of Boston, they state, "Gross does not recall meeting at operation a single instance of definite hypoplasia of the lung and feels that it must be very rare, or does not occur."

The 1957 publication my coworkers and me[1] attempted to point out and to address this dichotomy of literatures relating to congenital diaphragmatic hernia in the newborn. The glaring differences in both the incidence and frequency of this malformation and its lethality as viewed from obstetrical hospitals and units (infrequently reported) and from children's hospitals and large referral centers such as the Mayo Clinic[9] clearly required some efforts at clarification.

The obstetrical hospitals and units appeared to be the logical place to look despite the infrequency of reports from these units and institution. As frequency of congenital diaphragmatic hernia in newborn infants in obstetrical units ranged from one in every 1,196 births[10] to one in every 2,100 births,[11,12] many, many more infants were being born with congenital diaphragmatic hernias than were being seen for surgical care at children's hospitals where very few, if any, babies are born. The Evanston Hospital experience that 69% of babies born with congenital diaphragmatic hernia died in the first two hours after birth helps gain a clearer picture of the true gravity of congenital diaphragmatic hernia in the newborn, as does the University of Chicago Lying-In Hospital experience that only one of ten newborn infants born at that hospital with congenital diaphragmatic hernia lived past 6 hours of age. The site-of-birth hospital mortalities of 92.3%[10] and 100%[13] despite the availability of first rate surgical care further clarifies the magnitude of this problem which was only slowly appreciated by most major children's hospitals whose happy results only kept getting better.

Campanale and Rowland, in their important 1955 report and review of the literature, found that fewer than 6 cases of congenital diaphragmatic hernia had been reported in which operation had been carried out under 48 hours of age. My 1957 report[1] included three autopsy diagnosed cases and 13 operated upon in the first 90 hours of life, 11 under 40 hours of age at the time of operation. The autopsy diagnosed patients died at 45 minutes, two hours and six hours of age. The four youngest patients at the time of operation (4, 12, 14 and 14 hours of age) were all operated upon in the hospital of their birth with two deaths (50%) of respiratory insufficiency. Of the 11 infants operated upon under 40 hours of age six survived and five died (45.5% mortality). Eight of the 13 operated upon in the first 90 hours of life survived (62%).

At these early ages, the ipsilateral (left) lung in the great majority of cases was found to be small, collapsed and nonexpandable. No expansion of the left lung at the time of operation could be obtained in 8 of 11 cases in which this information was available (73%). Expansibility was minimal in two cases and moderate in one. Of particular interest were the repeated postoperative roentgen studies of the lungs in surviving infants whose lungs were resistant to any or the most minimal of expansion at operation. Over seven to 14 days following operation slow but progressive expansion of the formerly collapsed and nonexpandable left lungs occurred. Both the fatality and hazard of vigorous attempts to expand these small, collapsed and nonexpandable left lungs by positive pressure through an endotracheal tube at operation or by chest suction immediately following operation were emphasized. The last item in the summary section of this publication is as follows:

> It is urged that the possibility of employing some means of artificial oxygenation of the blood to support these infants with nonexpandable lungs during operation, and perhaps the early hours of life, be investigated.

Twenty years later, 1977, this "plea/ dream" was answered by the practical introduction of ECMO (extracorporeal membrane oxygenation) for neonatal respiratory failure by Robert Bartlett and associates.[14] With ECMO, an exciting new modality became available for both the treatment and the study of the central and most lethal component of congenital diaphragmatic hernia in the newborn—the small, nonexpansible so-called "hypoplastic" lung which was incapable of adequate blood oxygenation and of supporting life at birth and in the early neonatal period in the majority of cases.

The nature and magnitude of the congenital diaphragmatic hernia in the newborn problem was slow to dawn upon the world pediatric surgical community. A major component of this problem, as cited earlier in this Introduction, was that so few newborn infants with congenital diaphragmatic hernia made the trip from obstetrical unit to a children's hospital. More speedy diagnosis and transport led to a confusing increase, rather than decrease, in both morbidity and mortality.

Clifford Benson and Susan Adelman[15] in their 1976 article in the *Journal of Pediatric Surgery* lamented that "at the Children's Hospital of Michigan, the survival of infants with diaphragmatic hernias of the Bochdalek type steadily improved until 1970, then it deteriorated paradoxically just as our respiratory support measures grew more sophisticated." In their 1974 article in the *Journal of Pediatric Surgery*, Boix-Ochoa et al[16] of Barcelona (Spain) started their article on a similar note of frustration: "It seems rather paradoxical to see that the survival rates of recent large surgical series on diaphragmatic hernia is not much better than it was 20 years ago."

Also in 1974, Albert Dibbins and Eugene Wiener[17] reported that 20 newborns with left posterolateral diaphragmatic hernias were diagnosed and operated upon at the Children's Hospital of Pittsburgh before 24 hours of age with a 60% mortality (12 of the 20 died). Eight years later (1982), Wiener[18] reported from the same

Children's Hospital of Pittsburgh that of 66 infants with congenital diaphragmatic hernia operated upon at ages younger than 24 hours, 38 died (58%). In closing the discussion of his 1982 paper (before the Central Surgical Association), Wiener states, "I am afraid this study raises more questions than it actually answers, but such has been the history of this frustrating lesion."[18] Ten years later, 1992, Keith Georgeson[19] of the Children's Hospital of Birmingham (Alabama) in discussing a paper from Harvard and the Children's Hospital of Boston by Wilson et al[20] before the American Pediatric Surgical Association could still observe sagely, "I think the problem of diaphragmatic hernia and how to manage it is a matter of trying to hit a bunch of singles rather than to hit the home run. We've all tried to hit the home run and we have all felt foolish striking out."

Another 1992 presentation before a major surgical organization (the American Surgical Association) by Jay Grosfeld, Karen West and associates[21] from Indianapolis described an important experience in which delayed repair of diaphragmatic hernia and ECMO increased survival (from 43% to 67.4%) as compared with a prior pre-ECMO experience with repair only. This report also stimulated some interesting discussion.

Kathryn Anderson[22] (Washington D.C., then) cited the difficulties of comparing the heterogeneous groups of congenital diaphragmatic hernia patients at different children's hospitals at different times, "like comparing apples and oranges." She also repeated a prior observation of importance to the effect that "current predictors of high mortality in CDH patients are unreliable when ECMO is used"[23] by stating that "we have found no predictors of survival by any postnatal measurements".[22] She then made a particularly important statement as follows:

Our latest 10 patients who have gone on ECMO before operation have been operated upon only when the ECMO flows could be weaned to idling-that is, 10% of cardiac output only-and when their pulmonary hypertension is gone. This may take 3 weeks. Eight of these 10 patients have survived. So we believe that it is important to wait until pulmonary blood pressure is well below systemic values, operate on them, and get them off ECMO within 24 hours of surgery.[22]

Kathryn Anderson's discussion was followed by another discussion of great interest and significance by Arnold Coran[24] of Ann Arbor and the University of Michigan. He cited a remarkable survival of congenital diaphragmatic hernia patients managed at his institution with ECMO after diaphragmatic hernia repair between 1983 and 1990 with a survival of 35 of 39 patients (90% survival and 10% mortality). In the following two years, they began to see a different type of patient by establishing a high-risk obstetrical unit for delivery in their Mott Children's Hospital. These patients were diagnosed prenatally and transported to this unit still in their mother's uterus (the best of all membrane oxygenators). These were similar to the obstetrical unit experiences reported 25 years earlier where 69% of the liveborn infants with diaphragmatic hernia (9 of 13) died in the first two hours after birth.[10] These recent high-risk obstetrical unit babies with diaphragmatic hernia at the University of Michigan were essentially unresuscitable immediately after birth with conventional means and required emergency ECMO resuscitation within minutes to less than an hour after birth for survival. Only six of 14 consecutive neonates placed on ECMO emergently and then repaired survived (43%). This experience represented a massive and sudden increase in mortality for congenital diaphragmatic hernia, with all of the most sophisticated of modalities and experienced personnel available anywhere, from 10% to 57%.

I also discussed this paper[25] and reemphasized that children's hospital statistics do not now and did not (25 years ago)[1,10] reflect the magnitude and gravity of the congenital diaphragmatic hernia at birth problem and cited Arnold Coran's beautiful and dramatic discussion and recent findings as excellent illustrations of this important point which was presented rather forcefully in his 1957 publication.[1] This discussion also reiterated some of the more important of the 1957 publication observations and proposed a unique new approach to the management of congenital diaphragmatic hernia in utero which will be discussed in greater detail in the Challenges section.

Although all other aspects of the congenital diaphragmatic hernia problem at birth and later are dwarfed by the awesome and seemingly insoluble problem of disastrous respiratory insufficiency at birth, some of these items are worthy of mention and some limited discussion.

It is of utmost importance that left, right and bilateral diaphragmatic hernias be considered separately to obtain meaningful assessments of treatment and long term results. The most frequent and lethal of these hernias are, of course, left-sided. Right-sided diaphragmatic hernias must not be thrown into the same "pot" with left-sided ones.

I, in addition to my 1957 report which was all about left-sided diaphragmatic hernias, have also published a report and review of the literature concerning right-sided Bochdalek hernias.[26] This report appeared in the December 1973 issue of the *Journal of Thoracic and Cardiovascular Surgery* (66:969-973). Two cases of abdominal viscera incarceration in the right hemithorax managed successfully by surgery were reported. One case involved tension incarceration of the stomach and one involved incarceration of a large segment of the liver which required both right hepatic lobectomy and a large ventral abdominal hernia creation to close the diaphragmatic defect and the skin of the subhepatic abdominal incision.

In this report, 57 cases of surgically treated right-sided congenital posterolateral diaphragmatic hernia were collected from the literature. Forty-one of the patients (72%) were over 72 hours of age when operated upon. One of the author's two reported patients (the incarcerated liver case) was only seven hours of age when operated upon. The other with tension incarceration of the stomach was 14 months of age at the time of acute symptoms and operation. In 37 of the 57 reported cases of right-sided diaphragmatic hernia the contents of the hernia were specified and in 76% of these at least a part of the liver was protruding through the defect into the right hemithorax. Chronic cough or recurrent respiratory infections were the most frequent symptoms. These symptoms often were vague and a chest X-ray often was needed to indicate or to confirm the clinical diagnosis. In only two other cases was herniation of the stomach through the right-sided diaphragmatic hernia defect reported.

Campbell and Lilly[27] in 1982 reported four cases of right posterolateral (Bochdalek) diaphragmatic hernias and identified the common forms of presentation as respiratory distress, intestinal herniation, asymptomatic intrathoracic mass and progressive liver herniation after birth.

Congenital diaphragmatic hernia presenting beyond the neonatal period ("late") is plagued by many of the vague symptoms encountered with right-sided congenital diaphragmatic hernias cited above. In 1976, Osebold and Soper[28] from Iowa City called attention to the perplexing problem of congenital posterolateral Bochdalek hernia producing symptoms of confusing nature beyond infancy in a detailed and scholarly report. They credited Kirkland's 1959 report in the *British Journal of Surgery*[29] on congenital posterolateral diaphragmatic hernia in the adult with calling attention to this difficult diagnostic and therapeutic problem beyond childhood years. Kirkland had collected 35 patients from the Department of Pathology of the University of St. Andrews and the Royal Infirmary of Dundee (Scotland) with congenital posterolateral diaphragmatic hernia reported from 1953 to 1958. These patient's ages ranged from 12 to 72 years and only 13 of the 35 (37%) were diagnosed correctly before operation or autopsy. Osebold and Soper reviewed in considerable detail 27

additional cases including one of their own (a 16 year old). Nineteen of these 27 new patients were adults (70%) and eight were children (15 years of age or under). The ages ranged from four to 72 years. The complaints were gastrointestinal in 55.6% of these patients and respiratory in 44.4%. Only two of the patients were asymptomatic.

McCue et al[30] in 1985 reported six cases of posterolateral diaphragmatic hernia in older children. All six presented with acute symptoms, four gastrointestinal and two respiratory. X-ray interpretation was difficult and often misleading. The diaphragmatic defects tended to be small and most commonly associated with large bowel herniation and ischemia.

Newman et al[31] in 1986 reported from the Children's Hospital of Buffalo that 11 of 83 children with congenital diaphragmatic hernia became symptomatic beyond the neonatal period (13.3%). The ages of these 11 patients ranged from four months to seven years. Seven of the 11 (64%) presented with respiratory symptoms at a median age of 14 months, while four (36%) had gastrointestinal symptoms at a median age of 5 years. Eight of the hernias (73%) involved the left diaphragm and three the right. No sacs were encountered and the hernia contents ranged from the colon only to the entire bowel, spleen, liver and pancreas. Malrotation of the midgut was found in six of the 11 patients (55%). There was no mortality.

In 1988, Berman with Ein , Shandling and associates[32] from the Hospital for Sick Children in Toronto (Canada) recorded a 20 year experience with 26 cases of late presenting Bochdalek hernias in children. The majority (62%) were originally misdiagnosed. Four patients were misdiagnosed as having pneumothoraces and were subjected to inappropriate thoracenteses. Two of their patients were asymptomatic and of the 24 symptomatic patients, the symptoms were respiratory in two-thirds (16 cases) and gastrointestinal in one-third (8 cases). There were two deaths. They concluded that the signs, symptoms and radiologic findings of these patients were difficult to interpret and were associated with diagnostic delay, misguided therapy and a potentially fatal outcome. They found that the most useful (and safest) investigation toward a correct diagnosis was a plain chest and abdominal X-ray following passage of a nasogastric tube.

Malone et al[33] in 1989 recorded 22 patients from the Great Ormond Street Hospital for Sick Children of London ranging in age from one month to 11 years of age treated for late presenting diaphragmatic defects treated over a six year period. Ten of these patients had posterolateral foramen of Bochdalek hernias and five had central diaphragmatic defects. The remaining seven patients had eventrations (4) or foramen of Morgagni defects (3). It was of particular interest that the most frequently encountered presenting feature was failure to thrive. Abdominal pain, vomiting and respiratory difficulties also occurred. Three patients with right-sided defects were misdiagnosed as pleural effusions and chest tubes had erroneously been inserted prior to transfer of these patients to surgery. Seventeen of the 22 patients were symptomatic (77%) and were successfully treated surgically with relief of symptoms. The authors recommended a barium meal with follow-through to exclude malrotation and a transthoracic operative approach in those without malrotation.

Byard et al[34] in 1991 reported a tragic case of a four-year old boy who was admitted to the hospital with a two day history of listlessness, anorexia, left upper quadrant abdominal pain and vomiting which were followed by sudden cardiorespiratory arrest and death with autopsy identifying a left congenital diaphragmatic hernia with a herniated and perforated stomach filling the pleural cavity with gastric contents.

Also in 1991, Weber et al[35] from St. Louis reported 13 cases of congenital diaphragmatic hernia beyond infancy with ages ranging from two months to 26 years. Eight of their patients had left-sided hernias and four had right-sided hernias with one patient having bilateral hernias. Chronic respiratory tract infections were present in six

patients and vomiting and weight loss in six. Two patients were found to have severe failure to thrive difficulties and severe respiratory distress was encountered in three. Primary diaphragmatic defect repair was possible in 12 of the 13 patients and a patch was required in one. Although 12 of the 13 patients survived, gastric atony and retention remained severe postoperative difficulties in 7 of the 12 survivors which complicated postoperative recovery.

It would be of interest to know of the status of both lungs in late presenting cases, both symptomatic and asymptomatic cases, and the relationship of patient age and of abdominal or thoracic symptoms to these findings. Many years ago I had an interesting experience with a middle-aged man whose large left posterolateral diaphragmatic hernia had been asymptomatic for all of his life up to that point. It had caused trouble however when an army recruitment examination chest X-ray had been misdiagnosed as tuberculosis and has caused him to spend several years in a tuberculosis sanitarium. His first symptoms many years later were gastrointestinal and barium contrast studies revealed the extent of his diaphragmatic herniation. At operation, no functioning lung tissue remained. One lung was a tiny "nubbin" of nonexpansible tissue and the other was a moderate sized cyst with no discernible functioning lung tissue. His cecum and appendix were densely adherent to the superior sulcus area of the left hemithorax and had clearly been the source of prior inflammation. There was no sac. How many people today are wandering around with asymptomatic or minimally symptomatic congenital diaphragmatic hernias? How were they spared and how did they survive so long?

The gravity and magnitude of complicating factors such as prematurity and additional malformations are impossible to obtain from children's hospital data and will be dealt with in greater detail in the Challenges section.

Beyond death, the principal complications of surgical repair of congenital diaphragmatic hernia are recurrence of the hernia, gastroesophageal reflux and chylothorax. Surgical technique, the use and nonuse and size of patches as well as the relative discrepancy of the sizes of the herniated abdominal viscera and the capacity of the reduced-size coelomic cavity to accommodate these loss-of-domain viscera likely are factors in both hernia recurrence and in esophageal reflux.

Chylothorax is almost certainly thoracic duct and/or tributaries injury-induced during hernia repair. A major 1973 publication from Richmond (Virginia) by Wiener, Owens and Salzberg[36] in the *Journal of Thoracic and Cardiovascular Surgery* called attention for the first time to this important and potentially lethal complication. Their reported case was managed successfully by TPN (total parenteral nutrition)—another first. In 1983, Oshiro and Matsumura[37] from Japan reported a case of chylothorax following Bochdalek hernia repair in an infant (2 months of age) which was managed successfully by feeding with MCT milk (medium chain triglyceride milk). In 1986, Mercer[38] of Ottawa, Canada reported a case and made an important analysis of this problem from the published literature (his case and four others). All five of these patients survived and in all five the hernia was on the left side. It was of particular interest that a sac was present in all five and was excised in all five. TPN was used successfully in three of the four cases in which this information was available. The comparative frequency of this complication became apparent in 1989 when Capps, Kiely and Spitz[39] reported three cases from the Great Ormond Street Hospital for Sick Children in London in *Pediatric Surgery International*. All three cases were associated with chylous ascites and all three were managed successfully conservatively by external drainage and by TPN or MCT feeds.

CHALLENGES

1. The most overwhelmingly important challenge here is to provide the congenital diaphragmatic hernia patient (in utero at the very moment of birth) maximum blood oxygenation support simulta-neously with atraumatic and physiologically constructive ventilatory support and evaluation (without barotrauma) with rapid and atraumatic removal of abdominal viscera from their compressive intrathoracic position into a noncompressive extra-coelomic position (Shermeta bag).

This can only be achieved by prelabor Cesarian section and the use of best membrane oxygenator God could devise (the mother's placenta). Immediate newborn anoxia and cyanosis must be regarded as unacceptable and post-lung ischemia reperfusion injury as quite preventable and avoidable.[40] I set out this proposal and its rationale quite clearly in 1992 in my discussion[25] of the paper by West et al[21] before the American Surgical Association. This proposal is as follows:

One, mothers of diaphragmatic hernia babies, late in pregnancy and before the onset of labor, be subjected to Cesarian section delivery of the baby with care to avoid injury to the placenta or umbilical cord and with a stoked-up ECMO unit with operators at the ready in the delivery room.

Two, at birth and delivery from the uterus with placenta still intact and functioning-endogenous ECMO not requiring heparinization-the newborn infant is subjected to a supraumbilical midline laparotomy incision with care to avoid injury to the umbilical vein. The lung-compressing intrathoracic intestines will be promptly eviscerated and placed in a sterile, seamless Shermeta gastroschisis bag by the technique of Professor Dennis Shermeta, formerly of Johns Hopkins and the University of Chicago and now of Phoenix. This is a marvelous device and an ingenious technique, which requires about 5 minutes, and in this time both the lung compression and the small peritoneal cavity problems are solved.

Three, prompt endotracheal intubation will permit evaluation of lung expandability and gentle pulmonary resuscitation and the initiation of a battery of sequential lung function evaluations may be undertaken. Also prostaglandins may be used to maintain ductus arteriosus patency to avoid pulmonary hypertension problems during this period.

At least 4 to 6 hours of this approach may be consumed to get past the dead-by-2-hours barrier and hurdle.

The type and length of anesthesia, the ultimate need or nonneed for ECMO, the use of umbilical vessels-artery and vein-for ECMO, etc., etc. can be evaluated with experience.[25]

2. A particularly important two part challenge is to increase substantially the number (to absolute) of antenatal diagnoses of congenital diaphragmatic hernia with a massive expansion of high-risk obstetric units for delivery within children's hospitals as pioneered so brilliantly and effectively by Professor Arnold Coran[24] at the University of Michigan.

Although Professor Coran lamented the increase in mortality with and in this new high-risk delivery from to 10 to 57%, the central item of importance is that without it all of these 14 consecutive newborn infants almost certainly would have died within minutes, as the obstetric literature has clearly indicated for more than 25 years and as I have reiterated in print for 26 years.[1,25]

3. A serious and glaring deficiency over the years and an important current challenge involves the acquisition of valid and meaningful on-going data and statistics regarding the incidence of congenital diaphragmatic hernia, the incidence and nature of associated additional congenital malformations, its geographic and ethnic incidence and the number of "still births" and of live births that crash in minutes and contribute to the 69% dead-in-two-hours statistic of the early (and only) obstetric unit data where highly competent thoracic surgical talent was immediately available under the same institutional roof (Evanston Hospital and John Dorsey as the thoracic surgeon).[10]

The two-tier literature, massive from children's hospitals and almost nonexistent from obstetrical units and hospitals has created a major and quite important gap in this very important area.

In the past 26 years only one important publication addressing this major issue has appeared. It was published in the February 1984 issue of the *Journal of Pediatric Surgery* by Prem Puri and Freda Gorman[41] from the National Maternity Hospital of Dublin, Ireland and the Children's Research Center of Our Lady's Hospital for Sick Children of Dublin. In a 10 year period (1973-1983) 36 cases of congenital diaphragmatic hernia were encountered among 75,512 births in the Dublin experience for an incidence of one in 2,097 births—a figure almost identical to the one in 2,100 births from the Chicago Lying-in Hospital and not far above the one in 1,200 births at the Evanston Hospital from 1950's data.[1] Thirty-one percent of the births were still births and 69% were live births. Fourteen of the 36 infants were males and 22 (61%) were females. Nine of the 11 stillborns (82%) were female. The hernia was left-sided in 31 cases (86%), right-sided in four (11%) and bilateral (total) in one (2.7%). Fifteen of the 21 live birth patients died before transfer to a referral center (60%). Again not too far from the Evanston Hospital 1950s data of 69% of live births dead in two hours. All of the 11 still births had nonpulmonary lethal anomalies. Prematurity of less than 1,500 gm and more than 1,000 gm existed in one of the 15 neonates who died prior to transfer. Six of the 15 had trisomies, CNS or cardiac anomalies. Of the 15 who died prior to transfer, six (40%) died prior to 20 minutes after birth, nine of the 15 (60%) within 1 hour (60 minutes) of birth and all but one (14 of 15, 93%) within the first two hours (120 minutes) of birth. All were dead within $2^{1}/_{2}$ hours of birth. All 10 of the babies who arrived at the referral center were operated upon with six survivors and four deaths (40%). Of the 25 live births, the mortality was 19 of 25 (76%).

A greatly expanded achievement of antenatal diagnosis and use of high-risk delivery units in children's hospitals (à la

University of Michigan example), as well as careful scrutiny of large maternity unit statistics on a global geographic basis (considering possible teratogenic agents such as herbicides and pesticides) are needed to supply the critical sort of data involved in this Challenge.

The sort of data involved here is concerned both with very early (minutes) management, as well as potential prevention.

4. The anatomic nature and cause of the so-called "hypoplastic" lung and its potential for expandability, function and growth with time represents a challenge of the greatest magnitude.

The 1957 observations of my coworkers and me[1] strongly suggested a capacity for lung expansion and life-sustaining function within days after successful operation and were the basis for the suggestion of an urgent need for artificial oxygenation to tide the newborn infant with congenital diaphragmatic hernia over this critical early period.

Some recent publications have addressed the potential for lung growth and function if fatality and lethal barotrauma can be avoided. Vacanti et al[42] of Boston (Children's Hospital) in 1988 in an important report in the *Journal of Pediatric Surgery* stated: "Preliminary analysis of the lungs demonstrated significant iatrogenic damage, but showed some evidence of pulmonary growth. These data suggest that if support can be provided with less iatrogenic injury after ECMO, pulmonary vascular remodeling and growth may be sufficient for improved survival."

A 1992 report from this same group of Vacanti and associates[43] reviewed the pattern of lung growth of congenital diaphragmatic hernia patients who died from 1 to 391 days of age. All had had their hernias repaired. They concluded that significant lung growth does occur postnatally at the alveolar level after hernia repair and that there is postnatal vascular remodeling which results in larger and less muscular arteries which decrease the pulmonary vascular hypertension over time. This actually has been observed in a significant number

of patients on ECMO 3 weeks and less by Kathryn Anderson.[23] The important issue is that the pulmonary hypoplasia is reversible as I demonstrated 26 years ago.[1]

Price, Stolar and associates[44] of New York (Babies Hospital) have explored the concept that neonatal lung growth is controlled in part by mechanical forces. They cite studies showing that changes in thoracic volume[45-47] and unilateral diaphragm paralysis[48,49] have significant effects on respiratory mechanics and compensatory lung growth. They also cited studies in fetal models in which phrenic nerve section results in a reduction in both lung growth and in alveolar maturation.[50,51] In piglets, they demonstrated that phrenic nerve paralysis (ectomy) decreases lung cell size and cell numbers in lung quadrants closest to the impaired diaphragm and that restored lung volume contributes to neonatal lung growth.[44]

A 1993 report by this same Price et al[52] group provided additional evidence that thoracic volume relationships are important in establishing alveolar air space volume and growth in the neonatal period. Changes in thoracic volume were considered to be a vital stimulant of compensating lung growth. The results of their 1993 reported study indicated that restored thoracic volume relationships and diaphragmatic excursion are important contributors to postnatal lung and alveolar growth—and in a comparatively short time (one week). These are important observations as over 80 to 85% of alveolar formation and growth occur postnatally.[53]

In the closing discussion of his 1993 paper, Price[54] states that in the congenital diaphragmatic hernia situation, "by closing the diaphragm, you will probably stimulate the alveolarization process." He also stated that "a dramatic change" in spurring alveolar growth was observed in an interval as short as one week.

It takes little imagination to envision a marked postnatal depression in lung alveolar growth to occur with diaphragm motion freezing by stuffing a large amount of formerly intrathoracic normally intra-abdominal viscera into an abnormally small peritoneal cavity, hence the Shermeta bag application (see item 1 in this Challenges section).

Postnatal lung growth is a continuum of antenatal growth and factors influencing this at the anatomical level must be of the greatest importance in sorting out the mysteries of the congenital diaphragmatic hernia in the newborn problem.

5. Physiological components involving the pulmonary circulation in the so-called "hypoplastic" lung of congenital diaphragmatic hernia in the immediate and early newborn period and their reversibility and capacity for beneficial manipulation are of great importance as David Collins et al[55] of San Diego demonstrated and called attention to in their classic publication as the lead article of the April 1977 issue of the Journal of Pediatric Surgery.

Collins et al[55] correctly pointed out that the pulmonary hypoplasia theory could not explain the "honeymoon period" of adequate oxygenation which often is seen in children's hospitals after repair of the congenital diaphragmatic hernia. This "honeymoon period" of adequate oxygenation may last up to 24 hours before rapid anoxic death. They correctly reasoned that a dynamic pathophysiologic event must account for the terminal anoxemic effect following a period of adequate oxygenation rather than an absolute deficiency of lung parenchyma. They proposed pulmonary vascular spasm, pulmonary hypertension and right to left shunting (persistent fetal circulation) through the patent ductus arteriosus, foramen ovale and other potential intrapulmonary channels might account for these predominantly physiological rather than anatomical events and were able to demonstrate beneficial effects with pulmonary vasodilators (tolazoline, chlorpromazine, acetylcholine, bradykinin, etc.). Their studies demonstrated that the tendency to revert to a pattern of persistent fetal circulation (PFC) where pulmonary vascular resistance is high and pulmonary blood flow is diverted through the ductus

arteriosus and foramen ovale is reversible by pharmacological manipulation—at least for the short term. Their suggestion for management of this physiological component of early congenital diaphragmatic hernia lethality were (1) Inflation of the lung, (2) Oxygenation (high concentration if needed), (3) Avoidance of acidosis (including its correction when encountered), (4) Ligation of the patent ductus arteriosus and (5) Administration of pulmonary vasodilators. This approach came to be known as the "Collins Protocol".[56] Their earlier work in this important area was presented before the American Pediatric Surgical Association in 1974.

Dibbins[57] also has been an early and important worker in this critical area. His 1974 report with Wiener[17] also emphasized the exaggerated responses of the pulmonary vasculature in these infants to all stimuli and the need to control pulmonary hypertension by pharmacologic manipulation of pulmonary arterial pressure and the rate of ductal closure. Dibbins' 1976 publication[57] added dopamine to the list of suggested and employed pharmacological agents.

Pharmacological manipulation both to prevent and to treat the so-called "hypoplastic" lung of congenital diaphragmatic hernia is an exciting approach for the reasons cited above by Collins and by Dibbins but over the years has met with considerable frustration in the search for the "magic bullet". Exogenous surfactant therapy has recently (1992) been suggested by Glick et al[58] from Buffalo (New York) and prostaglandin D_2 by Ford et al[59] from the Adelaide Children's Hospital (Australia).

In a study by Ford et al,[59] involving antenatal production of diaphragmatic hernias in fetal lambs, these lambs and normal lambs when rendered hypoxic were found to have an increase in pulmonary artery pressure, a decrease in systemic arterial pressure and a decrease in pulmonary blood flow. The authors compared prostaglandins D_2, E, and I_2 (prostacyclin) with tolazoline and isoprenaline for the treatment of pulmonary hypertension. While all of the drugs altered the hypoxyic response cited above, none was consistently successful. Nonetheless, it was of particular interest that prostaglandin D_2 came closest to being the ideal vasodilator. It decreased the pulmonary artery pressure in all seven hypoxic lambs having a diaphragmatic hernia with a concomitant increase in pulmonary blood flow in six. In the remaining lamb, the decrease in pulmonary blood flow induced by the hypoxia was arrested. These are very exciting findings. The authors concluded that prostaglandin D_2 (PGD$_2$) is likely to be a useful drug (important endogenous substance, as well) for the treatment of patients with congenital diaphragmatic hernias and associated pulmonary hypertension.

Prostaglandin D_2 has been subjected to intense study in recent years with a major work by Hayaishi and associates[60,61] of Japan (Osaka) as a major producer of sleep in the mammalian brain (preoptical area site of action in the brain) with PGE$_2$ having an opposite effect, wakefulness producing, with action in the posterior hypothalamus. PGD$_2$ and PGE$_2$ are positional isomers[61] and it is of further interest that they appear to have opposite effects relating to the cellular immune response as well as to the CNS.[62]

This clearly is a fertile area for "helpful suggestions". I (in another 1993 published paper discussion[63] from the 1992 Colorado Springs meeting of the American Pediatric Surgical Association) suggested the use of nitric oxide (NO) as of potential value in the treatment of both the lung immaturity and the pulmonary hypertension of congenital diaphragmatic hernia of the newborn. At the May 1993 meeting of the same American Pediatric Surgical Association at Hilton Head, South Carolina, Butler, Stolar and associates[64] of New York (Babies Hospital) presented an important paper dealing with the differential effects of inhaled nitric oxide on normoxic and hypoxic isolated in situ neonatal pig lungs perfused by extracorporeal membrane oxygenation. Their model allowed reversible pulmonary hypertension in normal lungs. Their findings were of considerable

significance as they found that nitric oxide (NO) reduced pulmonary vascular resistance even in normoxic lungs with an even more exaggerated pulmonary hypertension reduction response in hypoxic lungs.

A report in the October 14, 1993 issue of *Nature* by Sekido et al[40] of Japan is of particular interest with respect to pulmonary "injuries" in the immediate postnatal period when the newborn infant with congenital diaphragmatic hernia is likely to experience a very severe ischemic period and then be "resuscitated" by various oxygenating devices which may, in turn, expose the already fragile lung ("hypoplastic"?) to reperfusion injury of the sort that reestablishing blood flow to ischemic tissues may cause greater injury than that produced during the ischemic episode. This may well be a factor in the sudden fatal collapse which so abruptly ends the delightful "honeymoon period" in postoperative congenital diaphragmatic hernia repair. The authors of this important and intriguing paper investigated the role of interleukin-8 in lung reperfusion injury in a rabbit model. They found that reperfusion of ischemic rabbit lung produced neutrophil infiltration and destruction of pulmonary structure and tissue as well as local interleukin-8 production. The authors reported that the administration of a neutralizing monoclonal antibody against interleukin-8 prevented neutrophil infiltration and tissue injury in this lung reperfusion injury model. They interpreted these findings as indicating a causal role of locally produced interleukin-8 in this model. From the findings of this study, the use of monoclonal antibodies against interleukin-8 may be of value in the study and possible therapy of lung damage in the immediate postnatal period in infants with congenital diaphragmatic hernia. In addition, Cesarian section delivery might avoid or diminish this immediate post-natal ischemia period and subsequent reperfusion injury in surviving patients.

6. *The development of appropriate animal models for the study of congenital diaphragmatic hernia both in utero,*

in the early postnatal period and in therapy has been a major challenge and has provided much useful information and insight and still remains an important and productive investigational tool.

The classic and ground-breaking study in this important area was presented before the Society of University Surgeons in 1967 and published in *Surgery* by Alfred de Lorimer and associates[65] of San Francisco and the University of California. This beautifully designed and carried out study duplicated both the antenatal anatomy and pulmonary pathology of congenital diaphragmatic hernia in humans and provided an outstandingly appropriate model for the continuing study of this condition by de Lorimer's group[66,68,69] and others.[67,70,71]

The extensive laboratory work on sheep which has included both the making and repairing of diaphragmatic hernia in utero has held high hopes for its successful use in humans in the repair of antenatally diagnosed congenital diaphragmatic hernia. These high hopes, however, have been difficult to bring to fruition. In the January 1990 issue of the *Journal of Pediatric Surgery*, Michael Harrison et al[72] reported a clinical experience with in utero repair of congenital diaphragmatic hernia in six cases. All six "fetal patients" died for a 100% mortality. The mothers, fortunately survived with only one complication. While this approach appeared comparatively safe for the mothers, despite two rather unrewarding major operations, it clearly was not safe for the "fetal patients". In the discussion of this paper[73] before the American Pediatric Surgical Association, a major early investigator in this field expressed concern regarding the appropriateness of the use of this approach in humans at this time and state of knowledge regarding the human condition of congenital diaphragmatic hernia.

In October of 1992, Harrison et al[74] presented an update on their clinical experience before the Surgical Section of the American Academy of Pediatrics meeting in San Francisco. Their report involved a recent three year experience (1989-1991) with 14 "fetal patients" in humans in which fetal repair was attempted. Ten of the 14 "fetal patients" died (71.4%). In their abstract for this presentation, they enumerated some "hard-earned lessons". These experiences do not suggest that the time is "ripe" yet for extended use of this approach to the management of congenital diaphragmatic hernia in humans diagnosed antenatally.

The fetal sheep model has provided some fascinating new information of a different source. Di Fiore, Wilson and associates[75] of the Children's Hospital of Boston have recently (1993) extended previous demonstrations of accelerated fetal lung growth by tracheal ligation in utero to explore the effects of this phenomenon in experimental diaphragmatic hernia produced in utero. They found that diaphragmatic hernia/tracheal ligation (DH/TL) animals had herniated viscera reduced from the chest by enlarged lungs. Histologically the DH/TL lungs were more mature and had increased alveolar numbers and surface areas as compared with either DH alone or control animals with neither DH/TL or DH. The DH/TL animals also had increased lung volume to body weight ratios as compared with the others. The DH/TL lungs were more compliant than DH alone lungs and had better gas exchange. These important and exciting findings suggest the potential for laparoscopy-fetoscopy to explore minimally invasive use of this remarkable and intriguing information.

The development and detailed study of a Nitrofen (herbicide)-induced in utero diaphragmatic hernia in pregnant rats by a combined Hamburg and Rotterdam group[76,77] is of particular interest and value. The timing of the Nitrofen administration and the relative effects on lung and diaphragm anlage development and on the development of other malformations by this teratogenic agent are of considerable interest and most worthy of continued study. Juan Tovar et al[78] from Spain have studied the effects of Nitrofen on other organs and caution against over-enthusiasm in exterpolating knowledge obtained from animal models to human disease. Caution also has been expressed concerning conclusions drawn from this Nitrofen diaphragmatic hernia by Professor Jan Molenaar[79] of Rotterdam.

Professor Patricia Donahoe, H-C Suen and associates at the Massachusetts General Hospital (Boston and Harvard) have employed this Nitrofen model to identify a number of biochemical parameters of lung immaturity in Nitrofen-treated neonatal rats with large diaphragmatic hernias.[80] They also, quite recently, have shown that antenatal glucocorticoid treatment corrects this pulmonary immaturity.[81]

7. *Use of laparoscopy-fetoscopy*

The potential use of laparoscopy-fetoscopy for investigative use in the in utero tracheal ligation/diaphragmatic hernia model of Di Fiore et al[75] was cited in the previous animal model Challenge section. The relative effects of in utero tracheal ligation and of occlusive intraluminal tracheal plugging could be investigated in this model and manner with some way-down-the-pike potential for human application.

CONCLUSION

There is no other area in all of pediatric surgery where there are so many and so persistent challenges as in congenital diaphragmatic hernia.

While attending the 1988 meeting of the British Association of Paediatric Surgeons in Athens, Greece, I was pleased and somewhat flattered to find his 1957 article in *Surgery, Gynecology and Obstetrics*[1] cited in a beautiful and scholarly poster demonstration by Jack Chang and John Barrington of Denver as a *Classic of Pediatric Surgery-Congenital Diaphragmatic Hernia* and one of three cited since 1950 (Fig. 9.1). It was an exciting experience to share space in such an attractive and scholarly poster demonstration with such eminent figures as Hippocrates, Galen, Ambrose Pare and Vincent Bochdalek, as well as Ladd and Gross. This was also somewhat of a surprise as I had long ago forgotten what I had said (important or not) in that publication.

The preparation of this chapter on Congenital Diaphragmatic Hernia has provided the author both an opportunity to "revisit" this 1957 publication both for past and present relevance and significance.

In the introductory paragraphs, the sharp divergence in obstetrical hospital and unit literature regarding congenital diaphragmatic hernia and that children's hospitals was clearly pointed out, as was the validity and importance of the obstetrical units' data regarding the frequency (high) and lethality (*very high*) of congenital diaphragmatic hernia. It has taken an incredibly long period for this crucial information to sink into the worldwide pediatric surgical thinking on congenital diaphragmatic hernia.

In retrospect, this personal clinical experience cited in the 1957 article uniquely involved the largest sometimes successful surgical experience with the repair of congenital diaphragmatic hernia in the early hours of life when nonexpansibility of lung ("hypoplasia") was a constant finding with an opportunity to observe and document progressive expansion of involved lung over time (7 to 10 days), as well as to observe early fatality from pulmonary insufficiency. This was the first observation of "hypoplasia" "correctability" in time (days) in surviving patients. This led to the final summary statement of an urgent need to provide artificial oxygenation for these patients with nonexpandable ("hypoplastic") lungs in the early hours of life who might by this temporary means be salvaged. The great importance of avoiding barotrauma to these fragile lungs was both stressed and documented by X-ray and photomicroscopic illustrations in this 1957 publication.

As for the future, Kathryn Anderson's observations[23] concerning the value of prolonged ECMO (up to 3 weeks) to permit pulmonary hypertension to subside before repair of the congenital diaphragmatic hernia on ECMO is one of the very most important observations in many years concerning the rational and minimally traumatic management of these fragile newborns with a highly lethal malformation.

I have outlined under the first Challenge in detail an approach which I feel strongly to be worthy of investigation. I felt that way when it was made before the American Surgical Association (a worthy

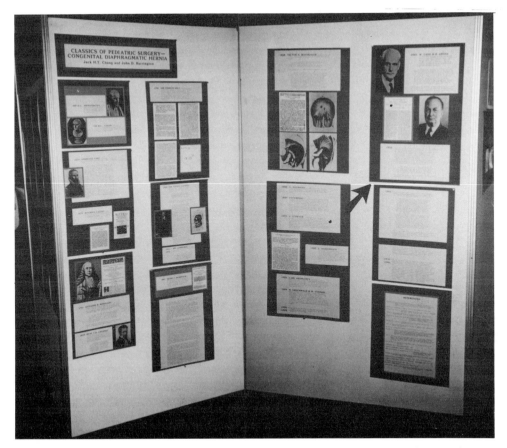

Fig. 9.1. Photograph of poster by Jack H.T. Chang and John D. Burrington of Denver shown at the 1988 meeting of the British Association of Paediatric Surgeons (BAPS) in the Greek coastal resort of Vouliagmeni (halfway between Athens and Cape Sounion). The title of the poster was "Classics of Pediatric Surgery: Congenital Diaphragmatic Hernia". I found my 1957 paper on congenital diaphragmatic hernia[1] listed as one of three "classics" cited since 1950 (arrow) and was sufficiently pleased and impressed to take this photo of the poster.

organization) in April of 1992[25] and I feel even more strongly today after the difficult and in-depth review of the past and recent literature necessarily to write this most challenging of chapters. This proposal also has the important feature of avoiding immediate post-"birth" anoxia and the serious hazard of accompanying reperfusion lung injury.

Laparoscopy-fetoscopy technology has a great future here and should be explored to the hilt in the laboratory and taken clinical when its value and safety have been firmly established.

REFERENCES

1. Moore TC, Battersby JS, Roggenkamp MW et al. Congenital posterolateral diaphragmatic hernia in the newborn. Surg Gynec Obstet 1957; 104:675-689.

2. Orr TG, Neff FC. Diaphragmatic hernia in infants under one year of age treated by operation. J Thoracic Surg 1935; 5:434-440.

3. Ladd WE, Gross RE. Congenital diaphragmatic hernia. New England J Med 1940; 223:917-925.

4. Ladd WE, Gross RE. Abdominal surgery of infancy and childhood. Philadelphia: WB Sanders Company, 1941:333-348.

5. Donovan EJ. Congenital diaphragmatic hernia. Ann Surg 1945; 122:569-581.

6. Koop CE, Johnson J. Transthoracic repair of diaphragmatic hernia in infants. Ann Surg 1952; 136:1007-1011.

7. Riker WL. Congenital diaphragmatic hernia. Arch Surg 1954; 69:291-306.

8. Gross RE. Congenital hernia of the diaphragm. Am J Dis Child 1946; 71:579-592.

9. Harrington SW. Various types of diaphragmatic hernia treated surgically. Surg Gynec Obstet 1948; 86:735-755.

10. Bowers VM, McElin TW, Dorsey JM. Diaphragmatic hernia in the newborn: Diagnostic responsibility of the obstetrician. Obstet Gynec 1955; 6:262-271.

11. Potter EL. Pathology of the Fetus and Newborn. Chicago: Yearbook Publ., 1952.

12. Potter EL, Adair FL. Fetal and Neonatal Death. Chicago: University of Chicago Press, 1940.

13. Campanale RP, Rowland RH. Hypoplasia of the lung associated with congenital diaphragmatic hernia. Ann Surg 1955; 142: 176-189.

14. Bartlett RH, Gazzaniga AB, Huxtable RF et al. ECMO in neonatal respiratory failure. J Thorac Cardiovasc Surg 1977; 74:826-833.

15. Adelman S, Benson CD. Bochdalek hernias in infancy: Factors determining mortality. J Pediatr Surg 1976; 11:569-573.

16. Boix-Ochoa J, Peguero G, Seijo G et al. Acid-base balance and blood gases in prognosis and therapy of congenital diaphragmatic hernia. J Pediatr Surg 1974; 9:49-57.

17. Dibbins AW, Wiener ES. Mortality from neonatal diaphragmatic hernia. J Pediatr Surg 1974; 9:653- 660.

18. Wiener ES. Congenital diaphragmatic hernia: New dimensions in management. Surgery 1982; 92:670- 679.

19. Georgeson K. Discussion of paper by Wilson JM et al. J Pediatr Surg 1992; 27:373.

20. Wilson JM, Lund DP, Lillehei CW et al. Delayed repair and preoperative ECMO does not improve survival in high-risk congenital diaphragmatic hernia. J Pediatr Surg 1992; 27:368-372.

21. West KW, Benston K, Rescorla FJ et al. Delayed surgical repair and ECMO improves survival in congenital diaphragmatic hernia. Ann Surg 1992; 216:454-460.

22. Anderson KD. Discussion of paper by West KW et al. Ann Surg 1992; 216:460-461.

23. Newman KD, Anderson KD, Van Meurs K et al. Extracorporeal membrane oxygenation and congenital diaphragmatic hernia: Should any infant be excluded? J Pediatr Surg 1990; 25:1048-1052.

24. Coran AG. Discussion of paper by West KW et al. Ann Surg 1992; 216:461.

25. Moore TC. Discussion of paper by West KW et al. Ann Surg 1992; 216:461-462.

26. Ban JL, Moore TC. Intrathoracic tension incarceration of stomach and liver through right-sided congenital posterolateral diaphragmatic hernia. J Thorac Cardiovasc Surg 1973; 66:969-973.

27. Campbell DN, Lilly JR. The clinical spectrum of right Bochdalek's hernia. Arch Srug 1982; 117:341- 344.

28. Osebold WR, Soper RT. Congenital posterolateral diaphragmatic hernia past infancy. Am J Surg 1976; 131:748-754.

29. Kirkland JA. Congenital posterolateral diaphragmatic hernia in the adult. Br J Surg 1959; 47:16-22.

30. McCue J, Bell A, Brereton RJ et al. Congenital diaphragmatic hernia in older children. J Roy Coll Surg (Ed) 1985; 30: 305-310.

31. Newman BM, Afshani E, Kark MP et al. Presentaiton of congenital diaphragmatic hernia past the neonatal period. Arch Surg 1986; 121:813-816.

32. Berman L, Stringer D, Ein SH et al. The late-presenting pediatric Bochdalek hernia: A 20 year review. J Pediatr Surg 1988; 23:735-739.

33. Malone PS, Brain AJ, Kiely EM et al. Congenital diaphragmatic defects that present late. Arch Dis Child 1989; 64:1542-1544.

34. Byard RW, Bourne AJ, Cockington RA. Fatal gastric perforation in a year old child with a late presenting congenital diaphragmatic hernia. Pediatr Surg Int 1991; 6:44-46.

35. Weber TR, Tracey T, Barley PV et al. Congenital diaphragmatic hernia beyond infancy. Am J Surg 1991; 162:643—646.

36. Wiener ES, Owens L, Salzberg AM. Chylothorax after Bochdalek herniorraphy

in a neonate. J Thorac Cardiovasc Surg 1973; 65:200-206.

37. Oshiro T, Matsumura C. Chylothorax following Bochdalek herniorraphy in an infant. J Pediatr Surg 1983; 18:298-299.

38. Mercer S. Factors involved in chylothorax following repair of congenital posterolateral diaphragmatic hernia. J Pediatr Surg 1986; 21:809-811.

39. Capps SNJ, Kiely EM, Spitz L. Chylothorax and chylous ascites following diaphragmatic hernia repair. Pediatr Surg Int 1989; 4:417-418.

40. Sekido N, Mukaida N, Harada A et al. Prevention of lung reperfusion injury in rabbits by a monoclonal anitbody against interleukin-8. Nature 1993; 365:654-657.

41. Puri P, Gorman F. Lethal nonpulmonary anomalies associated with congenital diaphragmatic hernia: Implications for early intrauterine surgery. J Pediatr Surg 1984; 19:29-32.

42. Vacanti JP, O'Rourke PP, Lillehei CW et al. The cardiopulmonary consequences of high-risk congenital diaphragmatic hernia. J Pediatr Surg 1988; 3:1-5.

43. Beals DA, Schloo BL, Vacanti JP et al. Pulmonary growth and remodeling with high-risk congenital diaphragmatic hernia. J Pediatr Surg 1992; 27:997-1001.

44. Price MR, Galantowicz ME, Stolar CJH. Mechanical forces contribute to neonatal lung growth: The influence of altered diaphragm funciton in piglets. J Pediatr Surg 1992; 27:376-380.

45. Davies G, Reid L. Effect of scoliosis on growth of alveoli and pulmonary arteries and on the right ventricle. Arch Dis Child 1971; 46:623-632.

46. Cowan MJ, Crystal RG. Lung growth after unilateral puneumonectomy: Quantitation of collagen synthesis and content. Am Rev Respir Dis 1975; 111:267-277.

47. Simnett JD. Stimulation of cell division following unilateral collapse of the lung. Anat Rec 1974; 180:681-686.

48. Arborelius M, Lija B, Senyk J. Regional and total lung function studies in patients with hemidiaphragmatic paralysis. Respir 1975; 32:253-264.

49. Ridgard JB, Stewart RM. Regional lung function in unlateral diaphragmatic paralysis. Thorax 1976; 31:438-442.

50. Wigglesworth JS, Desai R. Effects on lung growth of cervical cord section in the rabbit fetus. Ear Hum Dev 1979; 3:51-65.

51. Nagai A, Thurlbock WM, Jansen AH et al. The effect of chronic biphrenectomy on lung development and maturation in fetal lambs. An Rev Resp Dis 1988; 137:167-172.

52. Price MR, Butler M, Gil J et al. Altered diaphragm function modifies neonatal lung growth: Biologic morphometic assessment. J Pediatr Surg 1993; 28:478-482.

53. Langstein C, Kida K, Reed M et al. Human lung growth in late gestation and in the neonate. Am Rev Resp Dis 1984; 129:607-613.

54. Price MR. Closing discussion of paper by Price MR et al. J Pediatr Surg 1993; 28:483.

55. Collins DL, Pomerance JL, Travis KW et al. A new approach to congenital posterolateral diaphragmatic hernia. J Pediatr Surg 1977; 12:149-156.

56. Ein SH, Barker G, Olley P et al. The pharmacologic treatment of newborn diaphragmatic hernia—A 2 year evaluation. J Pediatr Surg 1980; 15:384-394.

57. Dibbins AW. Neonatal diaphragmatic hernia: A physiological challenge. Am J Surg 1976; 131:408- 410.

58. Glick PL, Leach CL, Besner GE et al. Pathophysiology of congenital diaphragmatic hernia: III. Exogenous surfactant therapy for the high-risk neonate with CDH. J Pediatr Surg 1992; 27:866-869.

59. Ford WDA, Sen S, Barker AP et al. Pulmonary hypretension in lambs with congenital diaphragmatic hernia: Vasodilator prostaglandins, isoprenaline and tolazoline. J Pediatr Surg 1990; 25:487-491.

60. Hayaishi O. Sleep-wake regulation by prostaglandins D2 and E2. J Biol Chem 1988; 263:14,593- 14,596.

61. Hayaishi O. Molecular mechanisms of sleep-wake regulation: Role of prostaglandins D2 and E2. FASEB J 1991; 5:2575-2581.

62. Moore TC. Neurovascular Immunology: Vasoactive Neurotransmitters and Modulators in Cellular Immunity and Memory. Boca Raton:CRC Press Inc. 1993; 358-374.

63. Moore TC. Discussion of paper by Suen H-

C et al. J Pediatr Surg 1993; 28:476.

64. Butler MW, Lazar EL, Smerling AJ et al. Differntial effects of inhaled nitric oxide on normoxic and hypoxic isolated in situ neonatal pig lungs perfused by extracorporeal membrane oxygenation. J Pediatr Surg 1994; 29:275-279.

65. de Lorimer AA, Tierney DF, Parker HR. Hypoplastic lungs in fetal lambs with surgically produced congenital diaphragmatic hernia. Surgery 1967; 62:12-17.

66. Starrett RW, de Lorimer AA. Congenital diaphragmatic hernia in lambs: Hemodynamic and ventilatory changes with breathing. J Pediatr Surg 1975; 10:575-582.

67. Haller JA, Signer RD, Golladay ES et al. Pulmonary and ductal hemodynamics in studies of simulated diaphragmatic hernia of fetal and newborn lambs. J Pediatr Surg 1976; 11:675-680.

68. Harrison MR, Jester JA, Ross NA. Correction of congenital diaphragmatic hernia in utero: I. The model: Intrathoracic balloon produces fetal pulmonary hypoplasia. Surgery 1986; 88:174-182.

69. Harrison MR, Ross NA, de Lorimer AA. Correction of congenital diaphragmatic hernia in utero: I. The model. Intrathoracic balloon produces fetal pulmonary hypoplasia. Surgery 1986; 88:174-182.

70. Pringle KC, Turner JW, Schofield JC et al. Creation and repair of diaphragmatic hernia in the fetal lamb: Lung development and morphology. J Pediatr Surg 1984; 19:131-146.

71. Soper RT, Pringle KC, Scofield JC. Creation and repair of diaphragmatic hernia in the fetal lamb: Techniques and survival. J Pediatr Surg 1984; 19:33-40.

72. Harrison MR, Langer JC, Adzick NS et al. Correction of congenital diaphragmatic hernia in utero: V. Initial clinical experience. J Pediatr Surg 1990; 25:42-55.

73. Haller JA. Discussion of paper by Harrison MR et al. J Pediatr Surg 1990; 25:56.

74. Harrison MR, Adzick NS, Flake AW et al. Correction of congenital diaphragmatic hernia in utero: VI. Hard-earned lessons. Abstract No. 44, Program, Section on Surgery, 61st Annual Meeting, American Academy of Pediatrics. 1992, page 92.

75. Di Fiore JW, Fauza DO, Slavin R et al. Experimental fetal tracheal ligation reverses the structural and physiologic effects of pulmonary hypoplasia in congenital diaphragmatic hernia. J Pediatr Surg (In press).

76. Kluth D, Kangah R, Reich P et al. Nitrofen-induced diaphragmatic hernias in rats: An animal model. J Pediatr Surg 1990; 25:850-854.

77. Tenbrinck R, Tibboel D, Gaillard JLJ et al. Experimentally induced congenital diaphragmatic hernia in rats. J Pediatr Surg 1990; 25:426-429.

78. Tovar JA, Alfonso LF, Aldazabal P et al. The kidney in the fetal rat model of congenital diaphragmatic hernia induced by Nitrofen. J Pediatr Surg 1992; 27: 1356-1360.

79. Molenaar JC. Discussion of paper by Suen H-C et al. J Pediatr Surg 1993; 28:476.

80. Suen H-C, Catlin EA, Ryan DP et al. Biochemical immaturity of lungs in congenital diaphragmatic hernia. J Pediatr Surg 1993; 28:471-475.

81. Suen H-C, Block KD, Donahoe PK. Antenatal glucacortacoid treatment corrects the pulmonary immaturity of congenital diaphragmatic hernia. J Pediatr Surg 1994; 29:359-363.

INVITED COMMENTARY

David L. Collins, M.D.
Pediatric Surgeon, Medical Group of San Diego
Clinical Professor of Surgery
University of California, San Diego

I think that all the principles described by the author are true. I believe there are some babies with congenital diaphragmatic hernias that do have pulmonary hypoplasia and cannot be salvaged with the present available technology.

However, as I have mentioned in the past, and as Dr. Moore so generously quotes, I believe there is a significant group who have sufficient lung to survive. Pulmonary vasospasm takes place, perhaps partly as a result of our surgical and ventilator therapy. At present, the best technique we have for relieving the spasm is to put the baby on ECMO, and allow it to relieve itself, which it will eventually do.

Nonetheless, I do believe that if a truly specific vasodilator for the pulmonary vasculature only were produced, that ECMO would become unnecessary. Nitric oxide at first appeared to be such an agent, but recent experience is less encouraging. I believe the search for an effective and specific pulmonary vasodilator will go on and will eventually be rewarded.

Arnold M. Salzberg, M.D.
Professor of Surgery and Pediatrics
Division of Pediatric Surgery
Medical College of Virginia, Richmond

The author's suggestion of a new approach to congenital diaphragmatic hernia (CDH) is worthy. The first step should be an orderly investigation of newborn animal surgery with intact placenta, including technical and physiologic problems for the mother and newborn and diaphragmatic closure which was omitted in the original proposal. The question then remains of pulmonary parenchymal recovery after months of intrauterine compression of lung by bowel. Although growth and development of newborn lung under these circumstances has been documented, a significant residual fails to expand and even with expansion, function is not optimal. Thus, must relief of CDH occur earlier in intrauterine life than near term? If so, fetoscopy with tracheal occlusion by a low pressure balloon is conceivable.

The fate of the ipsilateral lung under the best possible therapeutic circumstances near the time of birth will answer the questions of therapeutic timing. If pulmonary morphology and function are reasonably normal, then treatment efforts may be confined to this time frame. If pulmonary morbidity occurs, second trimester intervention by fetoscopy may assume importance.

What about the possibility of creating an iatrogenic gastroschisis alone or with tracheal occlusion at early fetoscopy and remove intrathoracic contents into an extra-coelomic position? Would lung expansion follow or would amniotic fluid in the pleural space create an incarcerating "peel"? The production of an iatrogenic anomaly to correct a more serious embryologic defect has occurred in the relatively recent history of congenital heart disease.

At more current levels of challenges, the relationship between ECMO and operation has yet to be resolved as well as the type of ECMO. Standard indications for veno-venous and veno-arterial methods should crystallize soon. The eventual place for ECMO, be it before or after operative correction, and if before how long, is the short-term challenge. So far, conflicting data is available.

======== CHAPTER 10 ========

ESOPHAGEAL ATRESIA AND FISTULAS

INTRODUCTION

Esophageal atresias and tracheoesophageal fistulas have provided one of the oldest, greatest and most exciting of all major success stories in pediatric surgery. Despite many years of frustrating assault on this dramatic and particularly challenging major congenital malformation in the newborn, the mortality remained fixed at 100%. The history of this long and largely unrewarding struggle is beautifully and vividly presented by Keith Ashcraft and Thomas Holder[1] in their classic article in the February 1969 issue of *Surgery* in an article titled "The Story of Esophageal Atresia and Tracheoesophageal Fistula." This outstanding historical review is strongly recommended to all interested in this topic.

The first definitive successful repair of this pesky malformation (fistula ligation and end-to-end esophageal anastomosis) was finally achieved on March 15, 1941 by Cameron Haight at the University of Michigan in Ann Arbor.[2] The early experiences at the University of Michigan are impressively presented by Professor Haight in his 1957 Presidential Address[3] before the American Association for Thoracic Surgery on the occasion of the 40th Anniversary of the founding of that distinguished association. His scholarly presentation covered multiple aspects of this malformation including its incidence, its occurrence in twins, types of the malformation, additional associated malformations (significant and not significant), the development of surgical treatment, operations and results, the physiology of the reconstructed esophagus, colon transplants for long gaps and the occurrence of fistulas without atresia. He didn't leave much out! His classification of the types of the anomaly is the best and simplest before or since. He had two major types—(1) Air in stomach-fistula present and (2) No air in stomach. This is a much more anatomical, straightforward and easy to understand classification than the earlier (1929) Vogt classification[4] and subsequent more complicated and confusing ones of massive and insignificant detail (including a 1976 classification with 97 types and subtypes).[5,6]

General and specific advances in the care of the newborn infant over the intervening years has reduced the mortality to nearly 0% in cases not involving clearly still lethal major additional malformations. Most of the long-time "controversies"/"challenges" in the management of these patients have faded over the years as the general neonatal care advances have progressively reduced mortality regardless of which of the "controversial" approaches advanced were employed (transthoracic or extrapleural approach, one layer anastomosis or two, end-to-end or end-to-side anastomosis, etc., etc.).

The 1983 publication of a 31 year experience with 500 cases of esophageal atresia in the *Journal of Pediatric Surgery* by Louhimo and Lindahl[7] of Helsinki (Finland) is one of the truly great classics of pediatric surgery relating to this topic. They split their three decade experience into five 100 case modules/sections, with no omissions. This article is a joy to read and full of useful and important information beautifully and clearly presented, as well as full of a great deal of good common sense and intelligent evaluation of their experience. Their article provides a real "feel" for the dynamic movement in the management of this one-time uniformly fatal malformation over the years with constructive and rational reevaluations in treatment.

There was a dramatic fall in mortality in each of the successive one hundred patient modules from 81% in the 1947 to 1956 period to 57% in the 1956 to 1960 period to 44% in the 1960 to 1965 period to 30% in the 1965 to 1971 period to 15% in the 1971 to 1978 period.

From their experience, they estimate the incidence of esophageal atresia at approximately one in each 3,000 births. The type incidence is almost totally into two types—the overwhelmingly frequent distal fistula "air-in-the-stomach" type of Haight and the "no-air-in-the-stomach" type with no fistula. Of the air-in-the-stomach cases, 99% were of the distal fistula type. Of the no-air-in-the-stomach type, 92% had no fistulas and were atresias without fistulas (largely long gaps).

The birth weight of their patients was over 2500 g in 349 patients (69.8%), between 1800 g and 2499 g in 118 patients (23.6%) and under 1800 g in 33 patients (6.6%).

Their overall incidence of additional congenital malformations in the total 500 patients was 40.6%. In the last 200 cases the incidence had increased to 51% with the incidence of cardiovascular anomalies increasing from 9% to 19.5% in the last 200 cases. In the last 200 cases, gastrointestinal-anorectal anomalies accounted for 14.5% with anorectal anomalies being the most frequent (8.5%). Urinary tract anomalies were found in 13.5% of the last 200 cases, with musculoskeletal anomalies in 15.5% and facial anomalies in 10.0%. Central nervous system anomalies were found in 6.5% and trisomies in 4.0%.

In the early part of their experience, the approach was mostly extrapleural whereas in the last (fifth) module of patients all were operated upon transpleurally. The mortality of the 138 extrapleural operations was 61% and that of the 258 transpleural operations was 31%. The Sulamaa[8] end-to-side anastomosis was employed only in the first module (26 cases) and was abandoned because of refistulation. In the most recent 100 case module, the single layer anastomosis was the most frequently employed (70%).

The principal methods of surgical treatment for patients with a distal fistula were primary anastomosis (thoracotomy and anastomosis within a few hours after admission and no routine use of gastrostomy) and delayed anastomosis (suction gastrostomy with or without jejunal feeding catheter with thoracotomy and anastomosis within a few days). Of these two principal methods, only the primary anastomosis method has been employed in the most recent three 100 case modules (240 cases).

Refistula was much less common than leaks and occurred in only one of the last 100 patients. The overall incidence of anastomotic leak was 16.6% with a slight decrease in each 100 patient module. The authors routinely fed their infants five days following operation. Only 6 of their 500 patients required stricture resection. Their incidence of no postoperative complications increased from 8% to 43% in the fifth 100 case module.

There were 41 patients without a distal fistula (no air in the stomach) and only eight of these were treated with esophageal anastomosis. There were 12 patients with fistulas only.

The authors conclude this beautiful presentation of a most impressive clinical experience with an informed statement of policy:

> Primary anastomosis is done within a few hours after admission. Single-layer end-to-end anastomosis via transpleural route is done whenever technically possible. The lower segment is not mobilized at all. Livaditis[9] myotomy is used to overcome an otherwise too long gap. Gastrostomy is not done, but a silicone nasogastric tube is passed through the anastomosis during operation and tube feeding is begun on the fifth day after operating. The pleural drain is kept on suction, until the feedings through the tube are started in order to detect a possible leak.

Additional confirmation of the soundness and validity of this approach is to be found in the 1985 publication in the December issue of the *Journal of Pediatric Surgery* by Bishop et al[10] from Detroit. They reviewed a 30 year experience at the Children's Hospital of Michigan in Detroit with 240 patients where the general policy had been prompt transpleural repair without gastrostomy in infants of all birth weights. Their operative mortality in this 30 year period (1951 to 1983), including staged as well as primary repairs, fell from 44% to 15% to 7% in each of the three decades and the mortality from anastomotic leaks decreased from 88% to 47% to 0% in each of these decades. Their incidence of stricture was 15% and that of refistula was 5%. Their incidence of the various types of additional congenital malformations was quite similar to that of the Louhimo and Lindahl report of 1983. Their incidence of anastomotic leak ranged from

15% to 20% in each of the decades. They routinely fed their patients between four to five days postoperatively.

An excellent 1988 report in the *Journal of Pediatric Surgery* by Professor Sture Hagberg and associates[11] of Göteborg, Sweden, follows a similar approach with outstanding results. They reported a 16 year experience (1967-1984) with 110 cases of esophageal atresia. Of these 100 had atresia with a distal fistula and seven had atresia and no fistula. One case each had a proximal fistula, double fistula and fistula with no atresia. A short or moderate gap (less than 2 cm) was encountered in 94 patients and 90 were managed by a right thoracotomy without gastrostomy within two to six hours after admission with ligation of the fistula and the creation of a single layer end-to-end anastomosis with 5-0 silk and by the transpleural route. Great care was taken not to damage circulation to the lower esophageal segment. A pleural drain and a transanastomotic tube were left in place in all patients. Feeding was begun on the third postoperative day by the transanastomotic tube.

In 51 of the 90 cases (57%) there were no complications. An anastomotic leak was identified in 24 patients (26%), a stricture (identified as requiring more than 3 consecutive dilatations) in 16 patients (18%) and gastroesophageal reflux in 5 (5%). Fundoplication was required in none of these and in only 1 of the 7 "long-gap" no fistula patients. There was no refistulation. Death due to the esophageal malformation in the two eight-year time modules fell from 15 to 2% and that from associated anomalies from 18 to 7%. The birth of their 110 patients was over 2500 g in 77 (70%), between 2000 and 2500 g in 19 (17%) and under 2000 g in 14 (13%).

Except for the incidence of early postoperative anastomotic leaks which may have been related to early postoperative feeding (3 to 5 days postop), these three excellent reports which are so detailed in so many important ways make essentially no commentary regarding gastroesophageal reflux postoperatively and the need for fundoplication postoperatively—major morbidity problems in so many other series.

In the December 1986 issue of *Chirurgie,* Professor Michel Carcassonne et al[12] of Marseille, France reported that they had omitted gastrostomy in the care of esophageal atresia with tracheoesophageal fistula since 1973 and commented that gastrostomy was no longer considered useful in patients in good condition.

Routine gastrostomy in distal fistula esophageal atresia and the retropleural operative approach have long been among the most cherished relics from the "early days" of surgical struggles to surmount the awesome esophageal atresia challenge. For a very long time, not to do a gastrostomy was akin to heresy.

In one of the most important and significant publications in the past 40 years relating to esophageal atresia and distal tracheoesophageal fistula problem appeared in the January 1987 issue of *Pediatric Surgery International* by Edward Kiely and Lewis Spitz[13] of the Hospital for Sick Children, Great Ormond Street, London (UK). This article addressed the gastrostomy issue in the most scholarly and scientific of ways—a prospective randomized study. The title of their article was "Is Routine Gastrostomy Necessary in the Management of Oesophageal Atresia?"

Their study involved a 34 month period and 51 infants with esophageal atresia and distal tracheoesophageal fistula studied at the Great Ormond Street Hospital for Sick Children in London. The infants were assigned to either gastrostomy or transanastomotic tube group. The transanastomotic tube was fine caliber (5 Fr) silastic tube passed through the nasal cavity to the site of the anastomosis by the anesthetist when the posterior half of the anastomosis was completed and then on into the stomach by the surgeon before completing the anterior layer of the anastomosis. The gastrostomy was of the standard Stamm type.

The two groups were similar in terms of birth weight, gestational age, risk group, associated anomalies and anastomotic tension.

This important study was triggered by a significant immediately prior experience with 89 infants undergoing primary repair of esophageal atresia (1980-1983). Of this group, 24% of patients subjected to gastrostomy subsequently required antireflux operation for intractable gastroesophageal reflux compared with only 5% of patients with a transanastomotic feeding tube.

In this prospective-randomized study, the incidence of significant gastroesophageal reflux was 72% in the gastrostomy group compared with 30% in the transanastomotic tube group. In addition, 44% of the gastrostomy group required antireflux surgery as compared with only 15% of the transanastomotic tube group. The authors concluded that routine gastrostomy is unnecessary in the management of infants with esophageal atresia and distal esophageal fistula and may actually be positively harmful in promoting gastroesophageal reflux. What a devastating study with respect to hallowed and cherished relics!

A study of great importance was published in the April 1992 issue of the *European Journal of Pediatric Surgery* by Cavallaro et al of Tourino (Italy).[14] This critical study was concerned with feeding troubles associated with and following delayed primary repair of esophageal atresia and brings to mind again the importance of early neonatal establishment (hours) of peripheral and brain (cortical) neurocircuitry for satisfactory function which was considered in such considerable detail in the first chapter of this book on Imperforate Anus.

Their investigation concerned five babies with long-gap esophageal atresia who underwent delayed primary anastomosis after spontaneous growth of their esophageal stumps from 12 to 16 weeks after birth and 20 babies managed by immediate, nondelayed primary esophageal anastomosis. Severe feeding problems with prolonged dysphagia and severe swallowing incoordination were encountered in the delayed anastomosis group as compared with those with nondelayed anastomosis. Bottle feeding, and later on the introduction of semisolid foods, were significantly retarded in the delayed anastomosis group with growth retardation. In addition, failure to complete feeds, dysphagia, vomiting, coughing and recurrent respiratory difficulties were more common in the delayed anastomosis group in comparison with the primary anastomosis group even in the absence of stricture. X-ray contrast studies showed that pooling of the contrast medium, retrograde flow and delayed clearing of the esophagus were more frequent in the delayed anastomosis group. Twenty-four hour pH monitoring studies also suggested a higher incidence of gastroesophageal reflux in the delayed anastomosis group. The authors concluded that the retarded start of oral feedings and the associated and related failure to achieve swallowing coordination were negative factors which contributed to the protracted dysphagia of the delayed anastomosis group and which represented a major problem for both family and hospital staff.

Two other recent publications also raise some serious questions regarding severe dysphagia problems associated with the surgical management of esophageal atresia with distal fistula (99% of the "air-in-the-stomach" type). Curci and Dibbins[15] in 1988 reported in *Archives of Surgery* an experience with problems associated with Nissen fundoplication following esophageal atresia repair. Fourteen of 31 patients with gastroesophageal reflux post-repair underwent fundoplication (45%). Five of these 14 (36%) experienced several dysphagia problems which required prolonged gastrostomy feedings.

In 1993, Wheatley, Coran and Wesley[16] of Ann Arbor reported a chilling experience with Nissen fundoplication for gastroesophageal reflux following esophageal atresia repair. They evaluated an experience with 67 of 80 patients seen between January 1974 and December 1988. A Stamm gastrostomy had been placed in 59 of the 67 infants (88%) either before or at the time of repair with a single or staged procedure. Gastroesophageal reflux was iden-

tified in 34 of the 67 patients (51%) and 21 of these 34 (62%) were managed by fundoplication. Only 8 of these 21 patients had an uncomplicated course with elimination of reflux and no postoperative dysphagia (38%). Fundoplication wrap disruption and recurrence of reflux occurred in 7 of the 21 with Nissen fundoplication (33%)—3.3 fold higher than the 10% occurrence of this complication in their 220 without esophageal atresia who received fundoplication at their institution. It was of particular interest and importance, in the light of the above observations, that postoperative dysphagia requiring prolonged gastrostomy feedings complicated eight otherwise successful initial or redo-fundoplications. The roles of gastrostomy, gastrostomy-induced reflux or gastrostomy-associated delay in prompt (hours) establishment of esophageal continuity and peripheral target to brain neurocircuitry remain to be established, but clearly are of importance in unraveling this and similar persisting esophageal atresia morbidities.

In 1987, Molenaar and associates[17] of Rotterdam reported an important retrospective study of 110 patients with esophageal atresia to assess postoperative morbidity. Their review included 77 of 87 surviving patients who had had primary end-to-end anastomoses. The postoperative course was completely uneventful in only 17 of the 77 patients (22%). Gastroesophageal reflux was identified in 42 patients (54%). In 30, it was spontaneous and in 12 it was produced on provocation. They found that gastroesophageal reflux played an important part in the occurrence of esophageal stenosis (anastomotic stricture), anastomotic leaks and esophagitis. Esophageal stenosis (49%) was encountered twice as often in patients with reflux as in those without. In addition, anastomotic leaks presented almost twice as often in patients with gastroesophageal reflux as in those without. Furthermore, gastroesophageal reflux was identified also as a contributing factor in a number of patients with respiratory problems. The authors stressed that more attention should be paid to the early detection and prevention in the early postoperative period.

As extraordinary progress has been achieved in the virtual elimination of mortality in esophageal atresia, troublesome problems in morbidity remain as addressed above. It is also important that studies of esophageal atresia should consider the two main types "air-in-the-stomach" (99% proximal atresia and distal fistula) and "no-air-in-the-stomach" (92% atresia without fistula) separately in evaluations of results and problems, including long-gap problems.

CHALLENGES

1. The overwhelmingly most important challenge in the management of esophageal atresia with distal fistula (air-in-stomach) is to achieve immediate (hours) transpleural ligation of the fistula and single layer end-to-end esophago-esophagostomy anastomosis and decidedly without a gastrostomy.

A Livaditis myotomy to elongate the upper pouch may facilitate this approach. The recently described Schärli gastroesophageal elongation procedure[18] may also be of value here. Delay beyond two or three days should be scrupulously avoided. The rationale for early establishment of somatic peripheral target neuronal circuitry areas to the brain somatic cortex in the initial critical postnatal period of just a few hours is presented in detail in chapter 1. The gastrostomy avoidance imperative is dealt with in the Introduction section of this chapter. The so-called "congenital" distal esophageal dismotility may be an iatrogenic "acquired" problem due to failure of proper anatomical and neuronal circuitry connection (operative) in the critical early postnatal hours—comparable to the incontinence achieved by greatly delayed repair of imperforate anus as illustrated in chapter 1.

2. The "long-gap" problem.

This largely is in the arena of the comparatively rare atresia with no fistula ("no-air-in-the-stomach") problem. Here again immediate post-natal correction is essential. This rules out the pouch "let's get together" delay approach by dilatations or by just waiting (see above). This leaves only three valid approaches. The gastric tubes are quick, easy and safe, but not so safe long-term with the high (approximately 30%) Barrett's esophageal problem[19] and its association with malignancy. The colon substitution approach is probably second best but a rather formidable challenge in the immediate neonatal period—and what about esophago-colonic brain neuronal connectivity? I published a major article on colon substitutes with Battersby in *Surgery, Gynecology and Obstetrics* in 1959[20] (reporting five cases) but haven't used it for years and years.

The new Schärli gastroesophageal elongation procedure[18] for the early neonatal period clearly is the front runner here and involved esophagus to esophagus anastomosis—the best way to go. There is little argument that the esophagus is the best esophagus "substitute" when possible.

3. The anastomotic leak problem.

Anastomotic leaks have been detected in from 15 to 25% of major series[7,10,11] employing early operation (sans gastrostomy) and primary anastomosis with a transanastomosis feeding tube, usually small silastic. Early postoperative feeding at three to five days postoperatively through the transanastomotic tubes may have contributed to this incidence of leaks as well as vigorous efforts to look for and detect leaks. I do essentially what these authors recommend with the exception of relying on total parenteral nutrition (TPN) through a neck jugular vein Broviac catheter placed at the time of the original operation (early) and no feeding by mouth or nasogastric transanastomotic catheter for at least 14 days following operations. A very small thin single lumen supple silastic catheter is left at operation as a nasogastric transanastomotic tube to act as a "guide/drain" for swallowed saliva which is enough immediate postnatal swallowing experience to contribute to early postnatal swallowing and esophageal neurocircuitry establishment in this early "critical" postnatal period for peripheral neuronal to brain somatic cortex functional neuroconnectivity. No effort is made to feed through this tube. It is removed with the chest tube after satisfactory oral feeding is established.

4. *Thoracoscopy and laparoscopy.*

This is probably one of the most interesting and potentially fruitful and revolutionizing use of these "new" modalities. "New" if one can overlook the 1976 publication by Bradley Rodgers and James Talbert[21] in the *Journal of Pediatric Surgery* and titled "Thoracoscopy for Diagnosis of Intrathoracic Lesions in Children". The potentials for simultaneous or sequential thoracoscopy and laparoscopy in the minimally invasive management of both types of esophageal atresia (with and without fistulas) is almost limitless with mobilizations, ligations, inter-cavity manipulations and alimentary tract transfers and anastomoses. Also with these approaches one may forget the deforming scoliosis problems which have plagued thoracic operations for esophageal atresia in infancy and childhood over the years.[22,23]

CONCLUSION

The conversion of esophageal atresia and fistulas from uniformly fatal to almost uniformly successful congenital malformations in the past five decades has reflected continuing improvements and advances in the care of newly born infants, often prematurely and with multiple additional malformations. Safer anesthesia, respiratory support, intensive care units, improved antibiotics, TPN, resourceful surgical innovations and careful studies and reports have been major contributing factors.

The current interest and major challenge has changed from mortality (largely solved) to morbidity. Gastroesophageal reflux and severe postoperative dysphagia remain major morbidity problems and likely are involved in and associated with postoperative stenosis, refistulation and pulmonary problems. The involvement of gastrostomy and of delayed primary repair anastomosis in these morbidities remain to be sorted out, but likely are quite important.

I prefer immediate (hours) postnatal transpleural ligation of fistula and single layer end-to-end anastomosis with a thin and small transanastomotic tube from nose to stomach with a chest tube for thoracotomy drainage and suction and a simultaneous neck Broviac for TPN with feeding by mouth deferred for approximately 14 days and appropriate antibiotic coverage. Gastrostomy is scrupulously avoided.

The Schärli esophago-gastric lengthening procedure[18] is an exciting new option for immediate newborn anatomic correction in long gap cases. The thorascopy and laparoscopy options also are quite exciting.

REFERENCES

1. Ashcraft KW, Holder TM. The story of esophageal atresia and tracheoesophageal fistula. Surgery 1969; 65:332-340.
2. Haight C, Towsley HA. Congenital atresia of the esophagus with tracheoesophageal fistula. Surg Gynec Obstet 1943; 76: 672-688.
3. Haight C. Some observations on esophageal atresias and tracheoesophageal fistulas of congenital origin. J Thoracic Surg 1957; 34:141-172.
4. Vogt EC. Congenital esophageal atresia. Am J Roentgenol 1929; 22:463-465.
5. Kluth D. Atlas of esophageal atresia. J Pediatr Surg 1976; 11:901-919.
6. El Shafie M, Klippel CH, Blakemore WS. Congenital esophageal anomalies: A plea for using anatomical descriptions rather than classifications. Editorial. J Pediatr Surg 1978; 13:355.
7. Louhimo I, Lindahl H. Esophageal atresia: Primary results of 500 consecutively treated patients. J Pediatr Surg 1983; 18:217-229.
8. Sulamaa M, Gripenberg L, Ahvenainen EK. Prognosis and treatment of congenital atresia of the esophagus. Acta Chir Scand 1951; 102:141-157.
9. Livaditis A. Esophageal atresia. A method of over-bridging large segmental gaps. Z Kinderchir 1973; 13:298-306.
10. Bishop PJ, Klein MD, Philippart AI et al. Transpleural repair of esophageal atresia without a primary gastrostomy: 240 patients treated between 1951 and 1983. J Pediatr

Surg 1985; 20:823-828.

11. Sillén V, Hagberg S, Rubenson A et al. Management of esophageal atresia: Review of 16 years experience. J Pediatr Surg 1988; 23:805-809.

12. Carcassonne M, Coquet M, Kreitmann B. Le traitement de l'atrésie de l'oesophage type III sans gastrostomie. Chirurgie 1986; 112:743-745.

13. Kiely E, Spitz L. Is routine gastrostomy necessary in the management of oesophageal atresia. Pediatr Surg Int 1987; 2:6-9.

14. Cavallaro S, Pineschi A, Freni G et al. Feeding troubles following delayed primary repair of esophageal atresia. Eur J Pediatr Surg 1992; 2:73-77.

15. Curci MR, Dibbins AW. Problems associated with a Nissen fundoplication following tracheoesophageal fistula and esophageal atresia repair. Arch Surg 1988; 123:618-620.

16. Wheatley MJ, Coran AG, Wesley JR. Efficacy of the Nissen fundoplication in the management of gastroesophageal reflux following esophageal atresia repair. J Pediatr Surg 1993; 28:53-55.

17. Leenderste-Verloop K, Tibboel D, Haze-broek FWJ et al. Postoperative morbidity in patients with esophageal atresia. Pediatr Surg Int 1987; 2:2-5.

18. Schärli AF. Esophageal reconstruction in very long atresia by elongation of the lesser curvature. Pediatr Surg Int 1992; 7:101-105.

19. Lindahl H, Rintala R, Sariola H et al. Cervical Barrett's esophagus: A common complication of gastric tube reconstruction. J Pediatr Surg 1990; 25:446-448.

20. Battersby JS, Moore TC. Esophageal replacement and bypass with the ascending and right half of the transverse colon for the treatment of congenital atresia of the esophagus. Surg Gynec Obstet 1959; 109:207-215.

21. Rodgers BR, Talbert JL. Thoracoscopy for diagnosis of intrathoracic lesions in children. J Pediatr Surg 1976; 11:703-708.

22. Gilsanz V, Boechat IM, Birnberg FA et al. Scoliosis after thoracotomy for esophageal atresia. Am J Roentgenol 1983; 141:457-460.

23. Jaureguizar E, Vazquez J, Murcia J et al. Morbid msculskeletal sequelae of thoracotomy for tracheoesophageal fistula. J Pediatr Surg 1985; 20:511-514.

INVITED COMMENTARY

Arnold M. Salzberg, M.D.
Professor of Surgery and Pediatrics
Division of Pediatric Surgery
Medical College of Virginia, Richmond

Esophageal atresia with distal fistula poses no serious challenge with transpleural esophagoesophagostomy and trans-anastomotic feeding tube. If approximation of the two segments is under tension, additional length of the distal esophagus can be obtained by division of one intercostal artery and further dissection of the anti-aortic wall. Additional intercostal vessel ligation may jeopardize healing of the anastomosis. If tension after limited mobilization of the distal esophagus is still a factor, the Livaditis maneuver can be done 1.5 cm proximal to the atretic esophagus over a distended Fogarty balloon with a right angled knife handle which may prevent an oblique myotomy produced by the straight handle blade.[1] If tension still persists, this maneuver can be repeated by a transcervical myotomy rather than a myotomy high in the thoracic cupula.[2] Accordingly, the neck should be prepped within the operative field to provide access for this exposure.

Atresia without fistula (long gap) is the challenge at the moment. Definitive procedures such as colon replacement, reverse gastric tube and the Schärli operation are formidable in the newborn and gastrostomy may be necessary but its location remains debatable. Gastrostomy at the greater curvature leads to reflux and a more difficult Heimlich-Gavrilu procedure. At the lesser curvature, gastrostomy makes the gastroesophageal elongation of Schärli cumbersome. Therefore, future operative steps must be visualized before committing to Stamm gastrostomy. It has been suggested by others that the Livaditis maneuver can be done on the distal esophagus when its wall becomes more robust, secondary to reflux from gastrostomy feeding. Personally, it has been done at three months but surely an earlier time is conceivable and should be forthcoming.

In the long gap defect, as Dr. Moore emphasizes, the Schärli operation is exciting and the thought occurs of ligating the left gastric artery at the time of gastrostomy in preparation for its early execution. To do a major reconstructive operation in the newborn in order to avoid gastrostomy is a moot point because mortality would be difficult to defend. The elongation procedure can be done within the first several months and hopefully the reverse gastric tube and colon interposition will be historic in the pediatric age group. This experience is conceivably extrapolated to the adult population with more extensive indications for esophageal replacement such as carcinoma.

Finally, the challenge of thoracoscopy and laparoscopy is epidemic and perhaps meaningful at present for tracheoesophageal fistula. Thoracoscopic ligation of the fistula or its endoscopic obliteration by tissue glue adhesive, fibrin glue or laser scarification is feasible. The technical problem of instrumentation, is today temporary and tomorrow solvable.

REFERENCES

1. Salzberg AM, Ducey K. Complications of pediatric thoracic surgery. In: Greenfield LJ. Complication in Surgery and Trauma. Chap 25. JB Lippincott Co.: Philadelphia, pg. 328.
2. Hoffman DG, Moazam F. Transcervical myotomy for wide gap esophageal atresia. J Pediatr Surg 1984; 19:680-682.

Professor Michel Carcassonne
Department of Pediatric Surgery
University of Marseille
Hôpital d'Enfants Timone, Marseille

In the matter of esophageal atresia, the only challenge that deserves discussion is the treatment of long gap type I esophageal atresia. About feeding troubles associated with delayed repair, my experience does not fit with Cavallaro's. In 1970 I controlled ten cases of primary anastomosis with esophageal electromyography. In all type III esophageal atresias even without any clinical trouble, a disconnected peristalsis and impairment in electro-muscular activity was observed in the distal segment (Text not published).

As the esohpagus is the best esophagus possible, since 1975 a delayed anastomosis was performed from 8 to 12 weeks after birth. A gastrostomy on lesser curvature associated with a Replogle tube in the proximal segment was done primarily. Neither esophagostomy, nor elongation was attempted. In all 16 cases, delayed anastomosis was possible, twice only a modified Livaditis procedure was necessary. Two leaks were observed resulting in two stenosis cured by some dilatations. In two cases, gastroesophageal reflux necessitated fundoplication. In a follow-up to 19 years, no patient had any serious feeding problem. All grew normally, without any immediate, secondary or late mortality.

Bradley M. Rodgers, M.D.
Professor and Chief, Division of Pediatric Surgery
Children's Medical Center
University of Virginia Health Sciences Center, Charlottesville

Dr. Moore offers a provocative commentary on the potential role of laparoscopy and thoracoscopy in the management of patients with congenital esophageal atresia, with or without fistula. I believe that these techniques of minimally invasive surgery may play a significant role in the management of some of the complications of correction of esophageal atresia, but I have considerable reservations about their utility in the primary repair. Although we have extensive experience with thoracoscopy in small children, this technique has proven to be very difficult to perform in infants less than approximately 3-4 months of age. These patients often will not tolerate unilateral ventilation to allow complete collapse of the ipsilateral lung during the procedure and it is therefore very difficult to achieve a sufficient pneumothorax to adequately visualize intrathoracic structures. To fully dissect the proximal and distal esophageal pouches in these small infants (usually less than 2.5 kg) would truly be a technical tour de force. I have considered the possibility that thoracoscopy could be used to divide an H-type tracheoesophageal fistula, however, these lesions often present somewhat later in life and I believe that it would be technically feasible to divide this fistula using thoracoscopic techniques. Whether this would prove superior to the relatively simple transcervical approach remains to be seen however. It is entirely conceivable that laparoscopic techniques will prove useful in the management of some of the more complicated anomalies. We, and others, have had experience with laparoscopy in small infants and this appears to be quite a feasible technique. Lobe and others have reported increasing experience with laparoscopic Nissen fundoplication procedures which Dr. Moore has quite properly indicated are helpful in many of these patients. Mobilization of a colonic segment for colonic segmental interposition could conceivably also be performed laparoscopically, avoiding some of the morbidity of a full laparotomy in these patients. As with many of the procedures proposed for laparoscopy and thoracoscopy, we will be faced with attempting to differentiate between that which *can* be done and that which *should* be done with these procedures. I personally am somewhat skeptical that either procedure will gain a great deal of acceptance in the management of these difficult patients.

Professor Ilmo Louhimo, M.D.
Professor of Pediatric Surgery
University of Helsinki
Children's Hospital of Helsinki, Finland

More than ten years ago we analyzed the results of treatment of 500 consecutive esophageal atresia patients (*J Ped Surg* 1983; 18:217). Since then, there have been some important changes both in the treatment and follow-up policy.

We continue to perform an early transpleural one-layer anastomosis without gastrostomy. Associated anomalies remain to be the main and practically the only cause of mortality. The development of neonatal heart surgery has decreased the deaths due to cardiac anomalies but not abolished them. Prematurity as a risk factor is today less important. Low birth weight is no longer an indication for a staged treatment in our unit.

As predicted ten years ago, the need for esophageal replacement because of atresia has practically disappeared. Patients with long gap atresia without fistula are treated with delayed anastomosis and this has been possible in every case among the last nine patients. This policy has not been without problems, however. All needed Livaditis myotomy and in the follow-up study of the living seven patients (two died of cardiac anomalies) all had fundoplication because of severe gastroesophageal reflux, three had also stricture resection. After a mean follow-up time of 4 years only one patient has normal esophageal mucosa in endoscopy, five have mild to moderate esophagitis and one definite gastric metaplasia (Barrett's esophagus).

The above findings indicate our main concern in the management of esophageal atresia patients today, which is the possible risk of late carcinoma. It is a well known fact that Barrett's esophagus is a precancerous condition, and endoscopic studies years after primary atresia repair reveal gastric metaplasia in surprisingly many patients. We studied 39 patients 2 to 11 years (mean 7.6) after esophageal anastomosis and found esophagitis in 22 cases. In five it was associated with Barrett's esophagus (*J Ped Surg* 1993; 28:1178).

Patients with esophageal replacement do not behave differently. Ten out of fourteen gastric tube patients had Barrett's esophagus when studied at about 10 years of age (*J Ped Surg* 1990; 25:446). Colon replacement patients had less metaplasia, but two out of eight studied patients (of 15 survivors) had aneuploid cell population in flow-cytometry—also a precancerous condition (*J Ped Surg* 1992; 27:859).

Early adenocarcinoma of the esophagus in atresia patients has been described (*J Ped Surg* 1989:24:741). We believe that all esophageal atresia patients should have a life-long endoscopic follow-up program. Early treatment of reflux is certainly indicated. Unfortunately, the results of fundoplication are not very consistent in esophageal atresia patients, late failures occurring in 30-40% both in our hands (J Ped Surg 1989; 24:985) and elsewhere (*J Ped Surg* 1993; 28:56).

CHAPTER 11

PYLORIC STENOSIS

INTRODUCTION

Congenital hypertrophic pyloric stenosis is one of the most pleasing and satisfying major surgical disorders in the pediatric age group to diagnose and treat. The classical symptomatology of bile-free vomitus beginning from two to four weeks of age and of progressive and increasingly projectile nature leaves little choice in the clinical diagnosis. The 100% certainty of a diagnosis on careful examination with the palpation of the "olive"/"tumor " is a never ending joy and challenge of clinical skill and the ultimate in cost saving and speed of diagnostic certainty. A speedy and precise assault on a clear objective through a bloodless classical Robertson incision consuming a maximum of 15 to 20 minutes never ceases to thrill and please as the offending olive opens like a rose with a few deft strokes of first the scalpel blade and then its blunt rear end. Additional satisfaction comes from an essentially zero morbidity and mortality with only a brief period of hospitalization. The absence of the prematurity and additional malformations problems which bedevil so many other congenital malformations in the newborn is a further blessing.

Hypertrophic pyloric stenosis is one of the most frequent major congenital malformations to occur and become symptomatic in the newborn period. With an incidence of approximately one in every 600 births and an approximate four to one greater occurrence in boy than girl babies, it appears to be more frequent in the Caucasian race and with only a slight familial incidence in the 3 to 4% range,[1-4] involving twins as well as siblings.[5-10]

Its cause remains a mystery and a challenge.

CHALLENGES

1. The greatest current challenge in congenital hypertrophic stenosis is in the diagnosis in terms of accuracy, appropriateness, speed, safety and cost.

The ultimate in diagnostic skill is to make the diagnosis by a careful physical examination with a high accuracy (100%), speed (minutes), safety and cost. In congenital hypertrophic pyloric stenosis, this is achieved by a careful abdominal physical examination to elicit the presence of the pyloric "tumor"/"olive". The examination must be in a quiet and unhurried atmosphere (examining room) with the examiner seated to the right of the infant on an examination table with no parent present. An assistant feeds the infant with a bottle and nipple containing 10% dextrose in water as the examiner uses his right hand to press on the left upper abdomen while simultaneously the left hand palpates the tumor lateral to the rectus muscle and through it. If a pyloric stenosis is present, the infant is starved and relaxes, as if under an anesthetic. The pyloric tumor, if present, may and should be palpated in 100% of the cases. Failure of the infant to relax during the examination suggests that a "tumor" is not present. If the infant has lost a significant amount of weight, quite infrequent these days, a gastric peristaltic wave may be seen to course across the epigastrium from left to right. If the "tumor" is not palpated or the infant fails to relax, a trial by nonparent (nurse) feeding may be attempted.

Of competing diagnostic approaches, the ultrasound is operator-dependent, unreliable, costly and unnecessary. The use of ultrasound technology was first described in 1977 in the *New England Journal of Medicine* by Teele and Smith.[11] Technical improvements in sonographic equipment and increasing experience have increased the accuracy of this method.[12-14] In the 1988 publication of Blumhagen et al[13] in the *American Journal of Roentgenology*, the authors recommend that of the three measurements (muscle thickness, muscle length and channel length), muscle thickness as the most reliable one should be the most discriminating and accurate one to use.

Upper gastrointestinal contrast study with barium has long been a back-up study to physical examination demonstration or nondemonstration of an "olive" where questions and uncertainty arise. Here exposure to radiation and the risk of vomiting and aspiration of barium are added to the cost and delay aspects. Narrowing and elongation of the pyloric channel are the most frequent and reliable findings.

2. The preferred and best operative approach to the hypertrophic pyloric stenosis remains a challenge.

The pyloromyotomy first described by Rammstedt[15] of Münster in 1912 has stood the test of time and remains clearly and overwhelmingly the preferred approach to relieving the hypertrophic pyloric stenosis at the present time. Attempts at medical (nonoperative) treatment and balloon dilatation have proved to be disastrous.[16-18]

While there is no controversy regarding the operative approach of Rammstedt to the hypertrophied pyloric muscle, some difference of opinion still exists to the preferred technical approach (incision) to reach the hypertrophied pylorus. I have long preferred and employed the Robertson muscle splitting incision (McBurney in type) described by Robertson[19] in 1940. This incision is fast, avascular, strong and permits excellent exposure and myotomy of the pyloric hypertrophied muscle. With this incision the operation is rapidly completed with minimal bleeding and muscle division and maximum strength of closure.

Other incisions have included the upper midline and the transverse rectus. A recent new incisional approach was reported by Tan and Bianchi[20] in 1986 and used successfully in a 1990 report by Fitzgerald et al.[21] This incision is a circumumbilical, umbilical fold incision.

3. The period of time following pyloromyotomy for the initiation of oral feedings is not widely agreed-upon.

Many prestigious institutions long have had rituals or scenarios of early and frequent post-operative feeding with cutbacks on vomiting. When feeding is given in the early postoperative period vomiting has been recorded to occur in 69, 72 and 85% of patients in larger series.[1,22,23]

A particularly important study relating to this problem was published in *Surgery* in 1968 by Schärli and Leditschke.[24] They obtained gastric motility tracings before and after pyloromyotomy in 25 patients. They observed that gastric waves disappeared for four hours after pyloromyotomy and remained depressed for an additional 16 to 24 hours. The administration of oral feedings during this period could produced high amplitude contractions and vomiting. At 24 to 36 hours postoperatively, a normal motility pattern had returned. The authors concluded that early, frequent feeding after pyloromyotomy was not logical.

Mackay and MacKellar[22] in 1986 reported that postoperative vomiting occurred in 72% of their 222 patients with early feeding and recommended that babies should be fasted for between 12 to 24 hours after pyloromyotomy.

My initial experiences with post-pyloromyotomy feeding was at an institution (Children's Hospital of Boston) which had an early and frequent postoperative feeding protocol. A short time later, at the Indiana University Medical Center in Indianapolis, I was exposed to the local wait 24 hours before feeding after pyloromyotomy protocol. In contrast to the Boston experience where vomiting after early feeding was frequent, in the Indiana experience, delay in 24 hours before feeding, resulted in no postoperative vomiting. Since that time, I have deferred feeding after pyloromyotomy for approximately 24 hours with no postoperative vomiting problem. This clearly is the superior approach. The beautiful 1968 study of Schärli and Leditschke[24] provides sound investigative support for this delay.

4. One of the most elusive challenges relating to congenital hypertrophic stenosis is its cause.

Much of the study of the possible cause or causes of congenital hypertrophic pyloric stenosis has focused on nerve cells and nerve fibers and neurotransmitters. In a 1986 report in the *Journal of Pediatric Surgery* by Malmfors and Sundler of Lund, Sweden,[25] a reduction in VIP and enkephalin in nerve fibers in smooth muscle in pyloric stenosis was found. No change was encountered in substance P and GRP (gastrin releasing peptide) in nerve fibers in pyloric stenosis. Similar findings were obtained in a 1990 report from China (Shanghai) by Shen et al.[26] They also made the important observation that there was neither a reduction of nerve cell bodies or fibers in pyloric stenosis.

A 1990 publication in *Pediatric Surgery International* by Wesley, DiPietro and Coran[27] from Ann Arbor, Michigan presented some interesting clinical experiences and provided in the Discussion some interesting data and suggestions regarding pylorospasm in the evolution of hypertrophic pyloric stenosis. Vanderwinden et al[28] of Brussels (Belgium) in the August 20, 1992 issue of the *New England Journal of Medicine* explored the pylorospasm thesis by identifying absence of nitric oxide synthase activity in the nerve fibers of the hypertrophied circular musculature of 9 hypertrophic pyloric stenosis patients (tissue obtained at operation)—a finding not encountered in control pyloric tissues. In a December 1993 publication in *Cell*, Solomon, Snyder and associates[29] at Johns Hopkins (Baltimore) report that mice lacking the neuronal nitric oxide synthase gene (homologous recombination) develop grossly enlarged stomachs with hypertrophy of the pyloric sphincter and the circular muscle layer.

A particularly important study addressing the relationship between the extent of muscle hypertrophy in pyloric stenosis and the age of the patient and duration of symptoms by Ukabiala and Lister[30] of Liverpool (UK) was published in the *Journal of Pediatric Surgery* in 1987. They assessed the degree of muscle hypertrophy by measurements of DNA in biopsy specimens. Their results indicated that the degree of hypertrophy is not age-related and that all patients tend to progress to approximately the same degree of hypertrophy, which then tends to remain constant regardless of the duration of symptoms. These important basic studies are in accord with clinical observations of the hypertrophied pylorus size at operation.

CONCLUSION

Congenital hypertrophic pyloric stenosis is one of the great all-time success stories in pediatric surgery. The 1912 break-through pyloromyotomy report of Rammstedt[15] converted a frequent and highly lethal major congenital malformation in the newborn into a comparatively easily and safely managed surgical triumph. In comparison with the Rammstedt contribution, all other challenges relating to congenital hypertrophic pyloric stenosis are relatively minor.

It is particularly important that a careful and skillful physical examination, which can identify a hypertrophied pyloric stenosis 100% of the time in experienced hands with its speed, safety, cost effectiveness and professional clinical satisfaction, will not be abandoned for imaging techniques which are unnecessary, time consuming, costly and, in some studies, hazardous.

The Robertson[19] incision of 1940 also has stood the test of time. In postoperation management, deferral of oral feeding for 24 hours will be rewarding by the elimination of vomiting following operation.

REFERENCES

1. Bell MJ. Infantile pyloric stenosis: Experience with 305 cases at Louisville Children's Hospital. Surgery 1968; 64:983-989.

2. Joseph TP, Raman Nair R. Congenital hypertrophic stenosis. Indian J Surg 1974; 36:221-223.

3. Schärli AF, Sieber WK, Kieswetter WB. Hypertrophic pyloric stenosis at the Children's Hospital of Pittsburgh from 1912 to 1967. J Pediatr Surg 1969; 4:108-114.

4. Tovar JA, Pellerin D. Hypertrophic pyloric stenosis: A study of a series of 530 cases. Ann Espan Pediatr 1973; 6:85.

5. Finsen VR. Infantile hypertrophic pyloric stenosis: Unusual familial incidence. Arch Dis Child 1979;54: 720-721.

6. Metrakos JD. Congenital hypertrophic pyloric stenosis in twins. Arch Dis Child 1953; 27:351-358.

7. Cameron AL. Familial occurrence of congenital hypertrophic stenosis. Arch Surg 1955; 70:877-894.

8. Spitz L. Congenital hypertrophic stenosis in triplets. Arch Dis Child 1974; 49:325.

9. Hicks LM, Morgan A, Anderson MR. Pyloric stenosis: A report of triplet females and notes on its inheritance. J Pediatr Surg 1981; 16:739-740.

10. Barmeister RE, Hamilton HB. Infantile hypertrophic stenosis in four siblings. Am J Dis Child 1964; 108:617-624.

11. Teele RI, Smith EH. Ultrasound in the diagnosis of idiopathic hypertrophic stenosis. New Engl J Med 1977; 296:1149-1150.

12. Keller H, Waldmann D, Greiner P. Comparison of preoperative sonography with intraoperative findings in congenital hypertrophic stenosis. J Pediatr Surg 1987; 22:950-952.

13. Blumhagen JD, Maclin L, Krauter D. Sonographic diagnosis of hypertrophic pyloric stenosis. Am J Roentgenol 1988: 150:1367-1370.

14. Forman HP, Leonidas JC, Kronfeld GD. A rational approach to the diagnosis of hypertrophic pyloric stenosis: Do the results match the claims? J Pediatr Surg 1990; 25:262-266.

15. Rammstedt C. Zür Operation der angebornen Pylorusstenose. Med Klin 1912; 8:1702-1705.

16. Rasmussen L, Hansen LP, Pedersen SA. Infantile hypertrophic pyloric stenosis: The changing trend in treatment in a Danish county. J Pediatr Surg 1987; 22:953-955.

17. Tam PKH, Carty L. Nonsurgical treatment of pyloric stenosis. Lancet 1989; 2:393.

18. Hayashi AH, Giacomantonio JM, Gillis DA. Balloon catheter dilatation for hypertrophic stenosis. J Pediatr Surg 1990; 25:1119-1121.

19. Robertson DE. Congenital pyloric stenosis. Ann Surg 1940; 112:687-689.

20. Tan KC, Bianchi A. Cicrumumbilical incision for pyloromyotomy. Br J Surg 1986; 73:399.

21. Fitzgerald PG, Lan GPY, Langer JC et al. Umbilical fold incision for pyloromyotomy. J Pediatr Surg 1990; 25:1117-1118.

22. Mackay AJ, MacKellar A. Infantile hypertrophic pyloric stenosis: A review of 222 cases. Aust NZ J Surg 1986; 56:131-133.

23. Bristol SB, Bolton RA. The results of Ramstedt's operation in a district general hospital. Br J Surg 1981; 68:590-592.

24. Schärli AF, Leditschke JF. Gastric motility after pyloromyotomy in infants: A reappraisal of postoperative feeding. Surgery 1968; 64:1133-1137.

25. Malmfors G, Sundler F. Peptidergic innervation in infantile hypertrophic pyloric

stenosis. J Pediatr Surg 1986; 21:303-306.

26. Shen Z-x, She Y-x, Wang W-c et al. Immunohistochemical study of peptidergic nerves in infantile hypertrophic pyloric stenosis. Pediatr Surg Int 1990; 5:110-113.

27. Wesley JR, DiPietro MA, Coran AG. Pyloric stenosis: Evolution from pylorospasm? Pediatr Surg Int 1990; 5:425-428.

28. Vanderwinden J-M, Mailleux P, Schiffmann SN et al. Nitric oxide synthase activity in hypertrophic pyloric stenosis. N Eng J Med 1992; 327:511-515.

29. Huang PL, Dawson TM, Bredt DS et al. Targeted disruption of the neuronal nitric oxide synthase gene. Cell 1993; 75: 1273-1286.

30. Ukabiala O, Lister J. The extent of muscle hypertrophy in infantile hypertrophic pyloric stenosis does not depend on age or duration of symptoms. J Pediatr Surg 1987; 22:200-202.

CHAPTER 12

DUODENAL OBSTRUCTIONS

IINTRODUCTION

Congenital duodenal obstructions in the newborn and in the early neo-natal period may be intrinsic in the forms of atresia or stenosis, with annular pancreas almost always coexisting with atresia when it is associated with newborn duodenal obstruction. External or extrinsic causes of duodenal obstruction in the absence of coexisting atresia generally result from complications of intestinal malrotation in the forms of Ladd's bands, midgut volvulus and pressure from superior mesenteric vessels overlying the duodenum and usually associated with some twisting or torsion which produces obstructive pressures on the underlying duodenum. These malrotation forms are discussed in greater detail in chapter 7 *(Midgut Volvulus)*. Annular pancreas and superior mesenteric vessel torsion may also cause symptoms of duodenal obstruction in adult years.[1-3]

In 1953, I,[4] with Stokes, published in *Surgery, Gynecology and Obstetrics* the results of a 25 year study (1928 to 1953) with 40 consecutive cases of congenital stenosis or atresia of the small intestine seen at the Indiana University Medical Center in Indianapolis. At this time the vast majority of reports were of isolated cases. Although congenital intrinsic duodenal obstruction was first described in 1733 by James Calder,[5] the first successful operation for congenital intrinsic duodenal obstruction (atresia) was not reported until 1916 by Ernst.[6] Successes nonetheless remained infrequent as O'Neill et al[7] in 1948 were able to find only 34 reported recoveries in cases of small intestinal atresia.

There was no significant difference between genders in this 1953 Stokes and me and an incidence of small intestinal atresia and stenosis was estimated to be one in every 6,000 births from the number of infants with atresia and stenosis born at this medical center. Of the 40 consecutive cases, the obstruction was duodenal in 23 and jejunal or ileal in 17. Because of significant clinical differences between duodenal obstructions and those in the ileal and jejunal area, we elected to consider duodenal and jejuno-ileal intrinsic obstructions separately in this publication. These differences included the number and gravity of additional malformations, the incidence of prematurity, the incidence of multiple atresias and stenoses, the gross anatomic appearance of the atresias and stenoses and the prognosis of operative repair.

Additional associated malformations were found in 11 of the 23 infants with duodenal atresia (48%) and tended to be quite serious and often (5 of 11, 45.5%) associated with prematurity. The most frequent (and serious) additional malformations were atresias elsewhere in the alimentary tract (anorectal and esophageal areas), congenital heart disease and mongolism. None of these malformations occurred in jejunoileal obstructions and abnormalities outside the midgut area were quite rare. Prematurity, on the other hand, was more frequent in jejunoileal obstructions (41% versus 22%). All 5 of the prematurely born duodenal obstruction patients had serious additional malformations.

Multiple obstructions, atresia and stenosis, did not occur in the duodenum but were comparatively frequent in the jejunoileal area. Six of 14 jejunoileal atresias (43%) were multiple and one of three stenoses (33%) was multiple. Duodenal obstructions, atresia and stenosis, tended to be a single diaphragm in appearance. Atretic areas in the jejunoileum varied considerably from a simple diaphragm, to fibrous band(s) linking atretic segments to complete discontinuity of atretic ends often associated with defects in the mesentery in the atretic discontinuity area.

There was a marked difference in the survival prognosis of operative repair of the obstructions. In the jejunoileal obstruction group, anastomotic union of the proximal and distal atretic segments was not attempted in five of the 14 atresia cases and all five died. It was attempted in nine cases with only one survival (11%). The results were much better in the operative repair of duodenal obstructions. Eight of the duodenal obstruction patients were in serious condition on admission to the hospital because of additional serious malformations, prematurity and delays in diagnosis and supportive therapy. All eight died. Definitive procedures to bypass the duodenal obstruction were carried out in 15 cases (duodenojejunostomy in 8, gastrojejunostomy in 6 and duodenoduodenostomy in 1) with 11 survivors with relief of

duodenal obstruction (73%). There was one late death at one month from a gangrenous intestinal obstruction due to an adhesive band.

This experience clearly set out the sharp differences between atresia and stenosis in the duodenum and atresia and stenosis in the midgut areas of the jejunum, ileum and proximal colon and emphasized the importance of considering them as separate entities for study, etiology and clinical management and assessment.

I returned to the problem of congenital intrinsic duodenal obstruction in 1956 in a publication in *Annals of Surgery*[8] in reporting an experience at the Indiana University Medical Center with 32 cases with emphasis on the findings in 21 cases managed by operation between 1942 and 1956. Eighteen of the 21 infants recovered (86%). Two of the three deaths involved premature infants with serious additional malformations and one infant died of a subarachnoid hemorrhage. In the group of 32 patients, additional malformations, in addition to annular pancreas, mongolism and congenital heart disease, included four cases of imperforate anus and two cases of esophageal atresia. All but five of the 21 patients managed operatively had symptoms of complete duodenal obstruction from birth.

The problem of isolated or limited numbers of cases reported was resolved in 1969 by the publication in *Pediatrics* of a review concerning 503 patients with congenital atresia and stenosis of the duodenum compiled from 65 hospitals by the Surgical Section of the American Academy of Pediatrics. This review was authored by Fonkalsrud, de Lorimer and Hays.[9] This was a 10 year review ending in August 1967. Atresia of the duodenum was present in 245 infants (49%). A diaphragm which caused partial obstruction was present in 206 patients (41%) and a stenosis in 50 (10%). The obstruction was preampillary in 99 patients (20%), postampillary in 331 patients (66%) and uncertain in 73 patients (14.5%). Four hundred and eighty-seven patients underwent primary repair of the duodenal obstruction with an overall early and late mortality of 36%. Prematurity and associated additional malformations were the major cause of mortality. Prematurity was found in 54% of the patients and additional malformations in 48%. Annular pancreas was considered an integral part of the obstructive malformation and was encountered in 106 patients (21%). It was complete in 73 patients and incomplete in 33 patients. It was considered to be a factor in the obstruction in 70% of the patients with complete annular pancreas and in only 15% of those with incomplete annular pancreas.

Down's syndrome was the most frequent additional malformation and was found in 150 patients (30%). Malrotation of the colon was the next most frequent additional malformation (19.5%) followed by congenital heart disease (17%), esophageal atresia and fistulas (6.8%), renal anomalies (5.2%), imperforate anus (3.4%), etc. Twenty-four percent of the patients had more than one additional malformation. In addition, maternal polyhydramnios was observed in 45% of the patients.

Another important 1969 publication by William Richardson and Lester Martin[10] of Cincinnati addressed the pesky problem of managing surgically the incomplete duodenal diaphragm. They described their 14 year experience with 21 patients with a diaphragmatic type of duodenal stenosis. They describe the "plunging" or "windsock" diaphragm described by Bill and Pope[11] and illustrate well the "nonbypassing" duodenojejunostomy in the presence of a "windsock" diaphragm.

A 1974 report by Girvan and Stephens[12] from the Hospital for Sick Children of Toronto presented a large experience of 20 years (1952 to 1972) with 158 infants with congenital intrinsic duodenal obstruction. Ninety-nine of the patients had atresia (63%) and 59 had stenosis (37%). Annular pancreas was associated with atresia in four cases (4%) and with stenosis in 15 cases (25.4%). Thirty-eight infants (24%) were not operated upon due to additional

serious malformations, Down's syndrome (failure to obtain parental consent) or failure to make the diagnosis before death. Of 120 infants operated upon, 67% survived. In the second of the two 10 year periods, the trend was strongly toward duodenoduodenostomy (62%) as compared with the earlier 10 year period (16%). The most frequent additional malformation was Down's syndrome (32%) followed by congenital heart disease (22%). Esophageal atresia and fistulas were encountered in 19 of the 158 cases (12%) and imperforate anus in 11 (7%). Urinary tract malformations were present in 17 infants (11%).

With the passage of time improved care of prematurity and the additional congenital malformations with parenteral nutrition and neonatal intensive care unit monitoring, survival of newborn infants with congenital intrinsic duodenal obstruction has greatly improved. In a 1987 report by Mooney, Lewis, Weber and associates[13] from the Cardinal Glennon Children's Hospital of St. Louis, 19 of 20 infants with congenital intrinsic duodenal obstruction were operated upon with 100% survival. A 94% survival of 105 infants with congenital intrinsic duodenal obstruction operated upon at the Childrens Memorial Hospital of Chicago was recorded in 1990.[14]

Early judgements regarding the presence of atresia or stenosis prior to direct exposure and opening of the duodenum in the days of duodenojejunostomy bypass operation likely were flawed to a significant degree. Also differentiating atresia (total obstruction) and stenosis (partial obstruction) on the basis of X-ray evidence of a small amount of air in the small intestine may also be misleading as the common bile duct may bifurcate into a "Y" terminus with one end into each duodenal segment, above and below the complete atresia, and thereby provide a bypass circuit for air to pass from the completely obstructed upper segment into the lower segment beyond the otherwise impervious atretic wall.

This has been described in two important recent publications. Knechtle and

Filston[15] from Duke University in 1990 described and illustrated (drawings) two cases in which anomalous biliary ducts permitted communication between proximal and distal duodenal segments in cases of complete duodenal atresia. They emphasize that air may be present in the distal bowel when anomalous bile ducts provide a conduit around the atretic segment. The authors describe in detail 11 cases recorded in the literature since the report of Karpa[16] in 1906. In 1992, Stringer et al[17] of London (UK) reported in the *Journal of Pediatric Surgery* the occurrence of this type of bile duct "Y" bypass between atretic segments in two of four cases of double duodenal atresia/stenosis (also well illustrated with drawings).

The antenatal diagnosis of duodenal atresia by ultrasound provides some interesting potentials for the study and management of duodenal atresia in utero including amniocentesis and the determination of chromosomal patterns and abnormalities. A recent, 1989, report by Hancock and Wiseman[18] of Winnipeg (Manitoba) describes an experience with antenatal diagnosis in 15 of 34 infants with congenital duodenal obstruction. In these 15 cases the diagnosis was made between the fifth month of pregnancy and term.

CHALLENGES

1. With the increasing frequency of antenatal diagnosis of duodenal atresia, a major challenge would appear to be to obtain chromosomal studies with amniocentesis to identify the most seriously disabled and compromised fetuses.

With a one in three incidence of mongolism/Down's syndrome and a high incidence of prematurity and very serious multiple additional malformations, often (25%) combined such as esophageal atresia, imperforate anus, severe congenital heart disease, renal malformations, etc., an antenatal option of pregnancy termination should be available. Despite an improving survivability of operated upon patients, an awesome morbidity from severe additional and multiple malformations, including a 30% incidence

of Down's syndrome, seriously compromises short and long-term quality of life.

2. In salvageable cases, every effort should be made completely to mobilize the duodenum from under the transverse colon to permit direct vision identification of the obstruction(s), biliary tract, pancreatic and possible overlying portal vein malformations and to identify the exact character of the obstruction(s) for their characterization and classification for proper anatomical correction and for data collection for subsequent analysis.

Prior to the almost universal use of duodenoduodenostomy, the duodenum in its entirety was seldom mobilized and exposed and the presence of atresia(s) and stenosis or stenoses was not identified as duodenojejunal bypass operations were carried out. Furthermore, misinterpretation of small amounts of air in the small intestine generally led to classification as stenosis when, in fact, a biliary tract communication "Y"-wise above and below an atresia might provide a bypass circuit for this air as discussed in the next-to-last paragraph of the Introduction section of this chapter 12.

3. Laparoscopy and Endoscopy

The combined use of laparoscopy and gastroduodenal endoscopy have an exciting potential for the management of duodenal atresia(s) and stenosis/stenoses in salvageable cases and particularly in those with "plunging" or "windsock" diaphragmatic obstructions.

CONCLUSION

In contrast to congenital hypertrophic pyloric stenosis as discussed in chapter 11, congenital intrinsic duodenal obstruction is one of the most miserable and depressing of newborn serious malformations to deal with. Despite improving operative survivability of salvageable cases, the long-term morbidity from Down's syndrome and serious and multiple additional malformations remains a difficult and awesome challenge. Successful addressing of the challenges identified above may improve the outlook of this condition for patients and family alike.

REFERENCES

1. Moore TC. Annular pancreas: Review of the literature and report of two infant cases. Surgery 1953; 33:138-148.
2. Moore TC. Annular pancreas, common-duct compression and cholelithiasis. Arch Surg 1956; 73:1050- 1054.
3. Moore TC. Vomiting during pregnancy due to midgut volvulus with duodenal obstruction. Am J Obstet Gynec 1957; 74: 1356-1360.
4. Moore TC, Stokes GE. Congenital stenosis and atresia of the small intestine. Surg Gynec Obstet 1953; 97:719-730.
5. Calder J. Medical Essays and Observations. Vol. 1, p. 203. Edinburgh, 1733.
6. Ernst NP. Congenital atresia of the duodenum treated successfully by operation. Br Med J 1916; 1:644-645.
7. O'Neill JF, Anderson K, Bradshaw HH et al. Congenital atresia of the small intestine in the newborn. Am J Dis Child 1948; 75:214-237.
8. Moore TC. Congenital intrinsic duodenal obstruction: Report of 32 cases. Ann Surg 1956; 144:159-164.
9. Fonkalsrud EW, de Lorimer AA, Hays DM. Congenital atresia and stenosis of the duodenum: A review compiled from the members of the Surgical Section of the American Academy of Pediatrics. Pediatrics 1969; 43:79-83.
10. Richardson WR, Martin LW. Pitfalls in the surgical management of the incomplete duodenal diaphragm. J Pediatr Surg 1969; 4:303-312.
11. Bill AH, Pope WM. Congenital duodenal diaphragm: Report of two cases. Surgery 1954; 35:482-486.
12. Girvan DP, Stephens CA. Congenital intrinsic duodenal obstruciton: A twenty-year review of its surgical management and consequences. J Pediatr Surg 1974; 9:833-839.
13. Mooney D, Lewis JE, Connors RH et al. Newborn duodenal atresia: An improving outlook. Am J Surg 1987; 153:347-349.
14. Raffensperger JG. Pyloric and duodenal obstruction. In: Raffensperger JG, ed. Swenson's Pediatric Surgery. 5th ed. Norwalk, CT: Appleton & Lange, 1990: 509-516.
15. Knechtle SJ, Filston HC. Anomalous biliary ducts associated with duodenal atresia. J Pediatr Surg 1990; 25:1266-1269.
16. Karpa P. Zwei Falle von Dunndarmatresie. Virchow's Arch 1906; 185:208-226.
17. Stringer MD, Brereton RJ, Drake DP et al. Double duodenal atresia/stenosis: A report of four cases. J Pediatr Surg 1992; 27: 576-580.
18. Hancock BJ, Wiseman NE. Congenital duodenal obstruction: The impact of an antenatal diagnosis. J Pediatr Surg 1989; 24:1027-1031.

CHAPTER 13

INTUSSUSCEPTION

INTRODUCTION

Intussusception is one of the great classical surgical disorders of the pediatric age group. Its quite characteristic history, symptoms and physical findings and rapid progression to a fatal termination untreated have given it a dramatic component unequalled in pediatric surgery. Details of successful treatments and nontreatments of intussusception have been shrouded in classical antiquity. Hippocrates had advocated the forced instillation of water (enemas) or air (bellows) into the terminal intestines as the treatment of ileus of all kinds, as did other ancients. The ancients however, did not differentiate intussusception from other types of intestinal obstruction. An occasional victim of intussusception, over the years, survived intussusception by sloughing and passing per rectum a necrotic and gangrenous intussusceptum, a rare occurrence.

It was not until the seventeenth century that the findings of astute observers such as Rauchin, Hildanus and Peyer led slowly and gradually to the recognition of intussusception as a pathological entity separate from other types of intestinal obstruction. The great John Hunter,[1] father of scientific surgery, in 1789 was one of the earliest to describe the clinical characteristics of this condition which he called "introsusception". This term was altered to "intussusception" in 1837 by Rokitansky[2] who also introduced the terms "intussusceptum" and "intussuscipiens". In 1873, Leichtenstern[3] published the first thorough analysis of the literature up to his time and described the various types of intussusception as enteric, ileocecal, ileocolic and colic—there wasn't much more to add!

Controversies over treatment have been long and sharp and had their origin before the turn of the century. In 1874, a year after Leichtenstern's publication, Johnathan Hutchinson[4] reported the first successful case of operative reduction of intussusception in a child.

Early efforts at nonoperative reduction in the "modern" era (mid to late nineteenth century) included the use by rectum of effervescent powders, sponge tipped bougies and quicksilver. The work of Hirschsprung in Copenhagen did much to consolidate and systematize the methods of nonoperative reduction. His first report was published in 1876[5] and by the time of his classic 1905 report[6] he had managed 109 patients between 1871 and 1904 by controlled hydrostatic reduction with the then remarkable mortality of 35%. Following Hirschsprung, considerable success with nonoperative techniques for the management and reduction of intussusception has been reported by Koch and Oerum,[7] Hipsley[8,9] and Monrad.[10] In 1912 Koch and Oerum[7] reported an experience with 400 Danish cases. In 1937, Hipsley[9] of Australia published in the first volume of *Surgery* an experience with 142 cases of intussusception treated by hydrostatic pressure. Sixty of his patients (42.3%) were reduced by hydrostatic pressure alone without mortality. An additional 30 patients treated by hydrostatic pressure were operated upon to verify reduction with one death (3.3%). Fifty-two patients were operated upon after failure to reduce the intussusception by hydrostatic pressure (35.2%) with six deaths (11%). The overall mortality in this experience was 7 of 142 (4.9%).

Although the barium enema was first used to diagnose intussusception by William E. Ladd[11] of Boston and Harvard in 1913, it was not until the 1920s that fluoroscopic reduction of intussusception by barium enema came into use. Retan[12] in 1927 was one of the first to report the use of this approach to the nonoperative treatment and reduction of intussusception. In 1948, Hellmer[13] of Lund (Sweden) reported an experience with the use of barium enema in the treatment of 162 cases of intussusception between 1933 and 1947 with a mortality of 4.9%. The clinical and experimental work of Mark Ravitch and associates[14-17] in the late 1940s and early 1950s at Johns Hopkins did much to establish the safety and "respectability" of barium enema reduction of intussusception in the United States and other parts of the world where the predominance of thinking and therapeutic approach was toward immediate and early operation.

During the period of improving results with nonoperative treatment of intussusception with hydrostatic pressure method, including barium enema, the results of surgical reduction of intussusception also were improving. This was dramatically demonstrated by the landmark 1948 lead article in the October 28 issue of the *New England Journal of Medicine* by Robert Gross

and Paul Ware[18] reporting experiences with 610 cases of intussusception. Their report included the period from 1908 until 1947. Their Figure 1 presented in graph form the striking and progressive reduction in mortality from 59% in the 1908 to 1912 period to 2.9 and 2.7% in the 1941-1945 and 1946-1947 periods. The sharpest reduction occurred in the period from 1908 to 1932. The speed of diagnosis and effective reduction of the intussusception clearly was the most important single factor in this improvement in results. From 1928 through 1947, 180 patients with intussusception whose duration of symptoms was under 24 hours were managed successfully by operation without mortality. After 24 hours, the mortality increased sharply in both the 1928 to 1939 and 1940 to 1947 periods, from 23 to 38% in the 1928-1939 period and from 9 to 15% in the 1940 to 1947 period.

"In the long history of clinical investigation and thought relating to intussusception, no single observation stands out more prominently than the importance of early recognition and treatment. It is to Clubbe[19] and his associates that we are indebted for the earliest practical demonstration of this fact on a large scale."[20] Thanks to an energetic and resourceful community-wide public information effort by Clubbe every mother in Melbourne, Australia in the early part of the century knew the classic symptoms of intussusception in their babies and the vital urgency of rapid and early diagnosis and treatment and that they, by a telephone call, could achieve this rapid diagnosis and save their babies lives. This was one of the most important and effective public appeal efforts in the history of medicine.

I reported in the February 1952 issue of *Annals of Surgery*[20] a 15 year (1935 to 1950) experience with 43 cases of intussusception at the Indiana University Medical Center in Indianapolis and paid particular tribute to Clubbe's monumental contribution to the care of infants and children with intussusception (see quote above). As in the Boston/Harvard experience of Gross and Ware, there were no deaths in patients treated within the first 24 hours after the onset of symptoms. Thereafter the mortality increased steadily from 28 to 50% and to 100% for treatment after 96 hours (one case). Barium enema reduction was attempted in 16 cases and was successful in only two (12.5%). It was fortunate that of the 14 patients operated upon after unsuccessful attempts at barium enema reduction all but one survived. This one fatal case at operation was found to have a gangrenous perforation of the ileum which required resection (unsuccessful). In this report by me, patients were divided into two groups, those under and over two years of age. Thirty-seven of the 43 patients (86%) were under two years of age. Thirty-six of the 43 patients (84%) were 12 months of age or younger. The average age in this group was six months and the peak incidence in age was at five months of age. A leading point of the intussusception was found in only three of these 37 cases (8%). In two of these cases the leading point was a Meckel's diverticulum and in one it was a duplication of the terminal ileum. Leading points were found in five of the six patients over two years of age (83%). Two of these patients had Meckel's diverticula, two had polyps and one had a lymphosarcoma.

At the time of my 1952 report, bowel resection in cases of intussusception carried a formidable mortality. In that 1952 report, two of the five patients requiring resection died (40%). McLaughlin[21] in 1948 was able to collect only 13 cases of successful resection for irreducible intussusception in patients under one year of age in a review of the literature from 1907 to 1948. The hazard of resection and primary anastomosis was well-recognized by Gross and Ware[18] in their 1948 report. In their experience, 18 patients were treated by resection and primary anastomosis with only three recoveries for a 83% mortality. This experience led them to adopt the two-staged Mikulicz double enterostomy technique which they termed the "closed, aseptic, Mikulicz resection". With this approach in

the most recent nine year period the mortality was reduced to 9% with 10 of 11 patients surviving. A year earlier, 1947, Clarence Dennis[22] had reported 100% survival of eight patients resected with primary anastomosis for irreducible intussusception. His anastomoses were achieved by a single layer presection mattress technique with fine silk. Gross and Ware[18] attributed a portion of Dennis' success to his stature as "a master in intestinal surgery"—which was indeed true. It was also true that this was a beautiful and superlative technique which I have used with only increasing satisfaction during the past 40 years and in all sorts of small bowel anastomoses and in all ages.

I concluded my 1952 publication with its most important message: "The speed with which intussusception is recognized and effectively treated is unquestionably the most important factor influencing the outcome."[20]

With the passage of time, intussusception has remained a challenge although treatment mortalities have fallen. The speed of recognition, diagnosis and definitive therapy have remained problems. In 1970, Auldist[23] of the Royal Children's Hospital of Melbourne (Australia) reported before an international pediatric surgical congress in Melbourne (Clubbe's old hometown) a recent seven-year experience with 203 cases of intussusception. Barium enema reduction was attempted in 148 cases (73%) and was successful in 86 cases (58% of those in which it was attempted and in 42.4% of the whole series of 203 patients). He presented contraindications to barium enema reduction to be ages under one month or over three years, a history of symptoms over 24 hours, abdominal distention, significant dehydration, shock, signs of peritonitis and recurrence.

In a 1980 report in the *British Journal of Surgery* by Hutchinson et al[24] a 10 year experience with 209 cases of intussusception was reported. Diagnosis was made within 24 hours of the onset of symptoms in only 44.6% of their patients. Even more frightening was the information that at least 72 hours had elapsed before the diagnosis in 25.4% of their cases. There were five deaths (2.4%) with three of the deaths being characterized as directly attributable to the intussusception. Barium enema reduction could be attempted in only 27.3% of their cases and was successful in only a little over on half of the cases in which it was attempted. Of those undergoing laparotomy, 21% had a resection with end-to-end anastomosis.

A 1987 report in *Surgery* by West et al[25] was of particular interest to me coming as it did 35 years after my 1952 publication in *Annals of Surgery* and from the same Indianapolis institution, the Indiana University Medical Center. This report concerned a 15-year experience with 83 patients with intussusception. It was distressing that the diagnosis was made in less than 24 hours in only 44.5% of the patients in comparison with 48.6% in the 1952 report. Symptoms were greater than 48 hours in 50.6% of the patients and greater than 72 hours in 30.1% of the patients. The authors of this 1987 report state in their publication that 55% of their patients had been evaluated in an emergency room or by an office based physician at least once before being referred to their medical center. They comment that the infants were lethargic and irritable on admission and that abdominal distention was found in 85% of the children on admission. Small wonder that the failure rate of barium enema reduction was 58%, that the operative irreducible rate was 31.3% of the 83 patients and that temporary stomas were required in 11 of 18 irreducible patients requiring resection (61.1%) rather than the preferred primary end-to-end anastomosis. The authors describe and document a significant morbidity rate which they justifiably attribute to delay in diagnosis (actually to delay in recognition and referral). With all of those obstacles and hurdles, the one truly remarkable part of this report is the 100% survival rate which can only be attributed to magnificent in house care, plus not a few miracles!

A 1988 report from Melbourne by Beasley, Auldist and Stokes[26] is of particular importance. This 15-year experience analysis of 630 patients admitted to the Royal Children's Hospital of Melbourne was carried out to determine the influence of the accuracy of the original patient assessment on the subsequent clinical course and patient morbidity. This report makes a fine, but disturbing, companion piece to the previously considered report of West et al[25] and its bearing on early *(and accurate)* diagnosis and definitive treatment of intussusception. The original clinical assessment and provisional diagnosis by the first medical practitioner (referring clinician or emergency room staff) was found to be at variance with the ultimate established diagnosis of intussusception in 318 of the 630 cases (50.5%). In those patients with an incorrect original diagnosis the incidence of abdominal distension, severe dehydration, fever and peritonitis ranged from two to five times as common as in those correctly diagnosed. Barium enema reduction was only 21% as compared with 43% in those correctly diagnosed originally. In addition, laparotomy was more frequent (79 vs. 57%) and resection was more frequent (24 vs. 12%) in the incorrectly diagnosed cases. Furthermore, necrosis/infarction and failed manual reduction were twice as common and local perforation was three times as common in the incorrectly diagnosed cases. Wound infection or dehiscence was three times as common in the incorrectly diagnosed group. Despite all of this morbidity (as in the Indianapolis experience), death of patients was only slightly more frequent (3 versus 2) in the incorrectly diagnosed cases in whom both diagnosis and treatment were delayed.

In 1986, two important, intriguing and impressive papers appeared in the *Journal of Pediatric Surgery* from China concerning the use of air/oxygen inflation "enemas" for the reduction of intussusception in infancy and childhood in a massive number of patients (thousands).[27,28] In the January 1986 issue of the *Journal of Pediatric Surgery*, Zhang Jinzhe et al[27] of Beijing (China) reported an extended experience with air/

oxygen inflation enemas in the management of intussusception in infants. Since 1973, oxygen inflation from a tank with controlled pressure had replaced air pumped from a hand balloon. The authors state that air rectal inflation reduction of intussusception has been widely practiced in China since its introduction in 1961 by Dr. She[29,30] of Shanghai. They also state that this method differs from the old rectal inflation method used in Western countries in the early years of this century in the use of both fluoroscopic control and adjustable pressure control. In 2,496 cases so managed from 1978 to 1983, a successful reduction rate of 91% has been achieved without mortality. Their contraindications to the use of this method are similar to those used in Western countries as contraindications to attempted barium enema reduction. These include a history of symptoms over 48 hours and evidence of intussusception irreducibility, necrosis and/or perforation.

The Shanghai experience was published in the December 1986 issue of the *Journal of Pediatric Surgery* with other papers presented from the May 1986 meeting of the American Pediatric Surgical Association. This paper was authored by Guo et al[28] and dealt with 6,396 cases of intussusception managed in a 13 year period at the Shanghai Children's Hospital—as many as 615 cases in a single year and 12 cases in a single night. They caution that the maximum safe air pressure is 110 mm Hg for older children and 80 mm Hg pressure for young infants. Cautious support of this approach was voiced in a discussion of this paper by Professor Robert Filler[31] of Toronto whose group had used this method in 15 cases of intussusception.

The use of air insufflation in the management of intussusception by prestigious Canadian and Australian groups (Toronto and Melbourne) hit the English radiological literature with hurricane force in 1988 with two major publications and one American commentary from Iowa in *AJR* (*Journal of the American Roentgen Ray Society*).[32-34] L. Gu of the Shanghai Children's

Hospital (China) was the first author of the Toronto publication which was awarded the John Caffey Award.[32] Air was used as the contrast medium for studies of the colon in 282 patients suspected of having intussusception with intussusception documentation in 118 of these patients. Reduction was achieved in 75% of these patients (89). Patients were selected by the same criteria employed for barium reduction efforts. The only absolute contraindications were peritonitis and shock. Twenty-nine patients in whom air reduction was unsuccessful were operated upon. In seven of these resection was required for devitalized bowel. Operative reduction was difficult in seven cases and easy in 12. It was of particular interest that no reductions by barium were achieved in patients in whom satisfactory trial with air had failed. Colonic perforation occurred in three of their 118 intussusception patients (2.5%). It was easily recognized fluoroscopically and fecal soiling of the peritoneal cavity at operation was notably absent and readily and easily managed with uneventful recovery and no late complications (adhesions, obstruction, etc.)—in sharp contrast to barium perforations. The average fluoroscopic time in experienced hands was less than 30 seconds, with an average total time for the procedure of five minutes in comparison with the 20 or more minutes for barium. The cleanup is easier and faster for obvious reasons and patient distress is less and radiation dose is lower. The authors concluded that air is a useful substitute for barium in the treatment of intussusception.

The Melbourne report of 1988 by Phelan, de Campo and Malecky[33] described an experience with oxygen insufflation of the colon for attempted intussusception reduction in 55 proved cases of intussusception since July 1986 at the Royal Children's Hospital. Successful reduction of the intussusception was achieved in 73% of the 55 cases (40). Resections were reduced from 18 to 8% and there were no perforations and no complications. Their results demonstrate a greater overall success rate with gas reduction than with barium with their success rate improving from 32% to 66%. The authors indicate the conservative nature of their approach to gas reduction of intussusception by reporting the use of pressures no greater than 80 mm Hg and the nonuse of premedication, antispasmatics or anesthesia. They conclude their report with the statement that "oxygen insufflation of the colon for therapeutic reduction of intussusception has superseded hydrostatic barium reduction at our institution."

Important follow-ups of the Melbourne experience appeared in the pediatric surgical literature in 1992.[35,36] They addressed the prediction of outcome with gas enema and the relative incidence of recurrence after gas reduction as compared to barium enema reduction. The article in *Pediatric Surgery International* by Renwick, Beasley and Phelan[35] presented important information regarding the incidence of recurrence of intussusception after gas/oxygen enema reduction as compared with barium enema reduction. Of 170 initial episodes of attempted gas enema reduction of intussusception in which 127 (75%) were successfully reduced, a recurrence occurred in 10 of the 127 cases for a recurrence rate of 7.9%. This was slightly smaller and compared favorably with an 8.9% recurrence rate after successful barium enema reduction. The authors concluded that gas enema reduction does not have a higher rate of recurrence than found with barium and that there is no significant incidence of incomplete reduction being unrecognized at the time of gas/oxygen enema reduction.

The publication by Beasley and Glover[36] in the *Journal of Pediatric Surgery* addressed the issue of the validity of previously adverse clinical features which in the pregas (barium) era predicted a low likelihood of successful reduction. The adverse features selected by them were four in number and were duration of symptoms over 24 hours, severe dehydration (greater than 5%), small bowel obstruction on plain abdominal X-ray and extremes of age for intussusception (less than 3 months of age or over 2 years of age). They concluded from their data that "for any given number of adverse

features, gas enema reduction is more likely to be successful than barium reduction and the presence of multiple adverse features in the absence of signs of peritonitis is probably not a contraindication to attempted gas enema reduction".

The long forgotten and much neglected major publication of 1959 in *Pediatrics* (a quite respected journal) by Eduardo Fiorito and Luis Recalde Cuestas[37] of Rosario, Santa Fe, Argentina has only recently received proper recognition in the burst of enthusiasm for gas enema reduction of intussusception. Their studies with air insufflation of the colon under manometric and fluoroscopic control began in September 1953. They termed their approach "controlled insufflation".[38] Poor results in their early experience between September 1953 and August 1954 happened because they had not used an occlusive catheter. In only four of 15 cases during this period was full reduction achieved (27%). From August 1954 to December 1958, 86 cases of intussusception were treated by their "controlled insufflation" method with successful reduction in 81 (94%). Of the five cases requiring operative reduction, the duration of symptoms in two had been more than 24 hours. If only cases of intussusception with symptom durations less than 24 hours are considered, the success rate of "controlled insufflation" in 84 cases rises to 96.5%—a truly remarkable achievement and in such a remote location (to most "mainstream" pediatricians and pediatric surgeons of the English speaking world) and at such an early time in the "modern" and sophisticated treatment of intussusception—especially by controlled, fluoroscopically monitored air insufflation enema. All of their patients were between three and 18 months of age. The device for "controlled insufflation" developed by them is pictured by a schematic drawing (Fig. 1) in their 1959 *Pediatrics* publication, as well as some beautiful roentgenogram illustrations of their air enema reduction of intussusception results. They also commented that Saenz and Paviotti,[39] employing their apparatus, had achieved similar results to theirs in the air enema reduction of intussusception in childhood. Saenz and Paviotti in 23 cases had obtained 21 full reductions of the intussusception (92%).

Some primitive and some less primitive attempts at air "enema" reduction of intussusception were published before the turn of the century. In a 1897 textbook of pediatrics L. Emmett Holt described how he reduced intussusception by an ordinary hand bellows successfully in 19 cases with the bellows connected to a catheter in the rectum and the buttocks held tightly together.[40] In 1899, H.S. Collier[41] in *Lancet* reported three cases of intussusception, clinically diagnosed, which were cured by enemas employing water in two and *air* in one.

In addition to barium and gas enema X-rays, ultrasonography also has been employed in the diagnosis of intussusception,[42] but lacks the potential for a simultaneous therapeutic effort in this condition in which time is of such critical importance between the onset of symptoms and diagnosis with prompt therapeutic reduction.

As cited earlier in this Introduction to chapter 13, infants and children over one year (12 months) of age and certainly over two years of age have a high incidence of "leading points" involved in their intussusceptions. In addition to a Meckel's diverticulum as the most common leading point, other leading points have included polyps, adenomas, duplications, eosinophilic granulomas, ectopic gastric mucosa and areas of submucous hemorrhage and hematomas associated with hemophilia and with Henoch-Schönlein anaphylactoid purpura. Intussusception in hemophiliac children is a rare but dangerous condition. David Collins and Kenneth Miller[43] reviewed this problem in 1968 and reported the second successful case. The intussusception was ileo-ileal in two cases and colocolic in one and all required resection for irreducible or perforated and gangrenous intussusception.

Henoch-Schönlein anaphylactoid purpura in childhood may provide significant diagnostic dilemmas. Surgical complications may include intussusception[44-46] as well as intestinal perforation and infarction. A major report and review of the literature by Bailey, Haase and associates[46] from the Children's Hospital of Denver appeared in the *Journal of Pediatric Surgery* in 1984. The authors reported a 10 year experience with 58 patients with Henoch-Schönlein purpura in which a surgical consultation was requested in 13. In seven of these, the clinical or radiological findings led to a laparotomy. An intussusception (ileocolic in two and ileoileal in one) was found in three children and a spontaneously reduced intussusception was suspected in two additional cases. The authors emphasize that abdominal pain may occur in approximately 50% of Henoch-Schönlein patients. Although they estimate significant surgical lesions in only 2 to 6% (12% in their experience), they caution that the same abdominal symptomatology may accompany a simple intestinal vasculitis or a catastrophic surgical lesion. Including their experience, they were able to find reports of 57 children with surgical lesions complicating Henoch-Schönlein purpura. These included six intestinal perforations, two bowel infarctions and 46 intussusceptions. Two thirds of the intussusceptions involved only the small bowel and at the time of surgical intervention 51 of the 57 children (95%) had already developed the pathognomic cutaneous rash.

Unusual types of intussusception have been encountered following operations and in utero. In both of these circumstances the intussusceptions have been almost exclusively small intestine into small intestine. Daniel Hays[47] of the Los Angeles Children's Hospital in a major 1961 publication in *Surgery, Gynecology and Obstetrics* was one of the first to call attention to the problem of intussusception occurring after an operation. Three of his nine cases were acute postoperative recurrences of intussusceptions previously reduced but six occurred following abdominal operations for unrelated conditions. He made the important observations that these intussusceptions are usually confined to the small intestine (five of the six cases), occur with equal frequency in both sexes, occur within five to 26 days of the original operation, are rarely associated with rectal bleeding or an abdominal mass and that nonoperative management should be brief and "conducted with recognition of the existence of postoperative intussusception as a significant clinical entity."

Raffensperger and Baker[48] in 1967 reported in *Archives of Surgery* a large experience with 47 instances of postoperative mechanical intestinal obstruction in 43 pediatric surgical patients seen in a seven year period at the Cook County Children's Hospital of Chicago. In 20 of their obstructions the postoperative interval was 30 days or less. They observed that children who developed intestinal obstruction soon after operation tended to have obscure signs and symptoms. Five of their patients had intussusception involving the small intestine and all within eight days of surgery. They state that their findings with postoperative intussusception confirm Hays' observations that these intussusceptions involve the small intestine only and that they rarely associated with a palpable mass or with rectal bleeding.

A cascade of publications on this topic occurred in short order. McGovern and Gross[49] of Boston in 1968 in *Surgery* reported 13 patients who developed postoperative intestinal obstruction in the initial 30 days postoperatively with the characteristic atypical findings. In 1973, Cox and Martin[50] of Cincinnati reported 16 cases seen in a prior 14 year period which always involved the small intestine. There were no leading points, no resections and no deaths. Dammert and Votteler[51] in 1974 recorded five cases seen in seven years at the Children's Medical Center of Dallas. All involved only the small intestine. In 1979, Mollitt, Ballantine and Grosfeld[52] in *Surgery* reviewed 119 cases of postoperative intussusception in infancy and childhood, including 14 cases of their own. Twenty-four patients (20%) had undergone retroperitoneal operations with 18 of these (75%) for tumors and 17 (14%) had had perineal pull-through procedures. Symp-

toms had begun within the first week following operation in 64% of the patients and within two weeks in 90%. The intussusception was limited to the small bowel in 86% of the patients. Simple operative reduction was successful in 95% and resection was required in only 3.4%.

The continuing hazard of postoperative intussusception in infancy and childhood is illustrated in a 1991 report from the Children's Hospital of Philadelphia by Holcomb, Ross and McNeill.[53] They encountered 14 cases in a prior four year period (3.5 cases per year) including two cases in one 24 hours period. They subtitled their report "Increasing Frequency or Increasing Awareness?"

In utero intussusception causing small bowel atresia also likely is more frequent than appreciated. My associates and I[54] have encountered two such cases at the Harbor-UCLA Medical Center in the past two years. Both atresias were in the distal ileum with a mesenteric gap in one case. One patient had perforation of the proximal segment with meconium peritonitis with calcification and free air on abdominal X-ray. Both patients were managed successfully by resection of the atretic ends and end-to-end anastomosis. In 1958, Parkkulainen[55] reported in *Surgery* an experience with three cases of intrauterine intussusception as a cause of intestinal atresia in a three year period at the Children's Hospital of Helsinki (Finland). Rowena Spencer[56] of New Orleans in 1968 in *Surgery* reported two cases of small intestinal atresia caused by intrauterine intussusception in a series of 53 patients with intestinal atresia (3.8%). Her article has a photograph (her Fig. 7) illustrating the gross appearance of the intussusception and atresia of one of these cases. As with postoperative intussusceptions, these atresia causing in utero intussusceptions are limited to the small intestine. They appear to occur quite late in pregnancy and are limited to the fibrous connecting cord and gap types.

Todani et al[57] of Okayama (Japan) in 1975 in the *Journal of Pediatric Surgery* also reported two cases of their own of intrauterine intussusception-induced intestinal atresia and also included details of 22 additional cases from Japan collected by questionnaire. All of their 24 cases involved only the small intestine. They estimated the incidence of intrauterine intussusception as a cause of intestinal atresia on the newborn from their data to be 7.4% (19 of 257 cases). The atresia was ileal in 16 of their cases and jejunal in eight. There was a gap in the mesentery in 13 cases and the atresia was of the cord-type in 11. There were no diaphragm or multiple atresias in this experience. The location of the intrauterine intussusception was in the distal blind end in all but one of the 24 cases where it was found in the proximal end. Most of these infants were full-term and without additional malformations.

It is of more than casual historical interest that one of the cases of intestinal atresia described by Jan Louw and Christiaan Barnard[58] in their landmark 1955 publication in *Lancet* proposing ischemic intrauterine intestinal catastrophes as a cause of intestinal atresia in the newborn was a case of intrauterine intussusception induced intestinal atresia.

Intussusception in Africa and in India has occurred in some unusual locations and with clinical pictures somewhat different from other parts of the world which have generated most of the reported cases of the four main types (first year of life classical picture, after two years of age with leading points, postoperatively and intrauterine as a cause of intestinal atresia).

Cole[59] in 1966 reported an experience with 100 cases of cecocolic intussusception in West Africa from the University Hospital in Ibadan, Nigeria in the *British Journal of Surgery*. Cecocolic intussusception was the second most common abdominal emergency treated at his hospital between 1958 and 1962. Fifty-two of the 100 patients were female and the majority were under 15 years of age with the highest incidence in the five to 15 years of age range. There was a seasonal incidence with most of the patients coming towards the end of the dry season, after the hot dry winds and cold

nights of January. Colicky pain in the umbilical area was the only symptom all of the patients experienced. Vomiting was not severe except in 16 patients who were clinically obstructed. Half of the patients had diarrhea and half passed some blood. Constipation occurred in 16 patients and in three of these after a period of diarrhea. Although the average length of illness was 18 days, half of the patients came to the hospital in the initial eight days of their illness. A mass was obvious in 66 patients. In 61, it was palpated on abdominal examination and by rectal exam in three, while in two it had prolapsed outside the anal opening. The mass hardened during spasms of pain.

The author emphasized the four characteristic radiological signs of this disease with particular attention to the unique importance of the last. They were (1) no cecal gas shadow, (2) a soft tissue shadow of the intussusception, (3) the apex of the intussusception visible against colonic gas and (4) a ground-glass appearance of the rest of the abdomen due to the exudate which was always present. As diarrhea and abdominal pain were the two principal symptoms, the author cautioned that dysentery from various causes often was blamed, resulting in a delay of diagnosis and treatment which has been surgical. In the 100 cases, resection was required in nine cases with manual reduction of varying degrees of difficulty being carried out in the rest of the cases. There were four recurrences and four deaths, all associated with bowel gangrene. Patients with symptoms of over two weeks duration tended to be over 10 years of age. The critical point of the disease was said to be the sigmoid colon. If the apex of the intussusception had passed this point, gangrene and mortality become dangerous possibilities. A dimple at the apex which arose from an area of not more than one square centimeter unfailingly was the starting point of the intussusception. The cause of this unique disorder was unknown and veiled in mystery, as was its unique geographical distribution with concentration to an area in

Western Nigeria of not more than 100 miles across.

In 1972, Margaret Mayell[60] of Cape Town, South Africa, described an experience with 223 cases of intussusception in infancy and childhood seen over a $9^1/_2$ year period at the Red Cross War Memorial Children's Hospital. Thirty-five of these intussusceptions (16%) were colocolic and only one of these was found to have local pathology. Five of the patients with colocolic intussusception had origins of the intussusception in the sigmoid colon and had prolapse of the intussusception through the anal opening. The colocolic intussusception tended to occur in children over one year of age. There were 50 resections in 215 patients operated upon (a resection rate of 23%). Four of the six deaths occurred in the resection group of patients for a resection mortality of eight%. The overall mortality of the 223 patients (6 deaths) was 2.7%. The two peaks in seasonal incidence occurred toward the end of summer and the end of winter which were peak periods of diarrheal and upper respiratory infections.

In 1973, Jennifer Chapman[61] published in the *Journal of Pediatric Surgery* an experience with intussusception in a slightly less "southern" area of Africa. Her report was from the Harari Central Hospital of Salisbury (Rhodesia) and was concerned with intussusception in a Rhodesian black population over a $4^1/_2$ year period (1967-1971). Three clinical features seen in this population in Rhodesia differed according to the author from those seen in other parts of Africa and in Europe. These included the age of incidence, the frequent occurrence of diarrhea and the mildness of the colic. Thirty percent of her 56 cases occurred in adults (14 to 60 years of age) and 27% in children ($1^1/_2$ to 4 years of age). The 24 infant cases (43% of the total) were clustered between three and 10 months of age with a peak incidence at 6 months. While the average duration of symptoms for infants and children was three to four days, for adults it had increased to 10 days. Diarrhea (61% of cases)

and vomiting (95% of cases) were the most frequent and diagnostically helpful symptoms. Colic was present in 90% of cases, but was frequent in other disorders as well. Diarrhea was an especially prominent part of the colocolic type of intussusception which (with the cecocolic type) occurred in 31% of the patients (17 of 55). Blood and mucus per rectum (73% of cases) and abdominal distention (48% of cases) were late symptoms. An abdominal mass (palpable in 68% of cases) was an important diagnostic feature and typically was tender in the line of the colon or in the right iliac fossa (7 cases—there were 7 cases of cecocolic intussusception in the infants and children age groups). The apex of the intussusception was palpable rectally in 27% of the cases. No clear cause was found in the majority of cases. In seven of 17 adult cases (41%), a tumor/largely acquired "mass" was encountered at the apex of the intussusception and was described as hemangioma, granuloma, fibroma/leiomyoma or "lipoma". The cecocolic type was also labeled the "Ibadan" type (see above findings of Cole[59]). Ileoileal intussusceptions were encountered in 10 of 55 cases (18%) and were concentrated in the adult population (80%, 8 cases). The overall mortality was 11%. The author commented that this was less than the University of Natal (Durban, South Africa) series of 67 patients with an overall mortality of 24% and an infant (ages 3 to 14 months) mortality of 62.5% (5 of 8 cases) as reported by Kark and Rundle[62] in 1960 in the *British Journal of Surgery*. Sixteen of their 67 patients were children ages 2 to 15 years (24%) and 42 (63%) were adults aged 16 to 76 years. This report was limited to black African and Indian patients. The low incidence of infant cases with intussusception (12% of the total) was striking.

Intussusception in infancy and childhood with emphasis on colonic intussusceptions at the Red Cross War Memorial Children's Hospital in Cape Town, South Africa (Rondebosch) was revisited in 1978 by Davies and Cwyes.[63] This multiracial hospital admitted children from birth to

13 years of age. In an eight year period (1968-1975) 197 patients were treated for intussusception and in 37 (19%) the intussusception was colonic. In a prior report from this hospital by Mayell[60] in 1972, 16% of 223 intussusceptions were colonic.

In a beautifully organized and presented report, the authors subdivided colonic intussusceptions into two main groups, presigmoid which included cecocolic and colocolic types and into the sigmoid/sigmoidorectal type. Presigmoid intussusceptions were the most frequent with 29 of 37 cases (78.4%) and were rather evenly divided between the two types with 16 cases of cecocolic and 13 cases of colocolic. These two types were similar in age ($3^3/_4$ and 4 years), symptoms (colic and vomiting in 80%) and physical findings (tender abdominal mass and blood in stools in 80 plus percent with abdominal distention rarely encountered). Their principal difference was in the duration of symptoms prior to hospital admission. The duration for cecocolic intussusceptions was nine days and that for colocolic was $1^1/_4$ days. The onset in colocolic cases was more acute and dramatic. Two of the cecocolic intussusceptions were reduced by barium enema and 14 were operated upon with one resection and no deaths. All 13 of the colocolic intussusceptions were operated upon with three resections and one death. Postreduction edematous "caputs" were found at the apex of intussusceptions in essentially all presigmoid types of intussusception and "traditional" leading points were quite rare.

The sigmoid/sigmoidorectal type of colonic intussusception was encountered in only 8 of the 37 colonic intussusceptions (21.6%). The average age of onset in this group was $1^1/_2$ years and the average duration of symptoms before hospital admission was 12 days. Transanal prolapse of the intussusception was found in five of the eight cases (62.5%) and in the other three cases the apex of the intussusception could be palpated on digital rectal examination. None of these patients had abdominal distention and an intra-abdominal mass was palpated in only one (left iliac fossa). Barium enema reduced one of these intussusceptions and manual reductions were utilized in seven with surgery in three with two resections and one death (gangrenous prolapsed intussusception at admission to the hospital). Two of these patients were white and 35 were characterized as "colored". No clear etiology of these colonic intussusceptions was identified. The authors speculated that contrast reductions might prove of greater value in future cases.

In 1992, Shekhawat et al[64] of Jaipur (India) reported in the *Journal of Pediatric Surgery* a 25 year experience with 230 infants and children with intussusception which included 31 children (13.5%) with chronic, ischemic intussusception which tended to occur in older children (all but five between the ages of one and 12 years) and with prominent clinical features which included pain of less intensity (75%) with diarrhea (40%) and vomiting (65%) being more frequent. Rectal bleeding and an abdominal mass were encountered in only one half of the patients. In 90% of the patients, the duration of symptoms prior to hospital admission ranged from five to 14 days. In four cases, the intussusception reduced "spontaneously" in association with a diagnostic barium enema and 27 children were operated upon with 25 easy reductions and two resections for difficult reduction and gangrene. The intussusception type was identified in four representative case reports but was not identified in the other 27 cases.

The above reports from Africa and India are presented in detail not only because they are "atypical" in relation to more voluminous reports from more climatically temperate and less tropical/subtropical areas but also because reports from these areas are so infrequent and these cases represent a distinct type of intussusception from important areas with large populations. In these areas, gastrointestinal infections and inflammations with their diarrhea and vomiting appear to be more frequent triggers of "idiopathic"/no-discrete-leading-point intussusceptions than the upper respiratory tract infections which are "incriminated" so often in more temperate regions of America and Europe.

CHALLENGES

1. The most important and serious current challenge in this important area of pediatric surgery is the urgent need to obtain earlier diagnosis and treatment of the most common first year of life (3 to 12 months of age) type of intussusception where the first 24 hours after the onset of symptoms are the most critical.

Increasing delays in diagnosis and treatment which are being reported by major and prestigious academic pediatric surgery centers[25,26] and in association with escalating morbidities and related hazards are most disturbing. These delays appear to be a failure to recognize the classical/ "telephone diagnosis" symptoms of intussusception in this age group by referring physicians and emergency room professional staff. A resurrection is much needed of the Melbourne/Clubbe[19]-type of public relations and indoctrination/instruction informing of parents (especially mothers) and referring physicians and pediatricians (private and emergency room) regarding the classical/ "telephone diagnosis" symptoms of intussusception and the *great urgency* of diagnosis and definitive treatment within the *first* 24 hours after the dramatic and characteristic onset and progression of symptoms. Current complacency and lack of information and awareness must be eliminated.

2. Another major and current challenge is determining the best, most effective, quickest and safest means of controlled contrast reduction of intussusception—air/oxygen insufflation "enema" or barium enema?

Recent publications from major and experienced pediatric surgery academic centers in North America (Toronto)[35] and Australia (Melbourne)[36] come down heavily in favor of air/oxygen insufflation reduction. Its only major hazard is tension pneumoperitoneum (rare) which is quickly and effectively managed by insufflation cessation and by prompt insertion of an 18 French needle into the peritoneal cavity in the midline between the xiphoid and the umbilicus. On all other scores, air/oxygen insufflation reduction is greatly superior (discussed in Introduction section of this chapter).

3. Another important challenge is the more frequent use of controlled contrast reduction of intussusception in tropical/ subtropical areas such as Africa and Asia where limited published information suggests the likelihood of a high frequency of reductions by this approach with barium (or air/oxygen insufflation) enema.[63,64]

This approach may also result in earlier diagnosis and treatment in cases which the index of suspicion should be high.

4. A worthy challenge may be accorded a closer look at midgut atresias in the newborn to see how often intrauterine intussusception is involved.

This may also open the possibility of more in-depth inquiry regarding late pregnancy triggering causes of these intussusceptions (fetal distress?, maternal distress or "stress"?, maternal drugs, activities, disease, etc.?)

5. A taxing and demanding (and at times frustrating) challenge is presented by the diagnostic difficulties and dilemmas encountered in acute abdominal pain and tenderness cases of Henoch-Schönlein purpura after the rash has appeared. (see discussion of this problem in Introduction section of this chapter).

6. More attention should be paid to the etiologic/? "infectious" causes of the most common types of intussusception without a clear-cut leading point (i.e. "idiopathic").

Past failures and frustrations should not deter the continuing search for clearly identifiable causes such as upper respiratory infections, gastrointestinal infections or infestations (viral, bacterial, parasitic, etc.), genetic, medications, etc.

CONCLUSION

When I started to write this chapter, I felt this would be a quick, brief, "ho-hum" undertaking as all major challenges relating to intussusception had long ago been resolved and solved. *Not so*, as the length and depth of this chapter will indicate! Each of the five major types of intussusception in infancy and childhood—first year of life and "idiopathic", after one year of age and leading point associated, postoperative, intrauterine and Africa/Asia tropical/subtropical are unique and distinct and require a different mind-set and clinical and investigative approach as the Introduction and Challenges sections of this chapter should clearly indicate. Intussusception remains not only one of the great classical surgical disorders of pediatric surgery with a great and illustrious past history, it also remains an area of great and significant current challenge.

REFERENCES

1. Hunter J. Works 1789; 3:587.
2. Rokitansky K. Med Jarhbuch d. Kaiserl. Konigh. oesterr. N.F. Staates. 1837; 14:558.
3. Leichtenstern. Prager Vierteljarschrift. 1873; 118:189.
4. Hutchinson J. A successful case of abdominal section for intussusception. Medico-Chir Trans. 2nd ser., 1874; 39:31.
5. Hirschsprung H. Tilfaelde af subakut Traminvagination. Hospital Stidende 1876; 3:321.
6. Hirschsprung H. Hundertsieben Fälle von Darminvagination bei Kindern. Mitt a.d. Grenzgeb. d. Med. u. Chir. 1905; 14:555.
7. Koch A, Oerum HPT. Intussusception in children: 400 Danish cases. Edinburgh Med J 1912; 9:227.
8. Hipsley PL. Intussusception and its treatment by hydrostatic pressure: Based on an analysis of one hundred consecutive cases so treated. Med J Australia 1926; 2:201.
9. Hipsley PL. The treatment of intussusception. Surgery 1937; 1:825.
10. Monrad S. A study of acute invagination of the intestine in small children. Acta paediat, Upps. 1926; 6:31.
11. Ladd WE. Progress in the diagnosis and treatment of intussusception. Boston Med Surg J 1913; 168:542.
12. Retan GM. Nonoperative treatment of intussusception. Am J Dis Child 1927; 33:765.
13. Hellmer H. Intussusception in children. Diagnosis and therapy with barium enema. Acta radiol, Stockh. suppl., 1948, lxv.
14. Ravitch MM, McCune RM. Reduction of intussusception by hydrostatic pressure: An experimental study. Bull Johns Hopkins Hosp 1948; 82:550-568.
15. Ravitch MM, Mc Cune RM. Reduction of intussuscpetion by barium enema: A clniical and experimental study. Ann Surg 1948; 128:904-917.
16. Ravitch MM, Morgan RH. Reduction of intussusception by barium enema. Ann Surg 1952; 135:586.
17. Ravitch MM. Reduction of intussusception by bairum enema. Surg Gynec Obstet 1954; 99:431-435.
18. Gross RE, Ware PF. Intussusception in childhood: Experiences from 610 cases. New Eng J Med 1948; 239:645-652.
19. Clubbe CPB. The Diagnosis and Treatment of Intussusception.New York: Oxford University Press, 1921.
20. Moore TC. The management of intussusception in infants and children: Report of 43 cases. Ann Surg 1952; 135:184-192.
21. McLaughlin CW. Surgical management of irreducible intussusception. Arch Surg 1948; 56:48-55.
22. Dennis C. Resection and primary anastomosis in treatment of gangrenous intussusception in children: Simple, one-layer silk anastomosis. Ann Surg 1947; 126:788-796.
23. Auldist AW. Intussusception in a children's hostpial. Proc Paediatric Surgical Congress, Melbourne (Australia) I:1-16, 1970.
24. Hutchinson IF, Olayiwola B, Young DG. Intussusception in infancy and childhood. Br J Surg 1980; 67:209-212.
25. West KW, Stephens B, Vane DW et al. Intussusception: Current management in infants and children. Surgery 1987; 102:704-709.
26. Beasley SW, Auldist AW, Stokes KB. The diagnostically difficult intussusception: Its characteristics and consequences. Pediatr

Surg Int 1988; 3:135-138.

27. Jinzhe Z, Yenxia W, Linchi W. Rectal inflation reduction of intussusception in infants. J Pediatr Surg 1986; 21:30-32.

28. Guo J-z, Ma X-y, Zhou Q-h. Results of air pressure enema reduction of intussusception: 6,396 cases in 13 years. J Pediatr Surg 1986; 21:1201-1203.

29. She Y, Ting W. Rectal inflation in the treatment of intussusception in children. China J Surg 1961; 9:318.

30. She Y, Ting W, Yeh H. Reduction of intestinal intussusctiton in infancy by colonic air insufflation. China Med J (Engl) 1964; 83:668-673.

31. Filler RM. Discussion of paper by Guo et al. J Pediatr Surg 1986; 21:1202-1203.

32. Gu L, Alton DJ, Daneman A et al. Intussusception reduction in children by rectal insufflation of air. AJR 1988; 150:1345-1348.

33. Phelan E, deCampo JF, Malecky G. Comparison of oxygen and barium enema reduction of ileocolic intussusception. AJR 1988; 150:1349-1352.

34. Franken EA. Nonsurgical treatment of intussusception. AJR 1988; 150:1353-1354.

35. Renwick AA, Beasley SW, Phelan E. Intussusception: Recurrence following gas (oxygen) enema reduction. Pediatr Surg Int 1992; 7:361-363.

36. Beasley SW, Glover J. Intussusception: Prediction of outcome of gas enema. J Pediatr Surg 1992; 27:474-475.

37. Fiorito ES, Recalde Cuestas LA. Diagnosis and treatment of acute intestinal intussusception with controlled insufflation of air. Pediatrics 1959; 24:241-244.

38. Fiorito ES, Recalde Cuestas LA. La "insuflación controlada" (baro-radioscópicamente), método de elección en el diagnóstico y tratamiento de la invaginación intestinal del lactante. Rev Soc pediat d litoral. 1953; 18:3.

39. Saenz AM, Paviotti RO. Diagnóstico y tratamiento de la invagincaión intestinal en la infancia por la método de la insufflacién controlada baro-radioscópicamente. Arch argent pediat 1956; 27:115.

40. Holt LE. Diseases of Infancy and Childhood. New York: D. Appleton and Company, 1897; 386-387.

41. Collier HS. An abstract of a clinical lecture on some details in the treatment of acute intussusception in infants. Lancet 1899; 2:551 (Aug. 26).

42. Reijnen JAM, Festen C, Joosten HJM. Chronic intussusception in children. Br J Surg 1989; 76; 815- 816.

43. Collins DL, Miller KE. Intussusception in hemophilia. J Pediatr Surg 1968; 3: 599-603.

44. Emanuel B, Lieberman AD, Rosen S. Intussuscepiton due to Henoch-Schönlein purpura: Case reports and a review of the literature. Ill Med J 1962; 122:162-167.

45. Noussias M, Blandy AC, Ward-McQuaid N. Intussusception in Henoch-Schönlein purpura: A report of two cases requiring operation. Br J Surg 1969; 56:503-504.

46. Martinez-Frontanilla LA, Haase GM, Ernster JA et al. Surgical complications in Henoch-Schönlein purpura. J Pediatr Surg 1984; 19:434-436.

47. Hays DM. Intussusception as a postoperative complication in pediatric surgery. Surg Gynec Obstet 1961; 112:583-589.

48. Raffensperger JG, Baker RJ. Postoperative intestinal obstruction in children. Arch Surg 1967; 94:451- 457.

49. McGovern JB, Gross RE. Intussusception as a postoperative complication. Surgery 1968; 63:507-513.

50. Cox JA, Martin LW. Postoperative intussusception. Arch Surg 1973; 106:263-266.

51. Dammert G, Votteler TP. Postoperative intussusception in the pediatric patient. J Pediatr Surg 1974; 9:817-820.

52. Mollitt DL, Ballantine TVN, Grosfeld JL. Postoperative intussusception in infancy and childhood: Analysis of 119 cases. Surgery 1979; 86:402-408.

53. Holcomb GW, Ross AJ, McNeill JA. Postoperative intussusception: Increasing frequency or increasing awareness? Southern Med J 1991; 84:1334-1339.

54. Lai E, Cunningham T, Moore TC. In utero intussusception producing ileal atresia and meconium peritonitis with and without free air: Report of 2 cases and a review of the literature. Pediatr Surg Int (submitted for publication).

55. Parkkulainen KV. Intrauterine intussusception as a cause of intestinal atresia. Surgery 1958; 44:1106-1111.

56. Spencer R. The various patterns of intestinal atresia. Surgery 1968; 64:661-668.

57. Todani T, Tabuchi K, Tanaka S. Intestinal atresia due to intrauterine intussusception: Analysis of 24 cases in Japan. J Pediatr Surg 1975; 10:445-451.

58. Louw JH, Barnard CN. Congenital intestinal atresia: observation on its origin. Lancet 1955; 2:1065-1067.

59. Cole GJ. Caecocolic intussusception in Ibadan. Br J Surg 1966; 53:415-419.

60. Mayell MJ. Intussusception in infancy and childhood in Southern Africa: a review of 223 cases. Arch Dis Child 1972; 47:20-25.

61. Chapman JA. Intussusception in Rhodesian Africans: A contrast with the accepted clinical picture. J Pediatr Surg 1973; 8:43-47.

62. Kark AE, Rundle WJ. The pattern of intussusception in Africans in Natal. Br J Surg 1960; 48:296-309.

63. Davies MRQ, Cwyes S. Colonic intussusceptions in children. South African Med J 1978; 54:517-519.

64. Shekhawat NS, Prabhakar G, Sinha D et al. Nonischemic intussusception in childhood. J Pediatr Surg 1992; 27:1433-1435.

INVITED COMMENTARY

Professor Sidney Cwyes
Head, Department of Paediatric Surgery
Red Cross War Memorial Children's Hospital, Rondebosch
University of Cape Town, South Africa

Although intussusception is a very common condition, there is still room for improvement with regard to early diagnosis. Air reduction has become very popular, with a decrease in the morbidity and an increase in the efficacy. However, who should do it—the surgeon, pediatrician or radiologist—the surgeon should certainly still control the overall management. There are still controversies with regard to the contraindications to attempted air, hydrostatic or barium reduction, and whether a second attempt at reduction should be performed if the first fails.

However, there are still many unanswered questions with regard to intussusception versus the etiology of intussusception where there is no obvious lead point pathology; and the higher incidence of colo-colic intussusceptions seen in Africa with, not infrequently, a perforation of the colon *distal* to the intussusception. Generally there is no obvious lead point in this type and some may in fact prolapse through the rectum. Laparoscopy may have a place in children after failed air reduction, just prior to laparotomy, as many are found to be reduced at surgery.

Surgeons in developing countries are faced with a dilemma. Without the availability of radiographic control, should they still attempt air or hydrostatic reduction or should they proceed to laparotomy reduction in all?

CHAPTER 14

OMPHALOMESENTERIC DUCT MALFORMATIONS

INTRODUCTION

Omphalomesenteric duct anomalies represent somewhat anomalous anomalies. While they constitute the most frequent malformation/ anomaly (Meckel's diverticulum type), they also are one of the least apt to cause symptoms (also Meckel's diverticulum type) and hence are rarely "pathological" in that removal is required or remotely justified for health reasons. They do represent a fascinating spectrum from the bizarre (sudden and unexpected massive intussusception/inversion prolapse of intestines onto the anterior abdominal wall through a seemingly tiny but patent omphalomesenteric duct) to the commonplace (a simple asymptomatic diverticulum).

As luck would have it, my first exposure to an omphalomesenteric duct malformation as a responsible and operating surgeon (chief resident), was in January 1951 and was to the most extreme of the bizarre type (prolapse/intussusception of *both* limbs of the intestinal tract) (Fig. 14.1). This riveting experience led to my first scholarly review of the literature and the publication of two cases seen and operated upon personally (one of them) by me. The other was photographed by me (single loop prolapse). These were published in the January 1952 issue of *Surgery*[1] and were submitted for publication when I was still a chief resident (June 7, 1951).

The 1952 publication represented the detailed case reporting of two recent cases at the Indiana University Medical Center involving me but also my first experience at a detailed and in-depth review of the literature involving one of my own cases. Peake[2] in 1811 was cited as the first to record this unusual occurrence in the literature. Excellent reviews by Cullen[3] and by Kittle, Jenkins and Dragstedt[4] (Fred, Hilger and Lester) of the University of Chicago were recommended to the readers of this exciting (to me) article. This Kittle et al article is a particularly scholarly and in-depth review of the problems and forms of the patent omphalomesenteric duct and is strongly recommended to the reader of this book. Their Figure 2 is an outstanding series of drawings picturing 16 types of patent omphalomesenteric duct and/or its remnants. The first long-term operative survival of this serious problem was reported in 1947 and concerned a patient operated upon in 1943 by Professor Lester Dragstedt and involved a resection of the intussuscepted mass and a side-to-side anastomosis. Bronaugh[5] in 1947 had described a successful resection of non-viable ileum and patent omphalomesenteric duct with an end-to-end anastomosis. In 1950, Arnheim[6] in *Surgery, Gynecology and Obstetrics* described a successful case in which 4 cm of ileum had been resected with the persistent and patent omphalomesenteric duct followed by a side-to-side ileal anastomosis. Death had occurred in all other cases treated by operation up to this time and also, certainly, in those not operated upon. This was an appallingly high mortality (89%) in recorded cases treated operatively up to this time and stimulated even more my enthusiasm to report these two successful cases,

in addition to the three previously reported successful cases in the literature.

This stimulating operative and literature searching and recording experience triggered an in-depth review of an 18 year Indiana University Medical Center experience with 46 omphalomesenteric duct malformations (symptomatic ones in adults, as well as children) for presentation at a 1956 meeting of the British Association Paediatric Surgeons (BAPS) spring meet in London at the Hospital for Sick Children at Great Ormond Street followed by an elegant black-tie dinner hosted by BAPS president, Sir Dennis Browne at the medieval Apothecaries Hall in a miraculously spared tiny segment of still rubble-strewn bombed out London. The study was put together in written form, accepted and published in the November 1956 issue of *Surgery, Gynecology and Obstetrics*.[7]

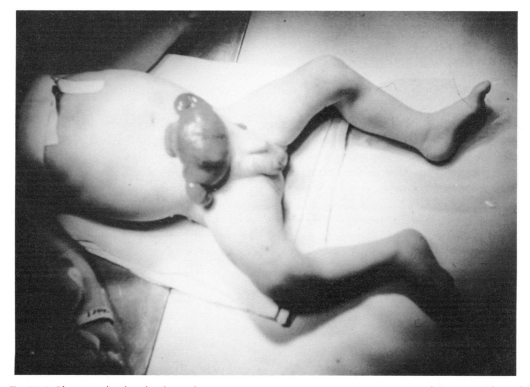

Fig. 14.1. Photograph taken by the author just prior to operation on January 28, 1951 showing a T-shaped prolapse of ileum (both proximal and distal limbs) through a patent omphalomesenteric duct onto the anterior abdominal wall. The patient was a 12 day old male who was admitted to the hospital for treatment of a large, discolored mucosa-covered mass which had prolapsed onto the abdominal wall eleven hours prior to admission. A fecal fistula at the umbilicus had occurred at seven days of age when the umbilical cord had sloughed away.

Cases with this malformation were divided into those with the omphalomesenteric duct patent from the ileum to the umbilicus and into those with diverticulum attached to the umbilicus by a fibrous band and those with an unattached diverticulum, a Meckel's diverticulum. Cases with a persistent omphalomesenteric duct to the umbilicus and open were subdivided into those with and without a prolapse/intussusception onto the anterior abdominal wall and into those without a prolapse. Cases with omphalomesenteric duct open to the umbilicus but closed at the umbilicus were divided into those closed with granulation tissue and those closed with skin. Meckel's diverticulum cases were divided into those with diverticulitis, those with bleeding producing melena and anemia, those acting as a leading point for an intussusception and into those in which an internal hernia orifice had been produced by attachment of the diverticulum (presumably inflammation induced) to an adjacent structure (usually mesentery or adjacent intestine). The distribution of these cases is shown in Table 14.1. Each category was illustrated by detailed case summaries. The chief complaints in each of these cases is presented in Table 14.2. The age at the occurrence of symptoms was under one year in 15 of the 46 cases (33%) and was between one and two

Table 14.1. Types of symptomatic omphalomesenteric duct malformations encountered in an 18-year experience with 46 cases

		No. Cases
Persistent omphalomesenteric duct		10
Intussusception of ileum through duct	5	
Duct open at umbilicus without prolapse	1	
Duct closed at umbilicus with granulation tissue	1	
Duct closed at umbilicus with skin	3	
Diverticulum attached to umbilicus with fibrous band		5
Meckel's diverticulum		31
Diverticulitis	12	
Bleeding	10	
Leading point of intussusception	6	
Internal hernia from attachment to adjacent structure	3	
Total		46

Table 14.2. Tabulation of chief complaints

		No. Cases
Intestinal obstruction		13
Intussusception	6	
Band to umbilicus	4*	
Internal hernia from Meckel's diverticulum attachment	3	
Abdominal pain		13
Melena and anemia		12
Invagination of ileum onto abdominal wall		5
Fecal fistula at umbilicus		1
Umbilical hernia		1
Associated anomaly (ileal atresia)		1
Total		46

*Volvulus of the diverticulum with ischemia and gangrene of the diverticulum had occurred in two of these cases.

years in another 5 cases bringing the onset of symptoms in the first two years of life in these 46 symptomatic cases to 44%. The onset of symptoms was between three and five years in one case, between six and 10 years in 8 cases and between 11 and 15 years in another 7 cases for a total of 36 of the 46 cases in the first 15 years of life (78%). In adult years, symptom onset occurred between 16 and 25 years in four cases and in 6 cases in patients over 25 years of age. Of the nonintestinal mucosas encountered, gastric was identified in 18 cases and pancreatic in two of 37 patients in whom a histological study of the anomaly was carried out (20 of 37 for 54%).

The prolapse/intussusception of involved mucosa covered ileum onto the anterior abdominal wall was described as the most dramatic and terrifying of the complications available to omphalomesenteric duct malformations. This occurred in five of these 46 symptomatic cases (11%). The prolapse of the inverted intestine was T-shaped with two orifices presenting in three cases and I-shaped with one orifice in two cases. In one of these cases, the T-shaped prolapse was discovered at birth on top of an omphalocele. All five patients survived operative reduction of the intussusception and resection of the omphalomesenteric duct. One death occurred later of congenital heart disease in an infant unable to survive outside an oxygen tent. In three of these five cases, a fecal fistula at the umbilicus prior to the intussusception prolapse onto the abdominal wall was found. The ages of these infants at the time of intussusception/ prolapse was one, two, 10, 12 and 30 days.

An opening of the duct at the umbilicus, with a fecal fistula, was encountered in one of the five patients with persistent omphalomesenteric duct without a prolapse. In this patient, a large umbilical cord had dropped off at one month of age followed shortly by a fecal fistula at the umbilicus. The persistent duct was resected promptly and successfully prior to the occurrence of an intussusception. The persistent duct was covered at the umbilicus by

skin in three cases and by granulation tissue in one case. The four covered at the umbilicus patients came to operation because of an umbilical hernia in one skin covered case and melena, anemia and umbilical area pathology (indurated umbilical mass in one skin covered case and bloody drainage umbilical granulation tissue in one granulation tissue covered case). The omphalomesenteric duct contained gastric tissue in both of these melena and anemia cases. All three of these patients were managed successfully by resection of the omphalomesenteric duct and umbilicus at five, 11 and 14 months. One patient was operated upon at five days of age because of an ileal atresia. The atresia was located in the ileum just distal to a completely patent omphalomesenteric duct covered with skin at the umbilicus. Resection of the ileal atresia and omphalomesenteric duct was followed by an end-to-end anastomosis. This infant did not survive. Nine of the 10 patients in this experience with patent omphalomesenteric ducts were male infants (90%). Thirty-seven of the 46 patients with symptomatic omphalomesenteric duct malformations were males (80%).

An intermediate type of malformation which consisted of a diverticulum which was attached to the umbilicus by a fibrous band was found in five of the 46 symptomatic cases (11%). Symptoms leading to operation occurred in the first decade of life in all but one of these five patients and were due to intestinal obstruction in four of the five. In two of these patients a volvulus of the diverticulum with gangrene had occurred. In one of these cases without obstruction, the diverticulum attached to the umbilicus by a fibrous cord arose from the side of the appendix which was involved symptomatically with an acute appendicitis with the inflammation also involving the diverticulum producing a diverticulitis. There was no gastric mucosa involved in this interesting case which had previously been reported in 1936 by Hadley and Cogswell.[8] Gastric mucosa was found in one of the volvulus and diverticulum gangrene cases but in none of the other five in this group. In the other gangrene/volvulus case the mucosa had been autolyzed by the ischemia gangrene and could not be identified as to type. All five of these cases were managed successfully by lysis of the band and resection of the diverticulum. Four of these five patients were male and all of those aged nine years and younger.

Symptomatic Meckel's diverticula were encountered in 31 of the 46 symptomatic cases of omphalomesenteric duct malformations (67.4%)—two in every three cases. Acute inflammation of the diverticulum was the most frequent cause of symptoms. It was found in 12 cases followed closely by melena and anemia in 10 cases. In some of these 12 cases the inflammation was of a nonspecific nature while in others it was presumably due to peptic ulceration resulting from the presence of gastric mucosa in the diverticulum. Gastric mucosa was identified in the diverticulum in five of the 10 cases and in an additional case the adjacent ileum was greatly inflamed distal to the diverticulum in a manner characteristic of peptic ulceration. As the mucosa of the diverticulum had been destroyed by the inflammation, the presence or absence of gastric mucosa could not be established. In two of the patients with gastric mucosa in the diverticulum, a perforated peptic ulcer in the diverticulum was found. The age range of the patients was considerably older than any other group in this study of omphalomesenteric duct malformations. Six of the 12 patients ranged from nine to 15 years and six were 21 years of age and older at 21, 24, 32, 34, 34 and 53 years of age. Although the sex distribution was approximately equal with five females and seven males, five of the six with established or strongly suspected (inflammation autolysis case) gastric mucosa (83%) were male. Resection of the inflamed diverticulum was carried out in all 12 cases and in two involved resection of involved ileum as well with end-to-end anastomosis. All 12 patients survived.

Severe melena and anemia dominated the clinical picture in 10 patients and in 8 (80%) was associated with the identified presence of gastric mucosa. In the other two, it likely was present but missed. Nine of these 10 patients were males (90%) and the ages ranged from four months to 69 years. Two of the patients were under two years of age and three ranged from four to eight years of age with two at 15 years of age (70% 15 years or under). Three patients were 21 years of age or older at 21, 30 and 69 years. The Meckel's diverticulum was resected in all 10 cases and in three of these cases additional resections involved inflamed ileum in two and an abscess mass with a perforated diverticulum (with gastric mucosa) in one. All 10 of these patients recovered.

In six cases, the Meckel's diverticulum was found to be the leading point of an intussusception. Four of these six patients were in their first 11 months of life and the other two were eight and 13 years of age. The intussusception was ileocolic in five and ileoileal in one. Four of the six had nonintestinal mucosa, gastric in one, pancreatic in one, both gastric and pancreatic in one and an adenomatous polyp in one (the 13 year old, a girl). Five of the six were males (83%). In five of the six cases, the intussusception was reduced with resection of the Meckel's diverticulum (perforated in one case) and in one case (9 months old male) resection of the intussusception with a gangrenous Meckel's diverticulum and end-to-end anastomosis was required. All six patients recovered.

In three cases, an incarcerated internal hernia through an intraperitoneal ring caused by attachment of a Meckel's diverticula to an adjacent structure had occurred. The attachment was to the parietal peritoneum 2 cm below the cecum in one, to the base of the mesentery in one and to an adjacent loop of ileum in one. The ages of these three patients (all males) were one month, 21 months and 10 years. All three died. Two of these three patients were in extremis on admission to the hospital and the diagnosis was made at autopsy. One of these infants (one month old) had been cyanotic since birth and at autopsy was found to have ileum herniated through a ring with strangulation, gangrene perforation and generalized peritonitis. The other in extremis patient also had a gangrenous ileal loop herniated. The third patient with this serious complication of a Meckel's diverticulum arrived in near extremis with fecal vomiting of four days duration and a temperature of 105°F. In this case, the diverticular attachment was to the base of the mesentery. The obstruction was relieved at operation and a gangrenous diverticulum was resected. This gravely ill patient died shortly after the operation. Only one had mucosal study and no gastric mucosa was found.

As omphalomesenteric malformations, including Meckel's diverticulum, in nonsymptomatic patients occur with equal frequency in males and females, the high male predominance in symptomatic cases and especially those with gastric (and pancreatic) mucosa is a mystery. In a 1956 report from Stockholm, Sonderlund[9] identified a 7 to 1 male to female ratio in 54 symptomatic cases of omphalomesenteric duct malformation while an equal ratio was found in 61 asymptomatic cases encountered at the same hospital as random findings (32 males and 29 females).

The high comparative and exclusive occurrence of pancreatic tissue in Meckel's diverticula acting as leading points for an intussusception also was of interest. A similar finding was reported in the *American Journal of Surgery* in 1948 by Migliaccio and Begg.[10] Twenty-one of their Meckel's diverticulum cases were symptomatic. Pancreatic tissue was found in the diverticulum in two cases and in both of them an intussusception had occurred.

It is difficult to gain a true picture of symptomatic cases of omphalomesenteric duct malformations from general hospital reports which are biased towards adult cases and from reports, adult and children's hospitals, which include large numbers of asymptomatic cases. It is for these reasons that I have devoted as much attention and space in this chapter to my 1950's publications which present much detailed information which is still revealing and rewarding many years later. Some reports also include cases in which the diverticula arise from the mesenteric border of the ileum and are more likely duplications than Meckel's diverticula which arise from the antimesenteric border of the ileum.

A 1968 report from the Toronto Hospital for Sick Children by Seagram et al[11] described the findings in 81 cases of symptomatic Meckel's diverticulum operated on in a 10 year period (8.1 cases per year). Histologic examination in 79 cases revealed gastric mucosa in 51 and gastric plus pancreatic mucosa in three for a gastric mucosa incidence in symptomatic cases of 68.4%. A 1987 report by Vane et al[12] from Indiana University Medical Center in Indianapolis, site of my 1952 and 1956 publications, described 85 symptomatic cases of omphalomesenteric duct malformations with presenting symptoms of bleeding in 48, obstruction in 28, pain in 5 and umbilical drainage in 4. Gastric mucosa was identified in all 48 bleeding patients and four of the five with pain.

In a review of a 20-year experience with 117 symptomatic cases of omphalomesenteric duct malformations from Montreal (Hôpital Sainte-Justine), St-Vil et al[13] described the most frequent complaint to be bowel obstruction in 49 cases (42%). The most common cause of obstruction was volvulus in 20 cases (41% of the obstructions) and intussusception in 19 cases (39% of the obstructions). Adhesions, internal hernia and kinking were found in 10 cases of obstruction (23% of the obstruction cases). The second most frequent complaint was bleeding and occurred in 45 of the 117 symptomatic cases (38%). Less frequent complaints were diverticulitis in 16 (14%) and umbilical pathology in 7 (6%). All of these patients were 17 years of age or under. The diverticulitis/pain group of 16 was of interest in that 10 of the 16 (63%) had evidence of diverticulum perforation with localized peritonitis or abscess formation. In two of these 16 patients, the diverticulitis was caused by a foreign body impaction at the base of the diverticulum. Patent omphalomesenteric duct malformations were found in seven patients and in five involved total patency with fecal discharge at the umbilicus. Of the other two, one had an umbilical granuloma and one an umbilical cyst. As in my 1956 report, diverticulitis patients tended to have their onset of symptoms later in childhood while those with patent omphalomesenteric duct malformations tended to have them earlier, in infancy. Ectopic pancreatic tissue was found in 10% of the 61% of resected specimens with ectopic tissue and gastric tissue in 91% (combined pancreatic and gastric tissue was found in 3% of these). We cautioned that pancreatic tissue in Meckel's diverticula predisposes to bowel obstruction by its mass effect and acts as a leading point for intussusception and volvulus. This hazard was pointed out in my 1956 publication and more recently by Artigas et al.[14]

Recent reports of intrauterine intussusception of an omphalomesenteric duct[15] or a Meckel's diverticulum[16] as the cause of ileal atresia in the newborn are of particular interest to me as antenatal and intrauterine intussusception of an omphalomesenteric duct was cited as a cause of ileal atresia in a newborn and one of five cases of symptomatic, persistent omphalomesenteric duct without prolapse[2] in his 1956 publication. In the 1987 report in *Pediatric Surgery International* by McMullin, Beasley and Kelley[15] of Melbourne a single-horned (I-shaped) prolapse onto the abdominal wall of a 1300 g newborn was found with an associated intestinal atresia to the midgut which had resulted from an intrauterine intussusception/prolapse of a completely patent omphalomesenteric duct, similar to my 1956 published case. Their case was quite remarkable in that careful surgical dissection permitted salvage of 55 cm of proximal small intestine. The 1990 report of Senocak et al[16] of Ankara (Turkey) contained an impressive photograph (their Fig. 1) showing a greatly distended distal segment of ileum with a Meckel's diverticulum led intussusception which had occurred in utero with a resulting mesentery gap type of atresia. Their patient was

managed successfully by resection and end-to-end anastomosis.

The most important contributions to the more effective and safer surgical care of omphalomesenteric duct malformations in the past 40 years were the introduction of the radionucleotide ^{99m}Tc-pertechnetate scan for the detection of gastric mucosa in Meckel's diverticula in 1970 by Professor Theodore "Ted" Jewett and associates[17] of Buffalo, New York in *Surgery* and the important, scholarly, perceptive and invaluable publication of Professor Alexander "Sandy" Bill with Soltero[18] in the August 1976 issue of the *American Journal of Surgery*. The technetium isotope scan for ectopic gastric mucosa in Meckel's diverticula has revolutionized the care of these malformations as the majority of symptomatic Meckel's diverticula contain gastric mucosa. It has been suggested that the sensitivity of these scans might be increased by the use of intravenous pentagastrin or oral cimetidine.[19,20]

The Soltero and Bill report[18] reviewed the natural history of Meckel's diverticulum and the relation of this history to the incidental (justified?) removal of asymptomatic Meckel's diverticula discovered accidentally at laparotomy for some unrelated condition. They reviewed the records of 202 cases at 26 hospitals in the Greater Seattle/Kings County area of the State of Washington with a population at that time exceeding one million. This was both the largest single series of symptomatic cases of Meckel's diverticulum to be reported in the literature up to that time (and since) and the first in which the incidence or likelihood of disease developing from a Meckel's diverticulum was calculated. With these calculations in place, the authors concluded their epic report as follows:

> Using previously unpublished mortality and morbidity figures, we calculated that to save one patient's life from the complications of Meckel's diverticulum, it would be necessary to remove approximately 800 asymptomatic Meckel's diverticula. This would be likely to incur a significant amount of postoperative morbidity

from intestinal obstruction and infection. We suggest that *the prophylactic removal of a Meckel's diverticulum is rarely, if ever, justified.* (italics added)

CHALLENGES

1. The most important challenge in the surgical management of omphalomesenteric duct malformations, in particular that of the quite common Meckel's diverticulum, is when if ever to remove an unsymptomatic Meckel's diverticulum discovered unexpectedly at operation for some other legitimate and presumably serious surgical condition.

From the important data of Soltero and Bill,[18] discussed just above in the Introduction section of this chapter, it is extremely unlikely that any patient with an asymptomatic and accidentally discovered Meckel's diverticulum would ever do the patient harm—unless it triggered an unnecessary and hazardous bowel resection in the face of some preexisting primary disease of sufficient magnitude and gravity to cause the "discovery" at laparotomy in the first place. I arrived long ago at a similar opinion from the findings of my 18 year study of the State of Indiana's only university hospital and only children's hospital experience reported in *Surgery, Gynecology and Obstetrics* in 1956. At any one time during this 18 year period, the 5,000,000 people in the State of Indiana with a 2% expected incidence of Meckel's diverticulum had 100,000 persons of all ages with a Meckel's diverticulum in their peritoneal cavities. With 31 cases of symptomatic Meckel's diverticulum found in 18 years for an average of 1.722 cases per year, the chance of a symptomatic Meckel's diverticulum per existing diverticulum would be approximately 1.722 to 100,000— hardly *an overwhelming likelihood*!

In the opening discussion of the Soltero and Bill paper at the 1976 meeting of the Pacific Coast Surgical Association, Professor Wiley F. Barker[21] of UCLA in his opening sentence stated, "Doctor Bill has combined his usual brilliant perception and ballistic reasoning as he and Doctor Soltero have shot down the myth concerning the hazard of the casually encountered Meckel's diverticulum."

This particularly important Soltero and Bill report provided the *coup de grâce* to the spurious existing doctrine supporting resection of the casually encountered and asymptomatic Meckel's diverticulum. From the time of their report, resections of casually encountered and asymptomatic Meckel's diverticula steadily decreased as the message got around with only one publication actually recommending it.[12]

In their 1991 publication, cited earlier, St-Vil et al[13] of Montreal record two significant morbidity complications of resecting asymptomatic Meckel's diverticula. These complications were a wound infections and a postoperative anastomotic leak which required a temporary ileostomy. They did not recommend asymptomatic Meckel's diverticulum resection unless there is a clear-cut indication for doing so such as ectopic gastric mucosa or a tethering fibrous band attached to the diverticulum.

In addition to anastomotic leaks, peritoneal cavity and wound infections and intestinal obstructions from adhesions following incidental (an unnecessary) resection of asymptomatic Meckel's diverticula, a further significant hazard (and deterrent) is to be found in the occurrence of postoperative intestinal obstruction in which the stump of the excised Meckel's diverticulum has served as the leading point of the postoperative intestinal obstruction.

In Daniel Hays'[22] landmark 1961 paper in *Surgery, Gynecology and Obstetrics* on postoperative intestinal obstruction, in three of the six postoperative intussusceptions occurring after abdominal surgery for superficially unrelated conditions the leading point of the postoperative intussusception was the stump of the excised Meckel's diverticulum (50%). In all three cases, the intussusception was characteristically ileoileal. The Meckel's diverticulum was asymptomatic in one case and symptomatic in two. The ileal closure had been in two layers in one case and in three layers in two cases.

In their important 1974 review of postoperative intestinal obstruction, Dammert and Votteler[23] of Dallas in *The Journal of Pediatric Surgery* reported five cases of postoperative intestinal obstruction in two of which the leading point was the stump of an excised Meckel's diverticulum (40%). One of these diverticula had been asymptomatic and one symptomatic. They reviewed 81 cases of postoperative intussusception collected from the literature, adding their own five cases. They found the most common lead point to be Meckel's diverticulum stumps (six cases) followed by appendectomy stumps (five cases). Additional cases of Meckel's diverticulum resection stumps acting as leading points for postoperative intestinal obstruction have been recorded by McGovern and Gross[24] and by Cox and Martin.[25] In a 1987 report by Bodycomb, Beasley and Auldist[26] of the Royal Children's Hospital of Melbourne (Australia), one of four postoperative intestinal obstructions recorded by them occurred six days after resection of an asymptomatic Meckel's diverticulum. The lead point of this intussusception was the suture line at the site of the previous excision of the Meckel's diverticulum. In a 1979 review of 119 cases of postoperative intestinal obstruction from the literature and their own experience, Mollitt, Ballantine and Grosfeld[27] of Indianapolis found that one third of the cases followed operations on distal ileum and included eight cases of Meckel's diverticulum resection.

I have long followed a policy of not resecting an asymptomatic Meckel's diverticulum unless gastric or pancreatic tissue is clearly present. This can reliably be determined by palpation as the consistency of gastric and/or pancreatic tissue differs sharply from ileal, jejunal of colonic mucosal lining. If a tethering band is present, simply divide and remove it with careful palpation of the remaining diverticulum as when no band is present. If the mucosa of the diverticulum appears to possess a thick and firm consistency, remove it by a staple device at the neck and get a frozen section and careful evaluation of the nature, loca-

tion and extent of any ectopic gastric or pancreatic ectopic tissues.

To counter the suggestion that an asymptomatic Meckel's diverticulum should be considered similar to an asymptomatic "casually encountered" appendix, Soltero and Bill[18] counter that the Meckel's diverticulum has a much broader base, no significant lymphatic tissue and is self emptying.

2. With reliable technetium scanning to detect ectopic gastric mucosa in omphalomesenteric duct malformations such as Meckel's diverticulum, the use of minimally invasive laparoscopy should be considered as it is with other intra-abdominal pathology.

CONCLUSION

The most pleasant and satisfying part of writing this chapter was the incentive for the first time in more than 40 years for the author to re-read with care the author's two major 1952[1] and 1956[7] publications on omphalomesenteric duct malformations. These publications with the superlative contributions of Ted Jewett and associates[17] and Sandy Bill and associate,[18] present a rather complete and comprehensive presentation and in-depth view of omphalomesenteric duct malformations as they exist today, including symptoms in all age groups.

Thanks to the work of Jewett et al[17] the preoperative diagnosis of most symptomatic Meckel's diverticula is far more accurate, safe and reliable and thanks to the work of Bill and Soltero[18] the plague and curse of unnecessary and hazardous resections of asymptomatic Meckel's diverticula has largely been eliminated as a proper and responsible part of surgical care.

REFERENCES

1. Moore TC, Shumacker HB. Intussusception of ileum through persistent omphalomesenteric duct: Review of the literature and report of two cases. Surgery 1952; 32:278-284.
2. Peake J. Case of preternatural anus found in a portion of ileum protruded at the umbi-

licus. Edinburgh Med Surg J 1811; 7:52.

3. Cullen TS. Embryology, Anatomy and Diseases of the Umbilicus Together With Diseases of the Urachus. Philadelphia: WE Saunders Company, 1916.

4. Kittle CF, Jenkins HP, Dragstedt LR. Patent omphalomesenteric duct and its relation to the diverticulum of Meckel. Arch Surg 1947; 54:10-36.

5. Bronaugh W. Herniation and extrophy of the ileum in the newborn incidental to adherent Meckel's diverticulum in the umbilical area. West Virginia Med J 1947; 43:126-129.

6. Arnheim EE. Surgical complications of congenital anomalies of the umbilical region. Surg Gynec Obstet 1950; 91:71-80.

7. Moore TC. Omphalomesenteric duct anomalies. Surg Gynec Obstet 1956; 103:569-580.

8. Hadley MN, Cogswell HD. Unusual origin of Meckel's diverticulum from the base of the appendix. JAMA 1936; 106:537-538.

9. Sonderlund S. Meckel's diverticulum in children: A report of 115 cases. Acta Chir Scand 1956; 110:261.

10. Migliaccio AV, Begg C. Meckel's diverticulum. Am J Surg 1948; 76:188-196.

11. Seagram CGF, Louch RE, Stephens CA et al. Meckel's diverticulum: A 10-year review of 218 cases. Canad J Surg 1968; 11: 369-373.

12. Vane DW, West KW, Grosfeld JL. Vitelline duct anomalies: Experience with 217 childhood cases. Arch Surg 1987; 122:542-547.

13. St-Vil D, Brandt ML, Panic S et al. Meckel's diverticulum in children: A 20-year review. J Pediatr Surg 1991; 26:1289-1292.

14. Artigas V, Calabuig R, Badin F et al. Meckel's diverticulum: Value of ectopic tissue. Am J Surg 1986; 151:631-634.

15. McMullin N, Beasley SW, Kelly JH. Prenatal intussuscpeiton of a vitello-intestinal duct in association with ileal atresia. Pediatr Surg Int 1987; 2:122-123.

16. Senocak ME, Büyükpamukçu N, Hiçsönmez A. Ileal atresia due to intrauterine intussusception caused by a Meckel's diverticulum. Pediatr Surg Int 1990; 5:64-66.

17. Jewett TC, Duszynski DO, Allen JE. The visualization of Meckel's diverticulum with ^{99m}Tc pertechnetate. Surgery 1970; 68: 567-570.

18. Soltero MJ, Bill AH. The natural history of Meckel's diverticulum and its relation to incidental removal: A study of 202 cases of diseased Meckel's diverticulum found in King County, Washington, over a fifteen year period. Am J Surg 1976; 132:168-171.

19. Ryan JW, Sephadari S. Detection of Meckel's diverticulum in an infant. Clin Nucl Med 1981; 6:193-195.

20. Cooney DR, Duszynski DO, Camboa E et al. The abdominal technitium scan. J Pediatr Surg 1982; 17:611-619.

21. Barker WF. Discussion of paper by Soltero MJ and Bill AH. Am J Surg 1976; 132:171.

22. Hays DM. Intussusception as a postoperative complication in pediatric surgery. surg Gynec Obst 1961; 112:583-589.

23. Dammert G, Votteler TP. Postoperative intussusception in the pediatric patient. J Pediatr Surg 1974; 9:817-820.

24. McGovern JB, Gross RE. Intussusception as a postoperative complication. Surgery 1968; 63:507-513.

25. Cox JA, Martin LW. Postoperative intussusception. Arch Surg 1973; 106:263-266.

26. Bodycomb JL, Beasley SW, Auldist AW. Postoperative intussusception. Pediatr Surg Int 1987; 2:108-109.

27. Mollitt DL, Ballantine TVN, Grosfeld JL. Postoperative intussusception in infancy and childhood: Analysis of 119 cases. Surgery 1979; 86:402-408.

CHAPTER 15

DUPLICATIONS AND MESENTERIC CYSTS

INTRODUCTION

Duplication of the alimentary tract and mesenteric cysts are rare congenital malformations both of which have multiple forms and types of presenting symptoms and physical findings. These add further to their diagnostic difficulties beyond their infrequent occurrences. Whereas the majority of duplications become symptomatic in the early months and years of life, mesenteric cysts tend to become symptomatic and detected more often later, including adult years. As the appearance, structure and symptoms of these two malformations differ sharply, they will be considered under separate Introduction headings.

DUPLICATIONS OF THE ALIMENTARY TRACT

I have had a long interest in both duplications of the alimentary tract and mesenteric cysts.[1-5] Duplications of the alimentary tract have smooth muscle walls and are lined internally by alimentary tract epithelium which may be that of adjacent alimentary tract or contain ectopic mucosa or gastric or rarely pancreatic tissue. In their most common location in the jejunum and ileum, the duplications occur on the mesenteric border of the adjacent small intestine, and often share a muscular wall with it as well as sharing a common blood supply. Mesenteric cysts, on the other hand, have extremely thin vascular-type endothelial walls which contain no smooth muscle layers and no alimentary tract epithelium. Both duplications and cysts are quite rare.

In a 1952 publication in *Surgery, Gynecology and Obstetrics*, the author with Battersby[1] recorded a 14 year experience at the Indiana University Medical Center in Indianapolis with 11 cases of duplication of the small intestine. Six of these duplications were symptomatic and five were asymptomatic and discovered at autopsy and tended to be small in size. Symptoms and operative findings in the six symptomatic cases were melena and anemia in three with associated inflammation in two of these, intestinal obstruction in two with inflammation in one of these and intussusception in one. All of the symptomatic duplications were located in the ileum. Four were tubular and two were spherical. All of the tubular duplications contained gastric mucosa and all but one communicated with the adjacent small intestine. In two the communication was distal only and in one it was both distal and proximal. Patient ages of symptomatic duplications were five, six and 16 months and 11, 15 and 67 years. All were managed by resection and all survived. All but one of the asymptomatic duplications were small (0.8 to 1.5 cm) and none contained gastric mucosa.

At the time of this publication, most reports of alimentary tract duplications were of single cases and successful resection cases were quite infrequent. Although Professor Sprengel[6] of Braunschweig (Germany) had reported the first successful resection in 1900 before the 29th Congress of the Deutche Gesellschaft für Chirurgie at Berlin, the mortality from reported resection as late as 1934 was 79% (11 of 14 cases).[7] At the time of my 1952 report, resection and anastomosis mortalities in then recently published "series" (two or more cases) had been 0 of 5 cases (1947),[8] 2 of 4 cases (1949),[9] 0 of 3 cases (1950)[10] and 4 of 23 cases (1952).[11] The 1947 report of Donovan and Santulli[8] was of particular interest in that their six cases of duplication of the gastro-intestinal tract had been encountered at the Babies Hospital of New York between April 1945 and November 1946 (17 months) and all six had been managed surgically without mortality (five by resection of duplication and adjacent intestine with intestinal anastomosis). Their paper included a beautiful and especially instructional color illustration (Plate I) of seven color photographs of gross specimens from five of their six cases. The Case 3 of H. Calvin Fisher[10] of Denver was a remarkable achievement of diagnosis and staged surgical resections of a large thoracoabdominal duplication.

It is also true that single case reports and small "series" fail to give reliable data regarding the wide anatomic distribution of alimentary tract duplications. The author, accordingly, has turned to five of the larger series of alimentary tract duplications (23 to 96 cases) to determine the anatomic

Table 15.1. Anatomic distribution of duplications collected from five large series[11-15]

	No.	Percent
Thoracic	51	18.2
Thraco-Abdominal	11	3.9
Abdominal	218	77.9
	280	100

	No.	Percent
Gastric	20	9.2
Duodenal	10	4.6
Jejunum-Ileum	128	58.7
Colon-Rectum	60	27.5
	218	100

distribution of alimentary tract duplications.[11-15] These findings are presented in Table 15.1. The great majority of duplications are abdominal in location (77.9%). Within the abdomen, the predominant location is the small intestinal area of the jejunum and ileum (58.7%) and in this area the greatest concentration of duplications is in the ileum and distal ileum. The five series utilized represented some of the world's largest and most active children's hospitals and extended for periods of 8, 18, 31, 32 and 37 years. The average number of alimentary tract duplications encountered per year ranged from 1.3 to 2.6 in the four series of 18 years and more.

The 1989 report of Holcomb et al[15] in *Annals of Surgery* from the Children's Hospital of Philadelphia (CHOP) is the most recent, longest (37 years) and largest (101 duplications in 96 patients) series to be reported. This series is representative of the collected five reports' experience with 20.7% of the duplications being thoracic (versus 18.2% for the collected experience), 3.0 being thoracoabdominal (versus 3.9% for the collected) and 76.2% being abdominal (versus 77.9% for the collected). Seventy-five of the 101 CHOP duplications were cystic and 26 were tubular in structure. Gastric mucosa was identified in 21 of the 101 duplications and pancreatic tissue in five. Of these 96 patients, the age at the onset of symptoms was less than one month in 36 (37.5%), between one and 24 months in 38 (39.6%) and over two years of age in 22 (22.9%).

The CHOP experience with regional duplications also was quite instructive. All of the 21 thoracic duplications were cystic and none communicated with adjacent esophagus. These duplications generally were found in the posterior mediastinum and in the area of the lower half of the esophagus. Seven of them also contained ectopic gastric mucosa (33%). Two additional statistics of interest were that five of the 21 patients with thoracic duplications also had separate and isolated intestinal duplications and that five patients also had vertebral anomalies with one duplication communicating with the spinal column.

The most common single location for duplications in this CHOP experience was the jejuno-ileum small intestine with 47 of 101 duplications (46.5%), with three-quarters (36 of 47) being in the ileal area. Sixteen of these 47 patients experienced symptoms in their first month of life (34%) and of these 13 (81.3%) presented with symptoms of intestinal obstruction with the symptoms being of vomiting in nine, abdominal distention in three and intussusception in one. Five of these patients had intestinal atresias at birth. In five patients, a volvulus was found at the site of the duplication. Rectal bleeding and intussusception were frequent presentations in older patients. Intussusception with cystic duplications occurred in three and eight patients with tubular duplications communicating with adjacent small bowel had bleeding. Two other ectopic gastric mucosa duplication patients experienced acute inflammatory complications which mimicked appendicitis.

Important contributions over the years have also come from single case reports. A particularly important one was the report of Earle Wrenn[16] of Memphis (University of Tennessee) in 1962, in which he described and beautifully illustrated his innovative technique of countering the ectopic gastric mucosa in tubular duplications

problem. These duplications may be too long and too closely attached to adjacent intestine to permit resection of intestine with duplication because insufficient normal small intestine would remain to sustain life. His gastric mucosa resection/stripping approach with multiple duplication incisions was a direct and successful approach to this difficult problem. An earlier (1958) report by Theodore Jewett[17] had reported in *Annals of Surgery* the successful use of resection of distal bleeding ulcer communications between the long and gastric mucosa lined duplication and adjacent intestine with anastomotic closure of the distal gastric mucosa containing end of the duplication, ileo-ileostomy and venting the duplication by a new and proximal "window" between the duplication and the stomach. The absence of ectopic gastric mucosa in the great majority of colonic tubular duplications makes possible the creation of a distal common lumen, as described by Robert Soper[418] of the University of Iowa (Iowa City) in *Surgery* in 1968.

In 1990, Gilchrist, Harrison and Campbell[19] of Portland (Oregon) reported in the *Journal of Pediatric Surgery* an experience with two cases of thoracoabdominal duplications with upper thoracic cyst termination in the spinal canal. They termed these duplications "neurenteric cysts" and discussed the importance of CT and MRI studies in facilitating removal of the entire cyst in one operation. They discuss the "split notochord theory" for the origin of these malformations which postulates an ectodermal-endodermal adhesion occurring in the middle of the split notochord resulting in both a vertebral column abnormality and a communication between the alimentary tract and the spinal canal. They attributed the coining of the term "neurenteric" to McLetchie et al[20] and the split notochord theory to Bentley and Smith.[21] The Holcomb et al[15] report of 1987 cited above described the occurrence of vertebral malformations in 25% of isolated thoracic duplications and a duplication-spinal canal communication in one case each of isolated thoracic duplication and of thoracoabdominal duplication.

The topic of thoracoabdominal duplications was reviewed thoroughly in 1982 by Pokorny and Goldstein[22] who reported two cases from the Children's Memorial Hospital (Chicago) and included a study of 23 additional cases from the literature. The onset of symptoms was in the first month of life in 48% of the cases and between one and 12 months in eight cases (32%) for a total of 80% in the first year of life. In newborn infants in the first month of life, respiratory distress and a chest mass on the right with upper vertebral anomalies should alert one to the possibility of a thoracoabdominal duplication. In older children, anemia with melena and/or hematemesis with substernal and epigastric pain are more frequent presenting symptoms. All 12 neonates presented with significant respiratory symptoms. The 10 children who had significant bleeding and the five with substernal and gastric pain had gastric mucosa in the duplicated segment. The site of communication in the reported cases of thoracoabdominal duplication was jejunum in nine, duodenum in four, ileum in two and cervical esophagus in one of those cases in which the site of communication was known. In eight no communication was recorded. Eight patients died and 17 recovered.

MESENTERIC CYSTS

Mesenteric cysts of sufficient gravity and symptomatology to come to the attention of surgeons, surgery and the surgical literature are even rarer than duplications. In 1957, the author of this book reported[2,3] a 20 year experience at the Indiana University Medical Center in Indianapolis with four cases of mesenteric cyst. Three were found to be symptomatic in children (4 months, 19 months and 9 years) and one in an adult woman of 32 years. All three of the pediatric age patients had progressive and marked abdominal distention of two, nine and 18 months and all were considered ascites of unknown origin. In the youngest infant of 4 months of age, after two months progressive abdominal swelling, a dumbbell shaped mass was palpated

in the right side of her abdomen. This triggered an operation in which a large cystic mass in the mesentery of the ileum required resection and end-to-end anastomosis with success. The other two children had experienced progressive, marked painless and nontender abdominal swelling for nine and 18 months. The 19 month old boy with nine months of progressive abdominal distention had a markedly protuberant abdomen as shown in Figure 4 of my 1957 *Annals of Surgery* publication.[3] On physical examination, his protuberant abdomen had a generalized doughy consistency without tenderness. At operation, a huge cyst of the ileal mesentery which also involved the ascending mesocolon was found and aspirated with 3,000 ml of serous fluid being recovered. Collapse of this very massive and very thin-walled cyst permitted its removal by enucleation.

The third child was nine years old and she had experienced six months of painless progressive abdominal swelling (soon to become 18 months of the same). At the time of her first admission to the University Hospital (James Whitcomb Riley Children's) she had been under the care of her family physician for six months following the paracentesis removal of a large amount of "ascitic" fluid and a diagnosis of ascites of unknown origin had been made. On examination, her abdomen was markedly enlarged and both shifting dullness and a fluid wave were demonstrated. No masses were palpated and there was no hepatomegaly or splenomegaly or evidence of peripheral edema. Her blood, urine and serology examinations were normal as were her cardiac, renal and hepatic function studies. She was discharged home on "supportive" therapy and remained on this rather unsuccessfully as a patient with ascites of unknown origin for the next 12 months until she was readmitted with the sudden onset of nausea, vomiting and abdominal pain. Her white and red blood counts were normal. Paracentesis revealed 1,300 ml of dark fluid which tested positive for occult blood. After two weeks of further observation and "supportive" medical treatment and study, she was *finally* operated upon. At operation a huge dumb-bell shaped cyst of the distal ileum was found and aspirated for better exposure. The central constricted portion of the cyst was intimately adherent to the blood supply of the adjacent ileum and required ileal resection (one foot) to remove the huge cyst. Ileal continuity was reestablished by end-to-end anastomosis. All three of these pediatric age mesenteric cyst patients were managed successfully with patient survival.

In this 1957 report, I cited Gross's[24] 1953 report of 16 cases of congenital cysts of the mesentery, mesocolon and omentum at the Children's Hospital of Boston. All 16 of these patients were 10 years of age or younger. Also cited in my 1957 article was the excellent and most informative 1954 report in *Annals of Surgery* by Handelsman and Ravitch.[25] They reported in detail four cases of chylous cysts of the mesentery in children. Their patients were three boys of three, four and four years of age from the Johns Hopkins Hospital (Baltimore) and a girl of 10 years from the Mount Sinai Hospital of New York. This experience fleshed out the clinical symptomatic spectrum of mesenteric cysts in infancy and childhood addressed by me in my 1957 report. In two of their four year old cases (Cases No. 1 and 3) symptoms were of colicky abdominal pain and of bowel obstruction. At operation, the bowel obstruction was due to a volvulus about a large (600 ml) ileal mesenteric cyst and in the other four year old, it was due to stretching and flattening of jejunum over an underlying large mesenteric cyst. Both of these bowel obstruction cases were managed successfully by bowel resection with mesenteric cyst followed by end-to-end anastomosis. The other two cases (three and 10 years of age) involved acute cyst inflammation associated with pain, nausea, vomiting, fever (102° and 102°) and leukocytosis (28,000 and 23,500). Large cystic masses were encountered in the ileum in one of these cases and in the jejunum in the other. Both required small bowel resection for inflamed cyst removal with end-to-end anastomosis with success in both cases.

These cases of Handelsman and Ravitch and of mine identified the major complications and clinical symptomatology of mesenteric cysts in infancy and childhood as progressive and painless abdominal distention with a misdiagnosis of "ascites" of unknown origin, of acute cyst inflammation ("cystitis") and of bowel obstruction by cyst-triggered volvulus or cyst pressure on overlying bowel.

The prolonged painless marked abdominal enlargement picture ("ascites") of a mesenteric cyst was recorded in a case report in 1959 by Arnheim et al[26] of New York and later, in 1975, by Gordon and Sumner[27] (Travis Air Force Base, California), in 1982 by Molander et al[28] of the St. Goran's Hospital and Karolinska Institute of Stockholm (Sweden) and in 1984 by Geer et al[29] of the University of North Carolina (Case 2).

The 1975 report of Gordon and Sumner[27] described a case of mesenteric cyst which presented as the sudden onset of bloody ascites. The correct diagnosis was suggested by abdominal sonography and confirmed by operative removal of a 30x15 cm, 4,000 g thin-walled bluish bi-lobed cystic mass which was found adherent to and partially compressing a loop of jejunum. Their patient was a six year old male who experienced tense abdominal swelling which occurred over a two week period. Both hemidiaphragms were elevated with decreased excursions. On examination, the abdomen was found to be tensely distended with a palpable fluid wave. Abdominal paracentesis revealed a serosanguinous fluid. Sonography revealed an echo-free smooth walled structure with good sound transmission shown by strong and multiple back wall echoes which the authors regarded as consistent with a cystic ultrasonic pattern. Multiline linear echoes were recorded and were considered by them as suggesting the presence of a bi-lobed cystic mass. Midline linear echoes were interpreted as representing reflections from the elongated and effaced jejunal loop. Their well illustrated publication includes an excellent photograph of the gross surgical specimen

(Fig. 3) demonstrating how accurate their interpretation was. They cited a prior (1960) report by Whittlesey et al[30] in which a mesenteric cyst mimicked chronic recurrent ascites.

The 1984 report of Geer et al[29] described the imaging findings in a five year old boy who presented to the University of North Carolina (Chapel Hill) with a three year history of protuberant abdomen which was "unresponsive" to diet. Ascites was suggested on physical examination. Extensive studies including upper gastrointestinal series, liver-spleen scan, liver and bone marrow biopsies were normal. A CT scan was interpreted as "ascites" and a peritoneal tap showed mesothelial "hypoplasia". One year after the CT scan and continuing ascites "treatment", an abdominal gray scale ultrasound demonstrated a large septated fluid collection displacing the bowel loops posteriorly. The ultrasound findings were considered compatible with a mesenteric cyst. This was confirmed at surgery and the patient *finally* made an uneventful recovery. The authors point out the superiority of ultrasound over CT scans in the diagnosis of mesenteric cysts which masquerade as "ascites"—a not infrequent occurrence.

In a 1978 publication by Haller et al[31] from Brooklyn (New York), a large omental cyst in a 3 year old boy (Case 2) was misdiagnosed for $2^1/_4$ years as ascites. Abdominal distention had been first noted at 1 year of age. There was marked bulging of the flanks and shifting dullness. Multiple sonographic studies were misinterpreted as supporting the clinical diagnosis of ascites. The diagnosis ultimately was made in the presence of persistently recurrent symptoms by a cream meal followed by paracentesis which yielded fat globules followed by surgery. Later reinterpretation of the sonograms revealed findings very unusual for ascites with septa and supine scans showing fluid anterior to the bowel (in defiance of gravity) and none posterior to the bowel or between the loops—"a very unusual distribution for ascitic fluid".

The superlative report of Molander et al[28] from Stockholm describes in most help-ful detail six cases of mesenteric and omental cysts in childhood. All of these six patients were seven years of age or younger. Two were seven years of age and the other four were 5 months, 12 months, 18 months and $4^1/_2$ years of age. Two of these six patients (ages 12 and 18 months) had painless and progressive abdominal distention and a misdiagnosis of "ascites". The first of these patients (Case 1) at one year of age had painless abdominal distention, a fluid wave on abdominal palpation and protein-rich fluid on paracentesis. One year later, this now two year old boy was surprisingly still healthy and well nourished but with increased abdominal distention. Liver function tests remained normal. Finally, an exploratory operation was carried out and a huge omental cyst was found and removed. The second painless "ascites" patient (Case 6) had a shorter wait prior to operation, thanks to ultrasonography which demonstrated a multitude of widespread, thin-walled cysts. At operation, a huge omental cyst was found and removed. One additional patient, a $4^1/_2$ year old boy had painful abdominal distention and an X-ray diagnosis of "ascites". At operation, this child was found to have a large multilocular cyst of the mesentery which required resection of 10 cm of small intestine for its removal. Pain, vomiting, fever and an abdominal mass or large cystic "tumor" at operation constituted the clinical picture in the other three cases. Mesenteric cysts were found at operation in two cases and an omental cyst in one. One patient with a mesenteric cyst required a bowel resection for its removal and the other cyst (ascending mesocolon) was removed without the requirement of ascending mesocolon resection. It contained opalescent foul-smelling fluid which cultured *E. coli*. The authors emphasized the hazard of roentgen and physical examination misinterpretation of findings as "ascites". They cited the flaccid consistency of the very thin-walled cysts and the tendency for the fluid to "flow out" and fill the dependent parts of the abdomen and to interpose between abdominal structures. They also pointed out that traction in the mesentery or omentum and compression or torsion (volvulus) of the small intestine may produce abdominal pain and partial or complete intestinal obstruction.

Mesenteric cysts also have been reported to produce small bowel obstruction in the early neonatal period, at 26 and 60 hours of age. The 1965 case of Capt. Jay C. Fish and associates[32] of Fort Benning (Georgia) involved a 26 hours old infant with bile stained vomiting, a palpable large mid-abdominal mass and a "double bubble" sign on X-ray. At operation, a large, soft multicystic mass was found in the mesentery of the upper jejunum. The jejunum was stretched around this cystic mass to the point of complete occlusion of its lumen. Resection of the large cyst and jejunum were carried out with an end-to-end jejunal anastomosis and patient survival. A similar but more complicated case was reported in 1987 by Kovalivker and Motovic[33] from Isreal (Tel Aviv University). Their patient was a 60 hour old newborn infant whose initial symptoms were of bile stained vomiting and abdominal distention and rigidity with X-ray evidence of intestinal obstruction. At operation, a hard, biloculated cyst of six cm in diameter was found in the mesentery of the lower jejunum with the bowel compressed between the two lobes of the cyst with a perforation in a necrotic area of the involved jejunum. The obstruction and ischemia producing cyst and involved jejunum were resected with end-to-end anastmosis and survival. Both of these papers[32,33] included excellent photographs of the resected cysts and bowel.

Literature reviews over the years of mesenteric (and omental) cysts have included largely adult cases and also retroperitoneal cystic lesions which have made the determination of features of mesenteric and omental cysts in infancy and childhood next to impossible.[34-40] In addition, the rereporting of already reported cases adds an element of potential confusion in literature reviews and evaluations.[3,41]

The published literature regarding mesenteric cysts in any age group appears to be in a disappearing mode. The last report referenced in the *Cumulated Index Medicus* was the 1987 report of Kovalivker and Motovic[33] from Israel. Furthermore, the citation of mesenteric cysts as a separate category in *Cumulated Index Medicus* has been dropped in recent years.

CHALLENGES

1. The most important single challenge involving both alimentary tract duplications and mesenteric (and omental) cysts is the achieving of a timely and accurate diagnosis.

The multiplicity of symptomatic presentations and their timing with respect to patient age have long posed vexatious problems for the clinician. A familiarity with these symptoms and their likely timing of occurrence during infancy and childhood and an on-going awareness of their potential involvement in differential diagnostic occasions is the most reasonable approach to this difficult and perplexing problem.

The diagnostic evaluation of symptomatic duplication containing gastric mucosa with bleeding, melena, anemia and pain has been greatly facilitated by the technetium scan for ectopic gastric mucosa in the abdomen introduced in 1970 by Theodore "Ted" Jewett and associates[42] of Buffalo (New York).

With respect to mesenteric and omental cysts, a quote from the closing paragraph of the outstanding 1982 publication from Stockholm by Molander et al[28] is in order:

> In cases with a history of large abdominal circumference or "ascites" without further symptoms or, with a history of repeated episodes of a low grade bowel obstruction, omental and mesenteric cysts should be included in differential diagnostic considerations. Ultrasonography is the best examination modality for further investigation. The presence of a large multilocular cyst is from a practical point of view pathognomic for the current lesion.

2. The second most important challenge in the area of these congenital malformations is the best surgical approach to the management of the very long, gastric mucosa containing tubular duplications of the small intestine (ileum and jejunum).

The gastric mucosa stripping operation described in *Surgery* in 1962 by Earle Wrenn[16] of Memphis (Tennessee) remains the most direct and definitive approach to this difficult problem. Recent advances in surgical electrocautery instrumentation should further simplify this approach. Several generations of pediatric surgeons schooled and experienced in the Soave intestinal mucosa stripping operation for Hirschsprung's disease should find this Wrenn operation considerably less of a challenge than it was 32 years ago when Wrenn first described it.

The 1958 reported approach in *Annals of Surgery* by Ted Jewett[17] of Buffalo (New York) would appear to be a solid secondary/back-up option in case of stripping failure or unsuitability. In this Jewett operation, the distal duplication and normal ileum junction is resected with duplication lower end closure and restoration of ileal single lumen continuity by ileo-ileostomy. The proximal end of the gastric mucosa containing duplication then is vented into the gastric mucosa containing stomach by an anastomotic connection.

CONCLUSION

While these two congenital malformations are comparatively rare and of unknown etiology, embryological or otherwise, they do constitute an ancient and fascinating component and chapter of Pediatric Surgery. Their elusive symptomatology and clinical pictures and their proper and timely surgical management remain as significant challenges to the most scholarly and talented of Pediatric Surgeons.

REFERENCES

1. Moore TC, Battersby JS. Congenital duplications of the small intestine: Report of 11 cases. Surg Gynec Obstet 1952; 95:557-567.

2. Moore TC. Congenital cysts of the mesentery. Quart Bull Indiana Univ Med Center 1952; 14:29-34.

3. Moore TC. Congenital cysts of the mesentery: Report of four cases. Ann Surg 1957; 145:428-436.

4. Gamal R, Moore TC. Massive acquired omental cyst as a complication of ventriculoperitoneal shunting. J Pediatr Surg 1988; 23:1041-1042.

5. Baumgartner F, Moore TC. Recurrent ventriculoperitoneal shunt pseudocyst in a nine-year old girl. Klin Wchnschr 1990; 68:485-487.

6. Sprengel. Ein angeobrene Cyst der Darmwand als Ursache der Invagination. Arch Klin Chir 1900; 86:1032-1047.

7. Hughes-Jones WEA. Enterogenous cysts. Br J Surg 1934; 22:134-141.

8. Donovan EJ, Santulli TV. Duplication of the alimentary tract: Report of six cases. Ann Surg 1947; 126:289-304.

9. Ripstein CB. Duplication of the small intestine. Am J Surg 1949; 78:847-852.

10. Fisher HC. Duplications of the intestinal tract in infants. Arch Surg 1950; 61: 957-970.

11. Gross RE, Holcomb GW, Farber S. Duplications of the alimentary tract. Pediatrics 1952; 9:449-468.

12. Basu R, Forshall I, Rickham PP. Duplications of the alimentary tract. Br J Surg 1960; 47:477-484.

13. Grosfeld JL, O'Neill JA, Clatworthy HW. Enteric duplications in infancy and childhood: An 18-year review. Ann Surg 1970; 172:83-90.

14. Hocking M, Young DG. Duplications of the alimentary tract. Br J Surg 1981; 68:92-96.

15. Holcomb GW, Gheissari A, O'Neill JA et al. Surgical management of alimentary tract duplications. Ann Surg 1989; 209:167-174.

16. Wrenn EL. Tubular duplications of the small intestine. Surgery 1962; 52:494-498.

17. Jewett TC. Duplication of the entire small intestine with massive melena. Ann Surg 1958; 147:239-244.

18. Soper RT. Tubular duplications of the colon and distal ileum: Case report and dis-

cussion. Surgery 1968; 63:998-1004.

19. Gilchrist BF, Harrison MW, Campbell JR. Neurenteric cyst: Current management. J Pediatr Surg 1990; 25:1231-1233.

20. McLetchie NGB, Purves JK, Saunders RL et al. The genesis of gastric and certain intestinal diverticula and enterogenous cysts. Surg Gynec Obstet 1954; 99:135-139.

21. Bentley JFR, Smith JR. Developmental posterior enteric remnants and spinal malformations: The split notochord syndrome. Arch Dis Child 1960; 35:76-80.

22. Pokorny WJ, Goldstein IR. Enteric thoraco-abdominal duplications in children. J Thorac Cardiovasc Surg 1984; 87:821-824.

23. Moore TC. Congenital cysts of the mesentery:Report of four cases. Ann Surg 1957; 145:428-436.

24. Gross RE. The Surgery of Infancy and Childhood. Philadelphia: WB Saunders Company, 1953:377.

25. Handelsman JC, Ravitch MM. Chylous cysts of the mesentery in children. Ann Surg 1954; 140:185-193.

26. Arnheim EE, Schneck H, Norman A et al. Mesenteric cysts in infancy and childhood: Review of the literature and report of a case. Pediatrics 1959; 24:469-476.

27. Gordon MJ, Sumner TE. Abdominal ultrasonography in a mesenteric cyst presenting as ascites. Gastroenterology 1975; 69:761-764.

28. Molander M-L, Mortensson W, Udén R. Omental and mesenteric cysts in children. Acta Paediatr Scan 1982; 71:227-229.

29. Geer LL, Mittelstaedt CA, Staab EV et al. Mesenteric cyst: Sonographic appearance with CT correlation. Pediatr Radiol 1984; 14:102-104.

30. Whittlesey R, Guenther H, Huntley W. Mesenteric cysts and chylous ascites. Arch Pediatr 1960; 77:357-363.

31. Haller JO, Scheider M, Kassner EG et al. Sonographic evaluation of mesenteric and omental masses in children. Am J Roentgenol 978; 130:269-274.

32. Fish JC, Fair WR, Canby JP. Intestinal obstruction in the newborn: An unusual case due to mesenteric cyst. Arch Surg 1965; 90:317-318.

33. Kovalivker M, Motovic A. Obstruction and gangrene of bowel with perforation due to a mesenteric cyst in a newborn. J Pediatr Surg 1987; 22:377-378.

34. Vaughn AM, Lees WM, Henry JW. Mesenteric cysts:A review of the literature and report of a calicfied cyst of the mesentery. Surgery 1948; 23:306-317.

3. Burnett WE, Rosemond GP, Bucher RM. Mesenteric cysts: Report of three cases, in one of which a calcified cyst was present. Arch Surg 1952; 60:699-706.

36. Ford JR. Mesenteric cysts: Review of the literature with report of an unusual case. Am J Surg 1960; 99:878-884.

37. Hardin WJ, Hardy JD. Mesenteric cysts. Am J Surg 1970; 119:640-645.

38. Walker AR, Putnam TC. Omental, mesenteric and retroperitoneal cysts: A clinical study of 33 new cases. Ann Surg 1973; 178:13-19.

39. Caropreso PR. Mesenteric cysts: A review. Arch Surg 1974; 108:242-246.

40. Kurtz RJ, Heimann TM, Bock AR et al. Mesenteric and retroperitoneal cysts. Ann Surg 1986; 203:109-112.

41. Mollitt DL, Ballantine TVN, Grosfeld JL. Mesenteric cysts in infancy and childhood. Surg Gynec Obstet 1978; 147:182-184.

42. Jewett TC, Duszynski DA, Allen JE. The visualization of Meckel's diverticulum with 99mTc pertechnetate. Surgery 1970; 68:567-570.

========= CHAPTER 16 =========

BLUNT ABDOMINAL TRAUMA

INTRODUCTION

In comparatively recent decades, major advances in both the biological sciences (infection and contagion control) and the physical sciences (development and mass production of motorized vehicles and the roads and highways they traverse with reckless abandon) have permitted trauma to forge ahead as the major killer of children, replacing the classical child killing scourges of antiquity.

A recent, 1990, report from my home State of Indiana by Vane et al[1] presents a current comprehensive picture of causes of childhood death in a representative state and the role and types of trauma involved. From June 1986 to May 1988, there were recorded 1,931 childhood deaths in Indiana. Of these, 806 were as a result of trauma (41.4% of all deaths). Blunt trauma accounted for the largest number of trauma deaths (54%). It was followed by asphyxia or drowning at 26%, penetrating trauma at 15%, electrocution at 3% and burns at 1%. Sixty percent of the deaths occurred in rural areas with 40% in urban areas. Statewide demographics define the population as 70% urban. Nonetheless, with the exception of Indianapolis and the northwestern corner of the state Chicago suburbs, there are no huge cities.

I spent the first 14 years of my life as a trained surgeon in the comparatively small home town of my birth, Muncie, Indiana with approximately 90% of my practice devoted to adult surgery with 10% to pediatric surgery. In both age groups, trauma was comparatively rare. The 1968 move to Southern California, Los Angeles County and the full-time faculty of the UCLA School of Medicine with an academic and clinical base at the Harbor-UCLA Medical Center (located at the junction of two of Los Angeles County's busiest freeways (the San Diego and the Harbor) was a real "eye-opener" with respect to the incidence and magnitude of trauma as an ongoing and increasingly serious "fact-of-life"—and death for children as well as adults.

The author's clinical responsibilities at Harbor-UCLA were limited to pediatric surgery and renal transplantation. The renal transplantation segment also involved direction of a metropolitan community-wide program of cadaver kidney harvesting and machine preservation (Belzer perfusion machines). Trauma became an important focus of both clinical responsibilities.

My first major clinical research project involved a 10 year review of blunt and penetrating trauma in childhood managed by major operation. This study was published in the April 1974 issue of the *Journal of Pediatric Surgery*.[2] This study included a 10 plus year period from October 1961 through April 1972. In this experience, there were 99 blunt injuries and 100 penetrating injuries. In blunt abdominal trauma, paracentesis and peritoneal lavage were the principal indications and triggers for laparotomy. In blunt trauma, the solid organs injured were spleen (43), liver (22), kidney (20) and pancreas (7). Sixty-one percent of the patients with blunt abdominal injuries had major associated injuries with 28 of them involving the head. Six of these head injuries were fatal. There were four patients with hepatic vein and vena caval injuries and all four (100%) exsanguinated on the operating table. Hollow viscera were less frequently subject to nonperforating injury, small intestine in three cases and urinary tract in seven.[2,3]

Perforating abdominal and thoracic injuries are largely gunshot and stab wounds and were largely concentrated in older childhood and adolescent age groups and their management did not differ significantly from those in the adult population, a situation quite different from that which appears to prevail in cases of blunt abdominal trauma.[2-8]

Another important report of a large experience with blunt abdominal trauma in childhood also appeared in 1974 in the *Journal of Pediatric Surgery*. This report by Hood and Smyth[9] from Belfast in Northern Ireland was concerned with 130 cases seen during a $14^1/_2$ year period between 1959 and 1973. This study was restricted to children under 15 years of age. There were 19 deaths for a series mortality of 14.6%. Uncontrollable hemorrhage from the liver and great veins was the most frequent cause of death in this series, accounting for 14 deaths in the 33 children with liver injuries (42.4%). Thirteen of 44 children with kidney injuries (27%) were considered to "require" nephrectomy.

The spleen and the liver are the principal intra-abdominal, nonretroperitoneal solid organs which may receive injury from severe blunt abdominal trauma in childhood. They also represent the historical break with adult routine operative approach to the management of these injuries, originating with the spleen.

The 1968 publication in *Surgery, Gynecology and Obstetrics* by Upadhyaya and Simpson[10] of the Hospital for Sick Children of Toronto, Canada provided the clinical rationale and support for nonoperative management of blunt trauma splenic injury in childhood. They reported an experience with 52 children with splenic injury admitted to their hospital between 1956 and 1965. The splenic injury was proven in 30 children by operation and in 10 by postmortem examination (death from other injuries). Twelve patients had classical signs, symptoms and history indicating splenic injury/rupture but were not operated upon because their condition improved within a short period of time and operation was not considered to be required. In the group of 30 children with operation, bleeding had stopped by the time of operation in 19 of 24 patients in whom this information was available (79%). There were no delayed splenic ruptures in those children managed without operation. The authors emphasized from this experience that there is a marked difference between splenic rupture in children and adults. In children there is a remarkable absence of clinical signs of significant blood loss and shock. They also emphasized that children in their study did not die of splenic rupture unless severe associated injuries were present. They concluded that isolated splenic injury is well tolerated in children and that spontaneous healing may occur after splenic rupture in childhood.

A 1971 report from this same Toronto institution by Douglas and Simpson[11] in the *Journal of Pediatric Surgery* provided data to support this nonoperative approach to splenic trauma. They described an experience with 32 children with suspected splenic rupture admitted to their hospital between 1948 and 1955. The diagnosis was confirmed in the six children on whom laparotomy and splenectomy were carried out. Twenty-five children were managed nonoperatively and all survived. Sixteen of these 25 children were selected for detailed clinical study because the severity of the trauma and the signs, symptoms and clinical course strongly indicated splenic rupture to be highly probable (despite the lack of operative confirmation of rupture). At this time, definitive diagnostic procedures such as splenic scans and angiography were unavailable. All children complained of abdominal pain and nine of these 16 patients also complained of shoulder pain. Significant abdominal tenderness and signs of cardiovascular instability were present in all 16. Associated extraabdominal injuries were encountered in seven children: extremity fracture in three, mild head injury in three and renal contusion in one. Nine of the 16 children received transfusions of 500 to 2000 ml of whole blood and two others received plasma (450 and 1000 ml). Significant abdominal signs persisted for two to 11 days and all received intravenous fluids. Their vital signs and hemaglobin determinations were monitored frequently. Hemaglobin determinations varied from 7.9 to 11.4% with a mean of 9.5%. A good correlation was noted between the disappearance of abdominal tenderness and the return of the pulse and temperature to normal. A left upper quadrant abdominal mass in two patients resolved with observation. Complete bed rest was continued for two weeks (at home or in hospital) and physical activities were restricted for an additional four weeks. This particularly important and significant experience was presented at the 1971 meeting of the American Pediatric Surgical Association where it was rather vigorously condemned and rather hesitantly defended. I consider these two reports and publications by Simpson and associates (Upadhyaya and Douglas) to be two of the great classics of pediatric surgical literature. The courage and persistence of the Toronto group has overcome sharp early and long continued criticism to achieve the current almost universal acceptance of this "conservative" nonoperative approach to splenic trauma and rupture in childhood.

By the 19th Annual Meeting of the American Pediatric Surgical Association in May 1988, the picture and reception had rather dramatically altered as the publication of the Toronto experience with nonoperative management of blunt abdominal splenic injury by Pearl et al[12] in the January 1989 issue of the *Journal of Pediatric Surgery* clearly indicated. In a five year period from 1981 to 1986, 75 patients were admitted to this hospital with a diagnosis of splenic injury. Sixty-five of the 75 children were managed nonoperatively and total splenectomy carried out in only three patients. Only 23% of patients treated nonoperatively required/received blood transfusions. In comparison with a prior 5-year period, the number of children managed nonoperatively was increased from 76 to 87%, those receiving blood transfusion decreased from 36 to 23% and those undergoing splenectomy decreased from 24 to 4%. The authors concluded that almost all children with splenic injury can be managed successfully without an operation and that the total hospital stay may be limited to seven days. In his closing discussion of this important report, Pearl stated that no patient had died of splenic injury at the Hospital for Sick Children in Toronto in the past 20 years. He also stated that they rarely did CT studies on abdominal injuries as they found clinical examinations and the use of blood products as very reliable indicators. They transfused patients, when needed, to stabilize them. Management decisions were based on physical findings plus blood availability and vital signs and had nothing to do with special tests or anything "magical". They estimated blood loss from the volume of blood products required to maintain normal vital signs, urine output and hematocrit.

The value of nonoperative management of blunt trauma liver injuries has been slower and more difficult to be achieved and accepted. In 1983, Karp, Cooney, Jewett and associates[13] at the Children's Hospital of Buffalo (New York) described in the *Journal of Pediatric Surgery* the successful use of nonoperative management of blunt liver trauma in 17 consecutive patients. Oldham et al[14] in 1986 made a particularly important report relating to blunt abdominal liver trauma in childhood. Of 188 consecutive children with serious blunt abdominal trauma, 52 patients (28%) were found to have hepatic parenchymal injuries, largely (51 of 53) by CT scans. Two patients operated upon emergently without CT scan study were found to have, at laparotomy, massive exsanguinating hemorrhage from hepatic vein and caval injury and both (100%) died. Forty-nine of their 53 patients with hepatic parenchymal injuries (92%) did not require operation for hemorrhage. Nonetheless, 11 children (21%) did require blood transfusions. The authors conclude that their large clinical experience demonstrates the ability of using nonoperative management of blunt liver trauma in children. They also reported that 97% of 28 splenic injuries were managed nonoperatively.

The Oldham et al[14] report stimulated me to publish an update on a nonoperative approach to all blunt abdominal trauma stimulated by the 1974 and subsequent experiences.[2-8] This update was published in *Surgery* in March 1987 in the Letters to the Editors section.[15] This update concerned the whole area of blunt abdominal trauma and all organs, solid and hollow, as did the 1974 report.[2] After referring to the 1974 report and experiences, the 1987 *Surgery* communication continued as follows:

> The high incidence of "negative" laparotomies in this study and a subsequent experience with a 10-year-old child—stable after transfusions who was promptly destabilized by a peritoneal lavage-induced laparotomy with speedy exsanguination from hepatic vein injuries—triggered an agonizing reappraisal of our approach to blunt abdominal trauma in childhood.

In the past 4 years (August 1982 to August 1986), peritoneal tapping or lavage for blunt abdominal trauma has been both abandoned and forbidden. The patients are managed quietly in our pediatric intensive care unit with careful and frequent monitoring of vital signs, abdominal girth and serial hematocrit determinations, with transfusions carried out when indicated. The stable or potentially stable child is not surgically treated or moved about. Since the majority of these children have multiple fractures, head injury, or both, movement about the hospital for CT and other imaging (except when indicated because of head injuries) is contraindicated—unduly hazardous, unpleasant and traumatic. With this approach, only one patient in 4 years has required an abdominal operation and that for proximal jejunal transection with free air in the peritoneal cavity. Associated with this 40-fold reduction in laparotomy for blunt abdominal trauma (as compared with our 10-year earlier study),[2] there have been no deaths from intra-abdominal causes.

The major intra-abdominal spaces or potential spaces, such as perirenal, peritoneal or retroperitoneal, are finite and comparatively readily filled with extravasated blood (easily replaced) with tamponade of bleeding sites. Since the major sites of major bleeding in blunt abdominal trauma in childhood are major veins, tamponade of these in closed spaces is comparatively easy with stabilization of the patient on blood replacement. Surgically opening these closed and finite spaces renders them infinite and the potential for blood loss equally infinite. It should be avoided at all costs. *Do not surgically destabilize a stable or potentially stable child with blunt abdominal trauma."*

A four year extension of this blunt abdominal injury nonoperative management protocol by my service increased the reduction in laparotomy to 80-fold with no mortality from intra-abdominal causes despite a steady increase in the admission of children with blunt abdominal injuries to our pediatric intensive care unit.

Exsanguination has remained an unresolved source of formidable mortality (80 to 100%) in blunt liver injury cases with hepatic vein and retrohepatic vena caval injuries submitted to abdominal operation. This was the sole intraabdominal source of mortality in two large series of blunt hepatic trauma cases reported in 1984 and 1990 from Toronto and Cleveland in which treatment consisted of a blend or combination of operative and nonoperative treatment.[16,17]

In a 1984 report from the University of Toronto by Giacomantonio, Filler and Rich,[16] an 8 year experience with 32 cases of blunt hepatic trauma was recorded. Fourteen children were managed nonoperatively with no mortality or complications and 18 were managed operatively. Seven of the 18 surgically managed cases died, five from uncontrollable bleeding and two from head injuries.

The 1990 report from Cleveland by Galant et al[17] from Case Western Reserve University recorded a 10 year experience (1979-1989) with 41 cases of blunt liver trauma. Twenty-six of the 41 patients were managed nonoperatively without mortality or serious complications. Seventeen of the 26 nonoperatively managed patients (65%) did not require blood transfusion. In nine of the 15 operatively managed children (60%), bleeding from the liver injury had stopped by the time of operation. Three of the 15 operatively managed children died, all (100%) from uncontrollable exsanguinating hemorrhage from injuries to the hepatic veins and inferior vena cava. The three operative cases with liver parenchymal injuries managed by resection of damaged tissue survived.

Moulton, Canty, Collins and associates[18] of San Diego, in a 1992 report, described their experiences with 21 cases of operation for blunt liver trauma. Nine of the 21 patients (45%) had major hepatic vein or retrohepatic vena caval injuries and seven of these nine (78%) died.

As with splenic injuries, the majority of hepatic blunt injuries have stopped bleeding by the time of operation. Cwyes and Millar[19]

in a major 1985 report in the *Journal of Pediatric Surgery* concerning nonoperative management of blunt liver trauma in children cite a 1977 report by Stone and Ansley[20] revealing that up to 70% of blunt hepatic injuries in children have stopped bleeding spontaneously by the time of laparotomy. The Cwyes and Millar report involved two sequential experiences first with operative and then with nonoperative management of blunt liver trauma in childhood. In the operative experience (1973 to 1977), 13 laparotomies were carried out for blunt hepatic trauma after initial resuscitation. In eight of the cases (62%) the bleeding had stopped and in an additional three simple suturing was all that was required. Since 1978 and based on this operative experience, of 23 consecutive children with blunt hepatic trauma, 19 were managed successfully nonoperatively (83%). Repeated and frequent clinical evaluations were the principal means of patient monitoring. They commented that peritoneal needle aspiration or peritoneal lavage were not a part of their routine patient monitoring as they did not regard free intraperitoneal blood as an indication for operation. Ultrasound, liver isotope scans and CT were employed to monitor healing progress of the injured liver. These authors clearly were on the right track and very early on.

A 1992 report from Padua, Italy by Amroch et al[21] describes an 8 year experience with the successful nonoperative management of blunt liver injury in 13 children with no complications.

A 1978 published lecture by Professor Alexander Walt[22] of Detroit puts the problem of operative management of major hepatic venous injuries in blunt hepatic trauma in refreshingly clear and candid perspective. His Founders Lecture before the Society for Surgery of the Alimentary Tract was published in the *American Journal of Surgery* and was titled "The Mythology of Hepatic Trauma—or Babel Revisited". In the section of his lecture on major venous injuries, he states:

Much has been written on the topic of hepatic venous injuries and there are probably more authors on the subject than survivors from the procedures described.

He goes on to "confess" that all nine of the patients with this sort of injury managed operatively at his university hospital died. In this section, he then quoted a statement of Charles Mayo that "experience can consist of doing the same thing wrongly over and over again." He concluded this section on major traumatic hepatic venous injury by the sage observation that:

> The stable nonexpanding retroperitoneal retrohepatic hematoma, even if large, may be left undisturbed as the tamponading effect will usually be sufficient to end the bleeding from the low pressure vena cava.

Of the retroperitoneal solid organs, kidneys and pancreas, the kidney has the longest history of nonoperative management. The renal nonoperative experience generated earliest from adult experience with renal traumatic rupture in which opening of Gerota's fascia led to almost certain loss of the kidney from uncontrollable hemorrhage. Superior results were achieved by maintenance of Gerota's fascial integrity and the continuance of hemorrhagic limiting tamponade.

A 1981 article from the University of Rochester by Mandour et al[23] in the *Journal of Pediatric Surgery* addressed some of the major problems of dealing with blunt renal trauma in the pediatric patient. Their report involved 90 patients 17 years of age and younger. Sixty-nine patients were managed successfully nonoperatively with only one death, and this from a head injury. Twenty-one patients were managed operatively. Six partial and three total nephrectomies were performed as delayed, elective procedures and there were four drainage procedures. Six patients were operated upon for other suspected or associated injuries. Three total nephrectomies were acutely

carried out. They presented five case reports to indicate features of the nonoperative management. One of a limited number (11) angiograms resulted in a femoral artery thrombotic occlusion which required a thrombectomy. Their goal was to maintain good health of the child while preserving the maximum amount of functioning tissue. The authors concluded that the majority of pediatric patients with blunt trauma renal injuries can be treated conservatively in the acute phase of their injury, and that surgical procedures that are necessary can be performed as elective procedures. The authors seriously doubt the possibility of successful revascularization when acute, complete, traumatic renal arterial occlusion has occurred (as *do I!*). They emphasize that "the time that elapses during transport of the patient, admission to the emergency department and completion of diagnostic studies often results in many hours between injury and the feasible time for surgery." This period is far beyond the maximum 20 minute warm ischemia time allowable for human cadaver kidneys harvested and preserved for transplantation.[24-26] I have observed one arterial angiographically nonperfusing, bluntly traumatized pediatric kidney managed nonoperatively to regain function on observation after a short period of mild systemic hypertension.

In a major 1991 report in the *Journal of Pediatric Surgery*, Bass, Semple and Cwyes[27] of the University of Cape Town (South Africa) report an 11 year experience with 91 demonstrated renal injuries in children ranging in age from six months to 13 years. They acknowledge that it is becoming increasingly apparent that conservative management is appropriate for the majority of renal injuries in children sustaining blunt abdominal trauma and that the majority of surgical explorations in these cases will result in nephrectomy (loss of the kidney). Seventy-eight of their 91 patients (84%) were managed conservatively nonoperatively with one death (severe head injury) and few complications (6.5%). Thirteen of their 91 patients (14%) underwent early laparotomy with a nephrectomy rate of 92%. The authors have abandoned arteriography in traumatic renal injuries because it is time consuming, invasive and carries a small but appreciable morbidity in children. They observe from their experience that the majority of blunt renal injuries sustained in childhood are contusions and lacerations that will heal on bed rest and broad-spectrum antibiotic coverage with a low complication rate. *They conclude that the best chance of renal salvage rests with nonoperative management.* Renal pedicle injuries in children are uncommon (between 0 and 5% of most published series). They seriously question the wisdom of attempted revascularization after blunt renal trauma in childhood. I agree with this assessment most heartily!

Blunt abdominal trauma injuries to the pancreas in childhood likely occur more frequently than recognized or documented, particularly in bicycle related injuries. Their nonintentional nonoperative management would appear successful in most cases. When recognized, the pancreas appears to have shared with other blunt trauma injured solid organs the additional trauma of overly aggressive surgical assault. In this environment, it is appropriate that the Toronto group at the Hospital for Sick Children would be one of the first, in a 1987 report by Gorenstein et al,[28] to record the successful use of nonoperative management of a serious complication of blunt abdominal trauma injury to the pancreas—pseudocyst. They reported that six of 10 post-traumatic pseudocysts resolved without surgical treatment.

A 1988 report from the University of Montreal by Bass et al[29] in the *Journal of Pediatric Surgery* also records successful nonoperative management of blunt pancreatic injuries in children. Five of 10 post-traumatic pancreatic pseudocysts resolved spontaneously and nonoperatively while another three were managed successfully (and nonoperatively) by percutaneous external drainage (PED). The authors observed that results with blunt pancreatic traumatic injury in children are better than in the adult population and that the likely

reason for this is the absence of primary pancreatic pathology which so often afflicts adults.

In 1981, I reported[8] the successful nonoperative management of a particularly severe blunt traumatic pancreatic injury resulting from the fall of a brick walk on a four year-old boy. Nasogastric suction, nothing by mouth and TPN (total parenteral nutrition) were employed for one month while the urinary amylase levels remained markedly elevated. Following their sudden return to normal, oral feedings were resumed and the child shortly was discharged to his home. Several weeks later he was readmitted with an acute small bowel obstruction which was found at operation to be due to fat necrosis adhesive obstruction of the mid-small intestine. Simple lysing of this adhesion was successful and this child had no further difficulties. More extensive and expedient use of nonoperative management of blunt trauma injuries to the pancreas would appear to be in order. Ultrasound monitoring[28] and percutaneous external drainage[29] would appear to be of value in this nonoperative approach for monitoring of fluid collection and its drainage from pseudocysts from the above cited experience of others.

Blunt abdominal trauma-induced intestinal perforation (largely proximal jejunal) may be detected by free air in the peritoneal cavity on cross-table lateral X-rays in the acutely traumatized child and dealt with accordingly with laparotomy.[2,3,7] A number of years ago, a preteen age boy on my service had received a severe blunt injury which rendered him unconscious for a week. He was maintained by nasogastric suction, intravenous fluids and antibiotics. At seven days post-injury, the patient suddenly awakened and equally suddenly complained of severe left upper quadrant abdominal pain. The marked local tenderness led to prompt laparotomy. At operation, the proximal jejunum was completely transected and the ends turned back and "matured" as established enterostomy stomas. There was no generalized peritonitis and only local inflammation of a mild degree. The "stomas" were excised and an end-to-end jejunal anastomosis was carried out. The postoperative course was quite uneventful and the patient was discharged home seven days following operation.

The principal cause of death in blunt trauma injured children is severe head injury. The management of blunt trauma abdominal injury and related blood loss and hypotension may impact in important ways on the outcome of severe head injuries. The Glasgow Coma Scale Score (Table 16.1) has proven to be the most useful means of assessing the severity of head trauma, following it and predicting outcome.[30,31] The score is influenced by additional factors including hypovolemia, hypoxia, cerebral swelling and intracranial pressure as well as intracranial hematomas. This Coma Scale Score has stood the test of time and has become an integral and anchor part of all other trauma scoring systems in children as well as adults.

A particularly important publication by Pigula et al[32] appeared in 1993 from Burlington, Vermont and the University of

Vermont concerning the effect of hypotension and hypoxia on children with severe head injuries. The authors cite that trauma is the leading (more than 50%) cause of death among children ages one to 14 with neurological injury present in approximately 90% of traumatized children and appearing to be the major (almost exclusive) factor affecting the outcome (especially in nonoperatively managed blunt abdominal trauma patients).[2,15] Several published studies have suggested that children recover from severe head injury better than adults and that the survival of children with Glasgow Coma Scale scores of less than 8 is better than adults, including the Pigula et al[32] University of Vermont study. Survival of normoxic and normotensive head injury children was increased four-fold over that of hypotensive and hypoxic patients. Employing National Pediatric Trauma Registry data to validate their own observations with a more limited number of children, they found that hypoxia alone was not associated with increased mortality in normotensive patients. On the other hand, hypotension significantly increased the mortality in these children even without coexisting hypoxia. The authors concluded that, in pediatric head injury, maintenance of systemic blood pressure is probably the most critical single factor affecting a favorable outcome (i.e. *survival*).

This data is of especial importance in the blunt traumatized child with both head injury and solid intraabdominal organ injury with bleeding when considering nonoperative versus operative management. The elimination of effective tamponade by anesthesia reduced tamponading abdominal muscle spasm and by open laparotomy may tilt the scales with respect to maintenance of adequate systemic blood pressure and its importance in the successful outcome of a severe head injury.

No consideration of trauma, blunt abdominal or otherwise, in childhood could come as close to the heart of the matter as Professor John Raffensperger's[33] heartfelt, beautifully expressed and very much to the point commentary in a Letter to the Edi-

Table 16.1. Glasgow coma scale scores

Eyes Open

Spontaneously	4
To speech	3
To pain	2
Never	1

Best Verbal Responses

Oriented	5
Confused	4
Inappropriate words	3
Incomprehensible sounds	2
Silent	1

Best Motor Response

Obey commands	6
Localizes pain	5
Flexion withdrawal	4
Decerebrate flexion	3
Decerebrate extension	2
No response	1

tor of the *Journal of Pediatric Surgery* which was published in the August 1987 issue and goes as follows (in its entirety):

> Dr. Harris's editorial on trauma in the January 1987, *Journal of Pediatric Surgery* failed to mention the subspecialist's role in pediatric trauma. Most children with major trauma suffer from head or orthopedic injuries. In fact, the most common cause of death in children with trauma is brain damage. The neurosurgeons at our hospital have treated 900 head injuries over the past 5 years. The role of the pediatric surgeon in these cases is to triage and resuscitate the patient, while the pediatric neurosurgeon is responsible for definitive care. We must, as pediatric surgeons, support our colleagues, the pediatric surgical subspecialists, particularly those in neurosurgery and orthopedics. There must be fellowships and residencies in these specialties that lead to certificates of special competence, just as we have in pediatric surgery. This is the best route to improved care of the injured child.

> Rather than be appalled by the small number of operations performed by applicants to the American Board of Surgery on patients with trauma, Dr. Harris should be pleased that surgeons are no longer doing needless operations on liver and spleen injuries. The experience of pediatric surgery residents in trauma is not measured by the number of operations performed, but by the patients who are evaluated, resuscitated, and successfully treated without an operation. Finally, I would argue with Dr. Harris about our knowledge of the epidemiology of childhood accidents. It is not rudimentary; childhood trauma is a social disease! Burns, gunshots, stabbings, and falls from high buildings are the consequences of poverty, carelessness and crowded living conditions! The worst possible injuries in children result from automobiles striking them on the street. Laws that rigorously punish careless or drunk drivers would reduce the mortality due these accidents. More playground facilities would keep children off the streets and bright orange vests would make children more visible on dark rainy nights. Preventative measures rather than bigger and better research programs are needed to reduce the morbidity and mortality of childhood trauma.

CHALLENGES

1. The most important challenge in the surgical management of blunt abdominal trauma in childhood is whether the principal and primary approach should be operative or nonoperative.

From my experience and from important recent publications, it is becoming increasingly clear and increasingly widely accepted that nonoperative management of blunt abdominal trauma in childhood is the best and safest way of preserving both life and vital, as well as critically important, organs. The liver and spleen are the principal sources of intraabdominal bleeding, and, in most operative cases, the bleeding has stopped by the time of laparotomy.

The almost universal abandonment of peritoneal lavage in childhood has eliminated a major laparotomy triggering stimulus. The increasing acceptance of the immunological importance of the spleen has greatly diminished the perception of the spleen as an "expendable" organ and sacrificable with impunity. The rather overwhelming evidence that laparotomy is the almost certain "kiss of death" in the presence of retrohepatic injury to hepatic veins and inferior vena cava with resultant rapid and overwhelming death from exsanguination should temper enthusiasm for laparotomy for hepatic injury. This is the almost exclusive cause of death from intraabdominal sources in blunt abdominal trauma.

Free air in the peritoneal cavity should be the only indication for laparotomy in cases of blunt abdominal trauma and this when the patient is resuscitated and hemodynamically stable. In cases of doubt or question, insufflation of air through the nasogastric tube may facilitate the identification on cross table lateral (or upright, if able) X-rays.

Prompt transfer of the blunt trauma injured child to the intensive care unit *after* rapid assessment of injury, cross table lateral X-ray for free air, admission blood work and type and cross match, placement of vascular access lines, placement of nasogastric tube and Foley catheter for gastrointestinal suction and for monitoring of urine output and appearance *is of the greatest importance.*

2. What is the most important approach to monitoring blunt abdominal trauma in childhood in the early posttrauma period?

Close and careful repeated clinical monitoring of vital signs, abdominal exam including palpation, auscultation and girth measurement, repeated hematocrit determinations, blood counts and amylase, etc. Hazardous movement about the hospital for unnecessary and potentially dangerous imaging and other procedures is counterindicated and condemned.

In commenting on a paper from Johns Hopkins before the American Pediatric Surgical Association in May of 1987 relating to the routine use of CT in abdominal monitoring of blunt trauma patients with head injuries, Professor John Raffensperger[34] of Chicago made some particularly sound and sage observations. He emphasized that

> you have to pay more attention to the physical examination" and went on to state that "unless there are positive findings either in terms of vital signs or change in the physical examination, there is probably no indication for laparotomy no matter what you find on your penetrating examination (i.e. peritoneal lavage) or on your CT scan.

3. How should transfusion requirements be determined and monitored in nonoperative management of blunt splenic and hepatic injuries in childhood(the major sources of significant intraabdominal/intraperitoneal cavity bleeding in blunt abdominal trauma in childhood)?

An especially sound and informative assessment and approach to this problem was presented in an important 1990 publication in the *Journal of Pediatric Surgery* by John Raffensperger and his associates[35] from the Children's Memorial Medical Center of Chicago (Northwestern University). They reviewed a clinical experience at their medical center with 37 children with blunt splenic or hepatic trauma treated by nonoperative management between November 1983 and September 1989. There was one death in a child with a lethal head injury. They found that the majority of those children with isolated injuries do not require blood transfusion and none required operation. Three children with multiple injuries underwent delayed laparotomy for reasons unrelated to active bleeding or blood loss. There were no late complications related to splenic or hepatic injuries. They found that two clinically distinct groups of 25 children received blood transfusions. One group consisted of eight patients with multiple injuries who were transfused during initial resuscitation when unstable or during early operation for other system (head or thoracic) trauma. These eight children were given a mean of 62.0 ml blood/kg of body weight. A second group of 17 children were transfused after initial resuscitation only because of decreasing blood counts. In this group, three patients with isolated spleen or liver injury received a mean of 16.5 ml blood/kg body weight and 14 stable patients with multiple injuries received a mean of 22.5 ml blood/kg body weight. Of the 12 children who received no transfusions, the hematocrit fell below 28% in four of these. In their discussion section of this publication, the authors state that "in retrospect, as many as 30% of the stable patients who were transfused after initial resuscitation would not be transfused by us today." The authors concluded that transfusion should be limited or withheld in hemodynamically stable children with blunt injuries to spleen, liver or both after initial resuscitation and that the hematocrit may decrease to 24 to 25% in these children without complications.

In the discussion section of their publication they emphasize that their review supports the safety of nonoperative management of children with blunt traumatic splenic and hepatic injuries. None of their nonoperatively managed patients required operation to treat a splenic or hepatic injury and none developed a late complication or died as a result of abdominal injuries. They make the particularly important point that "the condition of an acutely injured child with increasing intracranial pressure and/or pulmonary contusion may further deteriorate after an unnecessary anesthesia and surgery."

4. What is the proper role of imaging, scanning, etc. in the management of a child with blunt abdominal trauma?

They have no role, and indeed may be hazardous and consuming of critical away-from-intensive-care-unit time, in the acute and early management of children with blunt abdominal trauma with the exception of those with head trauma who should have head CT scanning only. Late identification of injured organs and extent of injury may be of value in determining periods of post-hospital periods of activity limitation. Ultrasound studies may be of value in later (nonacute) care in evaluating fluid collections around the pancreas or kidney.

In the discussion of the Raffensperger, Cosentino and associates paper on nonoperative management of blunt splenic and hepatic trauma in childhood cited above, Cosentino[36] states, "we usually follow them with serial hematocrits and serial examinations. We did not routinely get follow-up CT scans or ultrasound while they were in the hospital. *It all depended on their clinical course*" (italics by the author of this book).

5. Is some kind of anti-fulminant sepsis prophylaxis needed or advisable in children who lose their spleens as a result of blunt trauma.

The answer is emphatically yes! A 1952 report in the *Annals of Surgery* from the Department of Surgery of the Indiana University Medical Center in Indianapolis by Professors Harold King and Harris B.

Shumacker Jr.[37] recorded for the first time the occurrence of a high incidence of fatal bacterial infection in infants after splenectomy.

A 1980 article in the *World Journal of Surgery* by Leonard et al[38] has reviewed well the history of postsplenectomy sepsis and has stressed the gravity of this syndrome in adults as well as children. A major publication in 1982 by Holschneider et al[39] presented a follow-up series of 161 children who had undergone splenectomy for a variety of causes including trauma. The mean age at operation was 8 years. Since 1976, all patients received a three-year course of penicillin prophylaxis and, since 1979, vaccination against pneumococcal infections also has been given. Postoperative wound infection occurred in eight patients (5.3%) and peritonitis, pleuritis and bowel obstruction in another two. Twenty-four children (14.8%) acquired severe infections mainly due to pneumococcus (pneumonia, meningitis, sepsis) within four weeks following surgery. The overall mortality was 4.3%. However, 33.9% of the children with severe infections died. Forty-seven percent of the surviving children demonstrated leukocytosis while 50% were found to have lymphocytosis and 30% thrombocytosis following splenectomy. The authors strongly recommended preoperative pneumococcus vaccination and postoperative penicillin prophylaxis for three years.

Another 1982 publication, in *Surgery* by Mishalany, Mahnovski and Woolley,[40] addresses the sepsis problem, among others, in congenital asplenia infants. They reviewed the autopsy records of 36 patients with congenital asplenia (24 males and 12 females). The mean duration of survival was 13.8 months in males and 2.8 months in females. Twenty-eight children died in the first year, four between one and five years and three in adolescence. Thirty of the 36 deaths (86%) were due to sepsis.

A 1983 report in the *Journal of Trauma* by Caplan et al[41] presented evidence that pneumococcal vaccine can be administered early after splenectomy for trauma. In their study, 16 patients received polyvalent pneumococcal vaccine within 72 hours after splenectomy for trauma. At four weeks antibody levels were comparable to those of healthy controls.

The need for long-term prophylaxis in splenectomized children, as well as adults, has been recognized with increasing frequency in recent years. Although postsplenectomy infections occur most often in the first few years after spleen removal, the hazard of overwhelming and often rapidly fatal infection remains throughout life.[42,43]

A 1990 report by Murdoch and Dos Anjos[44] has clearly documented the need for long-term pneumococcus prophylaxis after splenectomy. The authors report an experience in which two children died from pneumococcal infection at extended periods postsplenectomy and post-stopping postsplenectomy prophylaxis with penicillin. One child had splenectomy for trauma at eight years of age. He was not vaccinated against pneumococcus and stopped taking prophylactic penicillin two years later. At the age of 13 he died of pneumococcal meningitis. A second child had splenectomy for trauma at four years of age. He was not vaccinated and had prophylactic penicillin which was stopped four years later at eight years of age. At the age of 12 he died of pneumococcal septicemia.

A 1992 report from Harvard and the Childrens Hospital of Boston reports the use of a conjugate vaccine against *Hemophilus influenza* type B polysaccharide encapsulated bacteria in children undergoing splenectomy.[45] This report is of the successful use of this conjugate vaccine. The authors emphasize that asplenic children are at risk for serious infection with polysaccharide encapsulated bacteria including *Hemophilus influenza* type B (HIB), *Streptococcus pneumoniae* and *Neisseria meningitidis*. HIB infection is the second most frequent organism after the pneumococci to cause postsplenectomy sepsis in younger children. Immunizations with polysaccharide vaccine are recommended for children undergoing splenectomy. In 1978, a 14-valent pneumococcal vaccine was licensed and in 1983 this was replaced by a 23-valent pure polysaccharide vaccine. Although older children respond to these pure polysaccharide vaccines, children under two years of age do not respond so reliably. Hence, the effort to achieve a conjugate vaccine. While the authors report the achievement of this conjugate vaccine for HIB, in the discussion of their paper, they state that the development of a pneumococcal conjugate vaccine, while in progress, is delayed by technical problems in linking all 23 serotypes to carrier proteins.

CONCLUSION

Blunt abdominal trauma in childhood represents one of the most critical and significant challenges in pediatric surgery. The early concept, derived largely from adult trauma experience, that early and emergent operation was the way to go had a dominant influence for many decades. A major trigger for operative intervention in pediatric blunt abdominal trauma was the peritoneal lavage. This operative intervention modality still is widely used in adult blunt abdominal trauma but thankfully has almost totally been abandoned and rejected by pediatric surgeons as both painful and frightening to an already injured child as well as misleading and unnecessary operation triggering.

I, from my personal experience and that of highly respected others, come down heavily in favor of nonoperative management of blunt abdominal trauma in childhood in the early and critical post-injury hours. The only indication for early operation in the stable child is evidence of intestinal perforation with free air in the peritoneal cavity.

None of the intraabdominal organs, spleen and liver, can be sacrificed by incision with safety and impunity. Although these organs are the major source of intraabdominal bleeding following major blunt trauma, in most cases the bleeding has stopped by the time of laparotomy. As operation for liver injury in the presence of retrohepatic lacerations of hepatic veins and inferior vena cava is almost always rapidly fatal from exsanguinating hemorrhage, operation here should scrupulously be avoided in favor of the much less hazardous nonoperative and do-not-disturb-the-beneficial-tamponade approach.

Retroperitoneal solid organs, kidneys and pancreas, also cannot be sacrificed with impunity and long-term responsibility in the case of the kidneys. Operative opening of Gerota's fascia in the presence of a ruptured kidney leads to almost certain loss of the kidney and should be avoided at all costs in favor of the much more satisfactory and organ preserving nonoperative approach. The pancreas is best observed and protected in the early post-traumatic period by nasogastric suction and TPN (total parenteral nutrition). It is more apt than the traumatized adult pancreas to heal spontaneously. Even post-traumatic pancreatic psuedocysts may heal spontaneously or require only percutaneous external aspiration drainage (PED).

The operative or nonoperative management of blunt abdominal trauma in childhood may have an important impact on survival in the presence of a serious coexisting head injury where an unnecessary anesthesia and operation may have a tamponade eliminating and hypotension inducing effect with accompanying aggravation of the head injury.

References

1. Vane D, Shedd FG, Grosfeld JL et al. An analysis of pediatric trauma deaths in Indiana. J Pediatr Surg 1990; 25:955-960.

2. Sinclair MC, Moore TC. Major surgery for abdominal and thoracic trauma in childhood and adolescence. J Pediatr Surg 1974; 9:155-162.

3. Sinclair MC, Moore TC, Asch MJ et al. Injury of hollow abdominal viscera from blunt trauma in childhood and adolescence. Am J Surg 1974; 128:693-698.

4. Sinclair MC, Moore TC, Asch MJ. Penetrating abdominal injuries in childhood and adolesence. Am Surg 1975; 41:342-346.

5. Moore TC, Peter M. Thru-and-thru gunshot penetration of distal abdominal aorta in a 4-year-old child managed by aortic transsection, debridement and reanastomosis with survival. J Trauma 1979; 19:537-539.

6. Asch MJ, Lachman RS, Lippmann M et al. Truck aerial impailment injury of the thorax: Report of a case in an 8-year-old boy. J Pediatr Surg 1974; 9:251-252.

7. Shabot MM, Asch MJ, Moore TC. Cecal perforation due to blunt abdominal trauma in childhood. Zeitschr Kinderchir 1979; 28:272-277.

8. Moore TC, Lachman RS. Distal mechanical small bowel obstruction as a sequelae of blunt trauma pancreatitis in childhood. Zeitschr Kinderchir 1981; 34:296-298.

9. Hood JM, Smyth BT. Nonpenetrating intraabdominal injuries in children. J Pediatr Surg 1974; 9:69-77.

10. Upadhyaya P, Simpson JS. Splenic trauma in children. Surg Gynec Obstet 1968; 126:781-790.

11. Douglas GJ, Simpson JS. The conservative management of splenic trauma. J Pediatr Surg 1971; 6:565-569.

12. Pearl RH, Wesson DE, Spence LJ et al. Splenic injury: A 5-year update with improved results and changing criteria for conservative management. J Pediatr Surg 1989; 24:121-125.

13. Karp MP, Cooney DR, Pros GA et al. The nonoperative management of pediatric hepatic trauma. J Pediatr Surg 1983; 18:512-518.

14. Oldham KT, Grico KS, Ryckman F et al. Blunt liver injury in childhood:Evolution of therapy and current perspective. Surgery 1986; 100:542-549.

15. Moore TC. Nonoperative management of blunt abdominal trauma in childhood. Surgery 1987; 101:380-381.

16. Giacomantonio M, Filler RM, Rich RH. Blunt hepatic trauma in children: Experience with oeprative and nonoperative management. J Pediatr Surg 1984; 19:519-522.

17. Galant JA, Grisoni ER, Gauderer MWL. Pediatric blunt liver injury: Establishment of criteria for appropriate management. J Pediatr Surg 1990; 25:1162-1165.

18. Moulton SL, Lynch FP, Hoyt DB et al. Operative intervention for pediatric liver injuries: Avoiding delay in treatment. J Pediatr Surg 1992; 27:958-963.

19. Cwyes S, Millar AJW. Blunt liver trauma in children: Nonoperative management. J

Pediatr Surg 1985; 20:14-18.

20. Stone HH, Ansley JD. Management of liver trauma in children. J Pediatr Surg 1977; 12:3-10.

21. Amroch D, Schiaron G, Carmignola G et al. Isolated blunt liver trauma: Is non-operative treatment justified? J Pediatr Surg 1992; 27:466-468.

22. Walt AJ. Founders Lecture. The mythology of hepatic trauma—or Babel revisited. Am J Surg 1978; 135:12-18.

23. Mandour WA, Lai MK, Linke CA et al. Blunt renal trauma in the pediatric patient. J Pediatr Surg 1981; 16:669-675.

24. Moore TC, Berne TV, Martin DC et al. Multi-institutional use of a mobile kidney preservation unit. Transplantation 1971; 12:526-527.

25. Moore TC, Berne TV, English TS. Use of mobile transplantation unit in a large metropolitan area. Am J Surg 1972; 124: 229-233.

26. Moore TC, English TS, Berne TV. Machine preservation of 302 human cadaver kidneys for transplantation. Surg Gynec Obstet 1974; 138:239-243.

27. Bass DH, Semple PL, Cwyes S. Investigation and management of blunt renal injuries in children: A review of 11 years experience. J Pediatr Surg 1991; 26:196-200.

28. Gorenstein A, O'Halpin D, Wesson DE et al. Blunt injury to the pancreas in children: Selective management based on ultrasound. J Pediatr Surg 1987; 22:1110-1116.

29. Bass J, DiLorenzo M, Desjardins JG et al. Blunt pancreatic injuries in children: The role of percutaneous external drainage in the treatment of pancreatic pseudocysts. J Pediatr Surg 1988; 23:721-724.

30. Grewal M, Sutcliffe AJ. Early prediction of outcome following head injury in children: An assessment of the value of the Glasgow Coma Scale Score trend and abdominal plantar and pupillary light reflexes. J Pediatr Surg 1991; 26:1161-1163.

31. Wisner DH. History and current status of trauma scoring systems. Arch Surg 1992; 127:111-117.

32. Pigula FA, Wald SL, Shackford SR et al. The effect of hypotension and hypoxia on children with severe head injuries. J Pediatr Surg 1993; 28:310-316.

33. Raffensperger JG. Letter to the Editor. J Pediatr Surg 1987; 22:797.

34. Raffensperger JG. Discussion of paper by Beaver BL et al. J Pediatr Surg 1987; 22:1121.

35. Consentino CM, Luck SR, Barthe PMJ et al. Transfusion requirements in conservative nonoperative management of blunt splenic and hepatic injuries during childhood. J Pediatr Surg 1990; 25:950-953.

36. Cosentino CM. Discussion of paper by Cosentino CM et al. J Pediatr Surg 1990; 25:953.

37. King H, Shumacker HB Jr. Splenic studies: I. Susceptibility to infection after splenectomy performed in infancy. Ann Surg 1952; 136:239-242.

38. Leonard AS, Grebink CS, Baesl TJ et al. The overwhelming postsplenectomy sepsis problem. World J Surg 1980; 4:423-432.

39. Holschneider AM, Kircz-Klimeck H, Strasser B et al. Complications of splenectomy in childhood. Zeitschr Chir 1982; 35:130-139.

40. Mishalany H, Mahnovski V, Woolley MM. Congenital asplenia and anomalies of the gastrointestinal tract. Surgery 1982; 91:38-41.

41. Caplan ES, Boltansky H, Snyder MJ et al. Response of traumatized splenectomized patients to immediate vaccination with polyvalent pneumococcal vaccine. J Trauma 1983; 23:801-805.

42. Wahlby L, Domellof L. Splenectomy after blunt abdominal trauma. A retrospective study of children. Acta Clin Scand 1981; 147:131-135.

43. Malangoni MA, Dillon LD, Klamer TW et al. Factors influencing the risk of early and late serious infection in adults after splenectomy for trauma. Surgery 1989; 96:775-783.

44. Murdoch IA, Dos Anjos R. Continued need for pneumococcal prophylaxis after splenectomy. Arch Dis Child 1990; 65: 1268-1269.

45. Ambrosino DM, Lee M-L C, Chen D et al. Response to *Hemophilus influena* type B conjugate vaccine in children undergoing splenectomy. J Pediatr Surg 1992; 27: 1045-1048.

INVITED COMMENTARY

David L. Collins, M.D.
Pediatric Surgeon, Medical Group of San Diego
Clinical Professor of Surgery
University of California, San Diego

I agree completely with the principles stated by Dr. Moore in that surgeons in general do too much unnecessary surgery, particularly for solid organ damage. The only true indication for a laparotomy is evidence of perforation of a hollow viscus.

As one of four or five pediatric surgeons on call for a busy trauma center to which all pediatric trauma cases are triaged from the entire San Diego County area, I have put in several consecutive years between cases on which I have operated.

The place of laparoscopy in the diagnosis of acute blunt abdominal trauma is yet to be defined, but it may have some application in detecting small bowel perforations, which sometimes leak fluid only. They are not diagnosable by plain X-rays.

Charles E. Bagwell, M.D.
Professor of Surgery and Pediatrics
Chairman, Division of Pediatric Surgery
Medical College of Virginia, Richmond

The magnitude of trauma as a cause of childhood death and injury can hardly be overemphasized. An approach to blunt abdominal trauma which emphasizes a nonoperative approach as advocated by the author is probably accepted by most pediatric surgeons currently. However, incumbent upon this nonoperative approach is some means for diagnostic assessment of intra-abdominal injury or injuries. Once these injuries are recognized, the child can be appropriately monitored in a setting which allows expedient resuscitation and/or surgical intervention should deterioration occur. Routine diagnostic testing is of little value based on mechanism of injury alone. However, the patient whose physical examination is unreliable due to associated injuries (rib fractures, severe abdominal wall contusions) or CNS alteration (injury, drugs or alcohol) should have diagnostic tests (in our institution, double contrast CAT scan) as should the patient with equivocal or suggestive signs of intra-abdominal injury.

While the presence of free air represents an absolute indication for surgical exploration, there is still a role for surgical intervention in the child with continued or massive hemorrhage in the face of directed transfusion of appropriate amounts. While such patients are uncommon, they continue to require the services of pediatric trauma surgeons; the occasional child with an injured spleen will still require laparotomy and splenectomy, even after timely attempts at splenic salvage.

Peritoneal lavage is now considered a test of diagnostic importance by only a small minority of pediatric surgeons since the presence of blood no longer serves as an accurate marker for intra-abdominal injury which requires operative intervention. Of greater concern, however, is the possibility of hollow viscus injury resulting in leakage of enteric contents

into the peritoneal cavity without pneumoperitoneum. Reports documenting such cases of intestinal perforation from blunt trauma with some
delay in diagnosis have not demonstrated an increased mortality or morbidity associated with this delay.[1] Of great concern to all pediatric trauma
surgeons is the dramatic rise in cases of penetrating abdominal wound in
children, especially those from gunshot. The improved results from
nonoperative treatment of blunt abdominal trauma pales in comparison
to the lethality of these injuries in children of all ages.

REFERENCE

1. Cobb LM, Vinocur CD, Wagner CW et al. Intestinal perforation due to blunt
trauma in children in an era of increased nonoperative treatment. J Trauma
1986; 26:461-463.

Professor Sidney Cwyes
Head, Department of Paediatric Surgery
Red Cross War Memorial Children's Hospital, Rondebosch
University of Cape Town, South Africa

Nonoperative management of splenic, liver and renal injuries, following blunt abdominal trauma in childhood, is practiced in most
paediatric surgical centres. Constant monitoring and assessment of these
patients is important for further bleeding and for bowel perforations which
are notoriously difficult to diagnose as so many of them do not exhibit
free air in the abdomen. So too occult spinal cord injury and diaphragmatic injury may be missed.

Although the nonoperative management of splenic, hepatic and renal injuries is the accepted form of treatment, one should question whether
under circumstances where there are no facilities for monitoring these
patients and where one does not have a sophisticated blood transfusion
system (as in developing countries), an initial laparotomy and repair of
the ruptured organ would not be a wiser form of treatment. (Blood transfusion risk, J.A.M.A. 1988)

The biggest challenge lies in the *prevention* of these accidental injuries. Child accident prevention centres have concerned themselves with
in-depth research into the causes of injury and then planned adequate
preventive strategies. Effective injury control means changing both the
environment and the people's behavior. In many countries there is a great
migration towards the cities and as urbanization progresses, more and more
children will be newly exposed to technological hazards in an over-crowded,
stressful and indeed violent environment, with inadequate safety awareness or precautions. I believe pediatric surgeons are in the forefront in
meeting this challenge.

John G. Raffensperger, M.D.
Professor of Surgery, Northwestern University
Surgeon-in-Chief, Children's Memorial Hospital, Chicago
Editor, *Swenson's Pediatric Surgery*

My experience with blunt abdominal trauma parallels that of Dr.
Moore. As a resident in the 1950's and up until about 1972, we regularly operated on children after blunt abdominal trauma when they showed
signs of abdominal tenderness or whenever we found free blood in the

peritoneal cavity. In spite of my repeated observation that often the bleeding was from a very minor laceration of the liver or spleen and that the bleeding had stopped and that occasionally there was free blood in the peritoneal cavity as a result of a retroperitoneal hematoma, we continued to operated for these indications. There was a time when we used liver/spleen scans and angiography to diagnose injuries of solid abdominal organs. I was horrified by the idea that injuries to the spleen could simply be observed. In spite of these early reservations, we have not operated on a ruptured spleen at the Children's Memorial Hospital in Chicago for twenty years. We have also observed children with major liver lacerations that were verified by CT scan. Until I read Dr. Moore's chapter, I still thought that we should operate on those children with blunt abdominal trauma who were unstable and who required massive blood transfusions. Upon reflection, however, I realized that all of those children in that category had not only severe liver lacerations but lacerations of the hepatic veins and inferior vena cava and they have all died. In retrospect, I believe these children would have been better served by continuing the blood transfusions without an operation. Perhaps if one does feel compelled to operate in this situation, one should wait until one has several large cannulas in place and perhaps even facilities for cardiopulmonary bypass. Then, combining a sternal splitting and midline incision, it might be possible to control the cava and the aorta and possibly repair the injuries. This, however, may very well be wishful thinking.

I do disagree with Dr. Moore about the treatment of pseudocysts of the pancreas. Yes, one can keep a child in the hospital for a month or two and treat them with nasogastric drainage and total parenteral nutrition. One can hasten their recovery, however, with a lateral, abdominal incision and then opening the lesser sac just in front of the spleen and placing several large suction drains. This external drainage will promptly allow the child to eat and leave the hospital. Percutaneous external drainage is not likely to be effective because the catheters used are too small to take care of the turbid fluid with fibrinous material and fat necrosis. Finally, when a transsected pancreas is identified on CT scan, the patient is best served by either a distal pancreatectomy or some type of a Roux-Y drainage procedure.

CHAPTER 17

APPENDICITIS

INTRODUCTION

Appendicitis is the most common major and serious surgical problem to be encountered in childhood years. Important reports in 1968 from Richmond (Virginia) by Salzberg and White[1] and in 1971 from Melbourne (Australia) by Fowler[2] addressed the crucial issue of mortality from acute appendicitis in a large series over extended periods of time. Salzberg and White reported a mortality of 0.33% (one case of 330 children) in a five year period (1961 to 1966) at the Medical College of Virginia. This death involved a patient with ruptured appendicitis and massive peritoneal cavity contamination. Their series incidence of perforation in childhood was 32%. Fowler reported a 20-year mortality at the Royal Children's Hospital of Melbourne of 0.2% (13 deaths in 5,566 patients with acute appendicitis). Mortality in the Fowler report was highest in cases involving perforation and generalized peritonitis and especially in children under five years of age with these complications. He considered antibiotics to have made the most important contribution to this reduced mortality in infancy and childhood appendicitis.

Several reports have focused upon the greater hazards and more difficult diagnosis in infants under two and three years of age. Snyder and Chaffin[3] of Los Angeles in 1952 in *Archives of Surgery* reported a mortality rate of 29% in children under two years of age with appendicitis. This was before the availability of antibiotics. Bartlett et al[4] in 1970 reported a 15 year experience from the Children's Hospital of Boston involving 40 infants under the age of two years with acute appendicitis. Ninety percent of these 40 infants were between the first and second years of life. The youngest patient was seven days old and only four infants were under one year of age. A perforation had occurred in 82% of the 40 patients. Lethargy, irritability and anorexia were the major symptoms noted by the parents and the majority had been under physician care for a diagnosis other than acute appendicitis with an average lag of four days from onset of symptoms to hospital referral and admission. Vomiting was a major early symptom and was observed in 36 of the infants (90%). Pain, difficult to evaluate in infants, was reported in 25 of the 40 (62.5%). Temperature elevation was found in 33 of the 40 (82.5%). On physical examination, 31 of the 40 (77.5%) appeared acutely ill, pale, dehydrated and in obvious distress. X-ray examination of the abdomen (flat and upright) in 21 patients studied was helpful in establishing or confirming the diagnosis in 18 (85.7%).[5] While there was no mortality, significant postoperative morbidity was experienced including prolonged or recurrent ileus in seven (17.5%).

Another experience with appendicitis in the first two years of life was reported in 1973 from the Children's Hospital of Columbus (Ohio) by Grosfeld and associates.[6] Their experience (1955 to 1970) involved 32 patients 24 months of age and younger with a mean age at admission of 17 months. Four of their patients were in the first year of life with three of them being neonates. The youngest was nine days of age. Sixteen of the 32 patients (50%) had been seen by a family physician or in the hospital emergency room at some time in the early course of their illness. All 16 patients were sent home with some diagnosis other than appendicitis. At the time of hospital admission 11 of the 32 (33%) were admitted to the pediatric medical service with an incorrect diagnosis. Of the 21 patients admitted to the pediatric surgery service, the initial diagnosis was acute appendicitis in only 10 of the 21 (47.6%) An additional 16 hour delay occurred between the time of admission to the hospital and operation.

Fever and vomiting were the most common symptoms and were found in 26 of the 32 (81.3%) in this Columbus experience. Other symptoms were irritability in 16 (50%), anorexia in 13 (40.6%), lethargy in 10 (31.3%), diarrhea in eight (25%), constipation in three, convulsions in two and scrotal swelling in one. At operation, perforation was found in 28 of the 31 patients who were operated upon (90.3%). There were three deaths (9.3%) and 50% of the patients had postoperative complications with prolonged adynamic (paralytic) ileus being the most frequently encountered complication.

A more recent (1988) 12 year experience (1972 to 1984) with acute appendicitis in the first three years of life was reported from the Adelaide Children's Hospital (Aus-

tralia) by Barker and Davey.[7] Their report included 13 cases with ages ranging from 16 to 36 months and a mean age of 25 months. The most frequently encountered symptoms were vomiting (85%) and abdominal pain (84%). All 13 patients were febrile and the abdominal X-ray was abnormal and helpful in diagnosis in 84% of the cases. At operation, gangrene and perforation were found in 70%. Postoperative complications included wound infection (15%) and bowel obstruction (15%). There were no deaths.

One of the most important developments in the management of perforated appendicitis in childhood in the past 20 years has been the recognition of the importance of anaerobic bacteria in the polymicrobial "mix"[8-10] and the search for the appropriate combination of antibiotic management to control a mixed aerobic and anaerobic population of enteric bacteria.[11,12] Professor Medad Schiller of Israel (Hadassah University Hospital, Jerusalem) and associates[12] in 1976 presented in the *Journal of Pediatric Surgery* a particularly interesting and important observation concerning antibiotic coverage in ruptured appendicitis in childhood. Their study was triggered by an observation during the October 1973 war that the use of clindamycin systemically was of value in the management of penetrating abdominal wounds. This observation and experience encouraged Professor Schiller and his associates to use clindamycin in colorectal surgery in pediatric surgical patients. Their report described their experience with a combination of gentamycin and clindamycin in a series of 25 pediatric surgical patients. In 9 of 11 patients with perforated appendicitis *B. fragilis* was isolated from the peritoneal cavity. "There was rapid clinical response to treatment in all cases", the authors reported.

In 1982, I returned from a four year clinical surgery hiatus to do first a research sabbatical and then a basic science Ph.D. in molecular immunology in England at the University of Cambridge to discover an almost miraculous change in the postoperative course of ruptured appendicitis in childhood. The routine use of "triple antibiotics" (ampicillin, gentamycin and clindamycin) both pre- and postoperatively appeared to be an important component of this "sea change" in the postoperative course of ruptured appendicitis in childhood. Other factors also were considered as a therapeutic protocol for acute appendicitis in infancy and childhood was set up and put in place. In addition to the use of "triple antibiotics" this included careful preoperative fluid and electrolyte resuscitation, prompt operation and appendectomy through a small (2-3 cm) lateral McBurney muscle splitting incision with Penrose drain drainage of the peritoneal cavity through the center of a primarily closed incision in cases of gangrene and/or perforation with scrupulous avoidance of peritoneal cavity lavage. This experience at $4^1/_2$ years with 230 consecutive cases of acute appendicitis was reported in the June 1990 issue of the *American Journal of Surgery*.[13] The incidence of perforation in this experience was 47% and 32% of the children were aged six years and younger. During this period 10 normal appendices were removed for a normal appendix rate of 4%. There were no deaths and a major morbidity of less than 1% in cases of both unruptured and ruptured acute appendicitis. The rapid transition from serious illness to near normalcy in a remarkably few number of hours was one of the most impressive and remarkable observations in this entire experience.

The factors involved in the continuing high morbidity in association with ruptured acute appendicitis in many comparatively recent reports will be considered in more detail in the Challenges section of this chapter.

CHALLENGES

1. The most important challenge in the management of acute appendicitis in infancy and childhood is achieving prompt diagnosis and effective therapy (appendectomy) and the elimination of perforation-inducing delay.

This is of particular importance in the early years of life where the symptoms and findings may be more confusing and "atypical" with respect to the more "traditional" findings associated with acute appendicitis in older children (and adults). This problem of acute appendicitis diagnosis in the first two years of life was vividly illustrated by the 1973 report of Grosfeld, Weinberger and Clatworthy[6] and discussed in some detail in the Introduction section of this chapter. It is also a continuing and increasing problem with children of all ages as the March 1993 report from Cleveland (Ohio) by Linz et al[14] tellingly illustrates. The title of their publication in the *Journal of Pediatric Surgery* is "Does the Current Health Care Environment Contribute to Increased Morbidity and Mortality of Acute Appendicitis in Children?" The answer to this important question was a resounding *yes*! Their study at the Rainbow Babies and Children's Hospital of Cleveland (Case Western Reserve University School of Medicine) was carried out "to determine whether the current 'gatekeeper' controls on health care lead to an increase in treatment delay and morbidity of acute appendicitis in children". They compared an earlier (July 1, 1978 to June 30, 1980) experience with a more recent (July 1, 1988 to June 30, 1990) one. The two groups were quite comparable with respect to major result and response factors such as age, race, sex, antecedent illness and negative appendectomy rate. A major difference in the two groups of patients was that more patients in the more recent group were seen initially in an emergency room or urgent care setting (62.2% versus 48.5%). In addition the accuracy of the initial diagnosis was significantly lower in the more recent group (p = 0.05). There was no difference in the two groups regarding the time to a physician. There was, however, a significant difference in the time to a surgeon (p = 0.04). There was no difference in time from surgeon to operation. These misdiagnosis-induced delays in surgeon referrals and operation resulted in an increased morbidity from 6.5% in the earlier group to 13.3% in the 10 year later and more recent group. Of particular importance was the finding that a more complex morbidity had occurred in the more recent group. *This included six patients with two or more complications and two deaths as compared with one patient with multiple complications and no deaths in the 10 year earlier group*! The authors of this very important communication concluded the summary of their publication as follows:

> In the interval of 10 years at a children's hospital, it now takes more time for patients with acute appendicitis to reach the pediatric surgeon, with a subsequent trend toward more frequent and complex morbidity. Factors in the current health care environment to account for these findings include changes in the initial physician-contact setting, greater misdiagnosis and delayed surgical referral. Greater physician and public education is necessary to deter these trends.

2. The second most important challenge involves the selection of the most effective and safest antibiotic coverage, before and after operation, in cases of gangrenous and ruptured acute appendicitis and the duration of this coverage and with emphasis on the control of both aerobic and anaerobic microorganisms in a complex and serious polybacterial setting.

My current and recent and more remote past experiences of the author of this book come down rather strongly in favor of the use of the "triple antibiotics" approach employing ampicillin, gentamycin and clindamycin (with metronidazole/Flagyl as an option for clindamycin particularly in cases with diarrhea where amebiasis is a possibility).

Two reports at different periods (1974 and 1982) from the Hospital for Sick Children of Toronto (Canada) are most revealing. A 1974 publication in the *Journal of Pediatric Surgery* by Shandling et al[15] explored the usefulness of antibiotics in the treatment of appendiceal peritonitis in children *and found none*. They concluded their

report with the following statement: "Antibiotics cannot supplant sound surgical principles and techniques in the treatment of perforating appendicitis." A subsequent, 1982, publication in the same journal from the same institution, but with different authors,[16] in a careful study of 300 children with gangrenous or perforated appendicitis concluded that "patients with local perforation or generalized peritonitis had a high incidence of infective complications if they were not treated with antibiotics. Children treated with ampicillin, gentamycin and clindamycin had markedly fewer wound infections and abscesses and were able to go home sooner than those receiving ampicillin and/or gentamycin."

In 1980, Brook[17] had reported in *Annals of Surgery* a significant study of 112 bacterial specimens from ruptured acute appendicitis in children from the Children's Hospital National Medical Center of Washington, D.C. Bacterial growth was found in 100 peritoneal fluid specimens. Anaerobic bacteria alone were encountered in 14 specimens, aerobes alone in 12 and mixed aerobic and anaerobic bacteria in 74 specimens. These findings clearly indicated the polymicrobial aerobic and anaerobic nature of peritoneal cavity fluid in children with perforated acute appendicitis.

King et al[18] of Columbus (Ohio) Children's Hospital in 1983 reported the results of a prospective, randomized, double blind clinical trial comparing the "triple antibiotics" combination of ampicillin, gentamycin and clindamycin (AGC) with a combination of ampicillin and gentamycin (AG) with an added placebo in patients with complicated appendicitis (gangrene or perforation). Thirty one patients were in each group. AGC patients experienced fewer therapeutic failures (3 versus 23%; p = 0.05), shorter durations of fever (2.9 ± 0.5 days versus 4.7 ± 0.9 days; p = 0.08). The authors concluded that "on the basis of this experience the routine use of gentamycin, ampicillin and clindamycin is recommended for all children with complicated appendicitis."

A 1980 report from Vancouver (Canada) in *Annals of Surgery* by Smith et al[19] had compared the effectiveness of metronidazole and clindamycin in the treatment of intra-abdominal sepsis in a prospective, double blind study. They found that the two antibiotics (each in combination with tobramycin) were of equal efficacy and that there was no difference with respect either to defervescence or the duration of infection.

3. The challenge to drain (Penrose drain) in cases of ruptured appendicitis and to bring the drain out through the center of a primary wound closure may be a problem to some.

But not to me, who prefers all of the above. In my 1990 publication in the *American Journal of Surgery*,[13] the experience of Professor John Raffensperger[20] of Chicago with drainage for ruptured appendicitis was cited. In his excellent text book of pediatric surgery (Swenson's Pediatric Surgery), Professor Raffensperger cites a Cook County (Illinois) Children's Hospital experience where three of four children who died of ruptured appendicitis did not have drainage. The institution then began to use drains routinely, with no deaths in the following 810 appendectomies. My own 12-year-old son almost died of an undrained ruptured appendicitis following operation in a far distant city near where my son was attending prep school. Promptly returning to Los Angeles with me, my son spent one month in the UCLA University Hospital under the superlative care of Professor William P. Longmire Jr. with multiple wound and pelvic abscesses, 20 pound weight loss, scoliosis, daily high temperature spikes, etc. One major operation and almost a second was required. Thanks to the outstanding skill and judgment of Professor Longmire he finally survived and left the hospital. This personal experience with drainage or nondrainage in cases of ruptured appendicitis in childhood reinforced my already strong opinion on this issue. In recent years, this opinion has further been reinforced by my personal operative experience with the use of extensive peritoneal cavity drainage with bilateral Penrose

drains in the "patch, drain and wait" approach to necrotizing enterocolitis in the newborn,[21] as well as to midgut volvulus with extensive necrosis.[22]

4. Another point of challenge (even controversy) is the issue of whether or not to employ peritoneal lavage in cases of ruptured appendicitis in childhood.

Here again the author of this book has some rather strong feelings based upon personal experience and this is strongly against lavage as of much more harm (rather than good) with respect to widespread dissemination of sepsis and abscess formations in areas remote from the perforation and initial peritoneal cavity septic contamination, generally relatively localized or drain localizable.

A 1990 report by Putnam et al[23] from Rochester (New York) in *Surgery, Gynecology and Obstetrics* involving 406 consecutive children operated upon for acute appendicitis with a perforation rate of 20.5% and "triple antibiotic" coverage with an aminoglycoside, ampicillin and clindamycin recorded that complications in ruptured appendicitis patients with generalized or extensive localized peritonitis managed by "complete peritoneal lavage" were double those of patients of this sort who had no lavage. Peritoneal lavage with saline was associated in 76 patients versus no lavage in 48 patients for perforated appendicitis with a complication rate of 19.7% versus 8.3%. In the crucial areas of small intestinal obstruction requiring operation for lysis of adhesions (4 cases) and prolonged paralytic ileus (4 cases), the incidence of complications was 10.6% versus 0%. They concluded that the lavage undertaking rather than the disease process was responsible for this greater incidence of postoperative complications in their children with ruptured acute appendicitis. It also was of interest that their rate of normal appendices was 1.7%.

The peritoneal lavage issue was also approachable through a recent 1993 report by Curran and Muenchow[24] involving a recent (1987-1988) two year experience with 656 emergency appendectomies at the

Los Angeles County-USC Medical Center in Los Angeles (sister hospital of the author's Los Angeles Country-Harbor UCLA Medical Center). Like the author's Harbor-UCLA Medical Center and location of his 1990 report,[13] the Los Angeles County-USC Medical Center is also a public/"county" hospital for poor and medically indigent patients. Their patient population included 394 children 12 years of age or less and in 227 of these patients with acute appendicitis the appendix was perforated or gangrenous (57%). This compared with a 47% perforation rate in the 1990 report of the Harbor-UCLA Medical Center experience with 230 consecutive cases of acute appendicitis in children 13 years of age or younger. Their patient population Hispanic rate of 83% was comparable to the Harbor-UCLA Hispanic child rate of 67% and overall perforation rate of 47% with a perforation rate of 57% in the Hispanic group of children.

Like the Harbor-UCLA experience, the Los Angeles County-USC Medical Center protocol and treatment involved perioperative antibiotics with gentamycin and clindamycin, appendectomy through a muscle-splitting incision and peritoneal drainage through the lateral aspect of the wound with skin closure. The only significant major difference in management at these two Los Angeles County hospitals was the use of peritoneal cavity lavage with saline at USC. Their complication rate was 19%, with 8% developing intraabdominal abscesses, 5% with bowel obstructions and 11% "minor" complications involving prolonged paralytic ileus and prolonged fever. These complications are substantially greater than the major complications rate of less than 1% in ruptured appendicitis without peritoneal lavage.

Four children at the Harbor-UCLA Medical Center were found to have intraabdominal abscesses in ruptured appendicitis after the close of the 1990 study.[13] On careful questioning of the involved residents, it was found that all four (three by one resident) had been subjected to peritoneal lavage.

5. A relatively minor challenge is whether any additional "high-tech" studies such as ultrasound, barium enema, CT scan or the use of technetium labeled leukocytes are needed or even worth doing in "establishing" more firmly the diagnosis of acute appendicitis beyond the traditional history, physical examination, abdominal X-ray and laboratory studies, especially the white blood cell leukocyte count.

The answer here is decidedly *no*! The most important single diagnostic point in acute appendicitis in childhood is right lower quadrant (McBurney's point) tenderness on palpation. The rest of the "traditional" points are helpful but without tenderness are suspect. A high fever, marked elevation of the leukocyte count, generalized abdominal tenderness, a fecalith and paralytic ileus findings on abdominal X-ray and a silent abdomen on careful auscultation point toward a ruptured appendicitis with likely extensive local or generalized peritonitis. All of this can be achieved by going and remaining "low-tech".

This has been well expressed recently (1990) by Burton H. Harris[25] of Boston: "The most sensitive, specific and predictive test for appendicitis is abdominal examination by an experienced pediatric surgeon. Since no one without peritoneal signs should have an operation for appendicitis, leukocyte imaging (and CT, barium enema, and ultrasound) are occasionally helpful, but there is no substitute for clinical diagnosis."

6. Laparoscopy

Minimally invasive laparoscopy has had considerable employment in acute appendicitis in childhood, especially in older children. The use of the very small (2-3 cm) very lateral McBurney-type muscle splitting incision as recommended, used and reported upon by me satisfies the minimally invasive small-incision(s) basis of laparoscopy. Indeed, the summation of laparoscopy incisions in childhood appendectomy is likely to be greater than the 2-3 cm single incision employed by me.

While it is true that incisions heal from side to side, it also is true that they *hurt from end to end.*

The most logical and appropriate use of laparoscopy for acute appendicitis in childhood is the older female child in the age groups where tubo-ovarian malfunction or inflammation may mimic acute appendicitis.

CONCLUSION

Acute appendicitis remains one of the most challenging and satisfying major and serious surgical problems and disorders of childhood years. It is particularly satisfying that the "art" of medicine still remains intact here and that the humble clinician and his years of experience cannot be replaced by some glamorous, awesome and *very, very* expensive "high tech" machine.

My 1990 publication in the *American Journal of Surgery*[13] reports the lowest incidence of major morbidity (less than 1%) after operation to be published for both nonperforated and perforated acute appendicitis. The use of preoperative fluid and electrolyte resuscitation with "triple antibiotics" (with ampicillin, gentamycin and clindamycin), small, lateral McBurney-type muscle splitting incision, prompt appendectomy, peritoneal cavity drainage with small soft Penrose drains placed both up and down, scrupulous avoidance of peritoneal cavity lavage, and wound closure up to the drain exiting in the central part of the incision may have contributed to these excellent results achieved by senior surgical residents operating under faculty supervision and under established management protocol.

REFERENCES

1. Salzberg AM, White NK. Current mortality for appendicitis in infants and children. Am J Surg 1968; 115:651-652.
2. Fowler R. Childhood mortality from acute appendicitis: The impact of antibiotics. Med J Aust 1971; 2:1009-1014.
3. Snyder WH, Chaffin L. Appendicitis in the first two years of life. Arch Surg 1952; 64:549-560.
4. Bartlett RH, Eraklis AJ, Wilkinson RH. Appendicitis in infancy. Surg Gynec Obstet 1970; 130:99-104.
5. Wilkinson RH, Bartlett RH, Eraklis AJ. Diagnosis of appendicitis in infancy: The value of abdominal radiographs. Am J Dis Child 1969; 118:687-690.
6. Grosfeld JL, Weinberger M, Clatworthy HW. Acute appendicitis in the first two years of life. J Pediatr Surg 1973; 8:285-292.
7. Barker AP, Davey RB. Appendicitis in the first years of life. Aust NZ J Surg 1988; 58:491-494.
8. Stone HH, Kolb LD, Geheber CE. Incidence and significance of intraperitoneal anaerobic bacteria. Ann Surg 1975; 181: 705-714.
9. Douglas B, Vesey B. *Bacteroides*: A cause of residual abscess? J Pediatr Surg 1975; 10:215.
10. Gorbach SL, Bartlett JG. Anaerobic infections. New Eng J Med 1974; 290:1177, 1237 & 1269.
11. Stone HH. Bacterial flora of appendicitis in children. J Pediatr Surg 1976; 11:37-42.
12. Berlatzky Y, Rubin SZ, Michel J et al. Use of clindamycin and gentamycin in pediatric colonic surgery. J Pediatr Surg 1976; 11:943-948.
13. Gamal R, Moore TC. Appendicitis in children aged 13 years and younger. Am J Surg 1990; 159:589-592.
14. Linz DL, Hraborsky EE, Franceschi D et al. Does the current health care environment contribute to increased morbidity and mortality of acute appendicitis in children? J Pediatr Surg 1993; 28:321-328.
15. Shandling B, Ein SH, Simpson JS et al. Perforating appendicitis and antibiotics. J Pediatr Surg 1974; 9:79-83.
16. David IB, Buck JR, Filler RM. Rational use of antibiotics for perforated appendicitis in childhood. J Pediatr Surg 1982; 17:494-500.
17. Brook I. Bacterial studies of peritoneal cavity and postoperative surgical wound drainage following perforated appendix in children. Ann Surg 1980; 192:208-212.
18. King DR, Browne AF, Birken GA et al. Antibiotic management of complicated appendicitis. J Pediatr Surg 1983; 18:945-949.

19. Smith JA, Skidmore AG, Forward AD et al. Prospective, randomized, double-blind comparison of metronidazole and tobramycin with clindamycin and tobramycin in the treatment of intra-abdominal sepsis. Ann Surg 1980; 192:213-220.

20. Raffensperger JG. Appendicitis. In: Raffensperger JG, ed. Swenson's Pediatric Surgery. 4th ed. New York: Appleton-Centery Crofts, 1980:815.

21. Moore TC. Management of necrotizing enterocolitis by "patch, drain and wait". Pediatr Surg Int 1989; 4:110-113.

22. Moore TC. Management of midgut volvulus with extensive necrosis by "patch, drain and wait" in early infancy and childhood. Pediatr Surg Int 1991; 6:313-317.

23. Putnam TC, Gagliano N, Emmens RW. Appendicitis in children. Surg Gynec Obstet 1990; 170:527-532.

24. Curran TJ, Muenchow SK. The treatment of complicated appendicitis in children using peritoneal drainage: Results from a public hospital. J Pediatr Surg 1993; 28:204-208.

25. Harris BH. Technetium scanning in suspected appendicitis. Pediatr Trauma & Acute Care 1990; 3:29-30.

CHAPTER 18

INGUINAL HERNIA

INTRODUCTION

Inguinal hernia in infancy and childhood is the most important and frequent congenital disorder providing a steady stream of challenging and technically demanding elective operative experience in the early years of life. There is no area in surgery of a frequent nature which requires such excellence and precision of fine operative technique throughout. It is fortunate such a high level of required operative skill is combined with the fascinating stimulus that no two cases of inguinal hernia in this age group are exactly alike. A high level of alertness results and boredom is never a problem. At my pediatric surgery service at the Harbor-UCLA Medical Center only very senior surgical residents (fourth year) rotate on pediatric surgery (just prior to their chief resident year) and only do inguinal hernia repairs with a faculty pediatric surgeon scrubbed and first assisting throughout the entire case.

It is strongly emphasized to residents and medical students that inguinal hernias in infancy and childhood are totally different disorders from inguinal hernia in adults in almost every area of importance, excluding only the anatomical site of occurrence and the common name of "inguinal hernia". Inguinal hernias in infancy and childhood are congenital rather than acquired as in adults, they involve only a sac and not a musculo-fascial defect (with incidental sac) as in adults, operative repair involves high ligation of a sac only with no musculo-fascial repair being required, recurrence should *never* occur (a recurrence must be accounted a technical error) whereas in adults recurrences are frequent regardless which of the many, many operations are employed as the preoperative causes (heavy lifting job, emphysema chronic coughing and straining for urine or stool) are still present postoperatively. In infancy and childhood operative repair is considerably more demanding in technical skill and fine, careful dissection and precise, gentle tissue handling. In addition, incarceration in adult years almost always requires emergency operative relief while in infancy and childhood it almost always may be relieved nonoperatively (sedation, ice packs, reverse Trendelenberg position and gentle pressure manipulation), and should be.

The diagnosis of an inguinal hernia by physical exam (thickened cord in the male and squishy mass possibly containing ovary in the female) is highly reliable and meddlesome and hazardous additional "tests" such as herniograms are not required. Outpatient repair is both economical and clinically justified and is one of the major advances in hernia repair in infancy and childhood in the past 40 years.

In 1990, Professor Prem Puri and Shun[1] of Dublin (Ireland) recorded an important and informative 15 year experience with inguinal hernia in the first 30 days of life in 70 patients. There was an overwhelming incidence of males (69 to 1) and in 87% of the cases the hernia was incarcerated. Reduction of the hernia without operation was achieved in 95% of those with incarceration followed by elective repair. The hernia was on the right side in 83% of the cases, on the left in 13 and bilateral in 4%. The age of the patients at presentation was within the first 10 days of life in 10% and 90% in the second 20 days of life with the highest incidence in the last five day period of 26 to 30 days (25 cases, 36%).

An interesting report by Gauderer and associates[2] of Cleveland appeared in the October 1992 issue of the *Journal of Pediatric Surgery* and concerned inguinal hernias in very low birth weight infants (<1,500 g). Although they conceded that the incidence of inguinal hernia was well known to be increased in prematurity, they made the important point that too little was known of its occurrence and related problems in the very low birth weight infant. In a 10 year period (1977 to 1987), 1,933 children with birth weights under 1,500 g were admitted to the neonatal intensive care unit of the Rainbow Babies and Children's Hospital of Cleveland (Ohio). Of these, 1,391 (72%) survived for at least 28 days and were followed until 20 months of corrected age. Inguinal hernia was found to have occurred in 16% of those surviving 28 days or more. Inguinal hernia occurred in 26% of the boys and in only 7% of the girls. The hernia incidence was right side in 19.8%, left side in 14.9% and bilateral in 61.7%. Of the 222 very low birth weight infants with inguinal hernia, 192 (86.5%) were operated upon at a mean postnatal age of 28 weeks (5 to 110 weeks).

Thirty-five (15.8%) were operated upon prior to neonatal discharge. One or more incarceration had occurred in 35 very low birth weight infants who were operated upon at their hospital. Only one infant had to be operated upon because of irreducibility of an incarcerated hernia (2.9%). There was no mortality and minimum morbidity.

The emergency room management of incarcerated inguinal hernias in infancy was addressed by Baguley et al[3] of Hamilton, Ontario, Canada in 1992 in *Pediatric Surgery International*. The authors describe the outcome of 94 infants less than one year of age who had an incarcerated inguinal hernia reduced in the emergency room. Fifty-six of the 94 infants were admitted to the hospital (60%) and 38 were sent home. Of the 56 infants who were admitted to the hospital, 12 (21%) reincarcerated prior to surgery. Of the 38 sent home, 28 (74%) reincarcerated. The mean time to operation in the admitted-to-the-hospital group was two days while it was 10 days in the sent-home group. The authors concluded: "Although it is safe to send infants home after emergency room reduction of an incarcerated inguinal hernia, definitive repair should be done within 72 hours to avoid an increased risk of incarceration." From their data, one might also conclude that it is safer and more prudent to have these sent-home infants admitted to the hospital and under professional nursing and pediatric surgical care and monitoring in the 72 hours intervening between emergency room reduction and elective/urgent operation. At my pediatric surgery service at the Harbor-UCLA Medical Center all incarcerated inguinal hernias in infancy and childhood are admitted promptly from the emergency room to the hospital where reduction is carried out and delayed repair undertaken at 48 to 72 hours post-reduction. In the past 11$\frac{1}{2}$ years, only one incarcerated inguinal hernia in infancy and childhood had to be repaired by operation because of nonreducibility. In a 1990 report in the *British Journal of Surgery* by Davies et al,[4] 35 of 85 children/infants under two years of age with incarcerated inguinal hernias (41%) had had a diagnosis of an inguinal hernia made prior to the occurrence of the incarceration. The authors concluded that prompt referral for surgery should be made once a diagnosis of inguinal hernia in the first two months of life had been made. At my Harbor-UCLA pediatric surgery service, all are placed on the "urgent" out-patient operation schedule. Nonetheless, an occasional infant has incarcerated the hernia before his elective/urgent out-patient scheduled operation time comes up.

The currently mildly "burning" issues of contralateral operation for unilateral hernias and routine hospital admission following outpatient hernia repair of one-time premature infants will be addressed in the Challenges section of this chapter.

CHALLENGES

1. Whether or not to do a bilateral inguinal hernia operation when only a unilateral inguinal hernia had been identified clinically?

The proposal and concept of routine exploration of the opposite groin in the infant or child with a unilateral inguinal hernia has generally been attributed to a 1955 report in *Surgery* by Rothenberg and Barnett.[5] Although this approach has received strong support over the years both in publication[6,7] and in practice, strong opposition had continued on the grounds that this additional operation is both unnecessary and hazardous. Some might even suspect that the indications for this approach are as much economical as clinical (you get paid more).

A 1980 report in the *Journal of Pediatric Surgery* by Chester McVay and associates[8] of Yankton, South Dakota recommended against this approach on the grounds that a number of unnecessary procedures would be performed and that the risk of bilateral testicular trauma is too great.

In addition to the testis, there also are the vas deferens and the blood supply to the testis to consider. In 1981 and 1982,

Shandling and Janik[9,10] of Toronto provided important experimental research laboratory evidence to indicate that even comparatively mild operative trauma to the vas deferens could cause serious immediate and long-term functional and anatomical damage and that mosquito clamp clamping was comparable to actual traumatic cutting or pulling division of the vas. In a 1989 report from Ottawa (Canada), Given and Rubin[11] report an experience with 904 unilateral inguinal hernia repairs at the Children's Hospital of Eastern Ontario during a recent three year period (January 1985 to December 1987). The unilateral repairs involved 758 boys and 89 girls. They found the subsequent occurrence of a contralateral hernia to be 5.6% (5.7% for boys and 4.7% for girls). The relative risk in boys for a right hernia following left hernia repair was 8.5% and that for a left hernia following a right hernia repair was 4.3%. They concluded that "Because of the low incidence of contralateral hernia and its complications and the possible negative effects on fertility, we suggest that contralateral exploration should not be routine." They concluded the abstract of their paper by stating: "Neither sex nor laterality should be considered as an indicator for contralateral exploration in children with a clinical diagnosis of unilateral hernia."

I have never done a contralateral exploration when the clinical diagnosis is of a unilateral inguinal hernia only in infancy or childhood, and furthermore *never intend to do so*!

2. The issue of whether or not to admit to the hospital overnight for bradycardia and apnea monitoring after outpatient repair of inguinal hernia of infants who were prematurely born and are at risk in these areas is an important and a significant challenge in the area of judgment.

A substantial opinion in favor of hospital admission for observation for up to 24 hours has developed over the past 10 years.[12-16] In a recent report before the American Pediatric Surgical Association and published in the February 1992 issue of the *Journal of Pediatric Surgery*, Schwartz, Tyson and associates[17] of Sacramento, California (UC Davis School of Medicine) reopened this issue by suggesting that sending these infants home after operation without hospital admission might be safe and supported this with the data from their university hospital. An important component of their experience was that none of their patients received pre- or intra-operative narcotics and only 14% of their patients were given muscle relaxants. This report was not received with great enthusiasm (perhaps the avoidance of narcotics and muscle relaxants was overlooked by the multiple discussants). Professor Donna Caniano[18] of the Children's Hospital of Columbus, Ohio (Ohio State University) discussed this paper and commented upon an experience with 62 premature infants operated upon for inguinal hernia at her institution. She described two problems which occurred. In the recovery room there was a 28% incidence of significant apnea and bradycardia which required vigorous stimulation for control. In addition, 20% of the preterm infants experience a significant apneic event up to 4 to 10 hours following operation. I feel that there is no point in pushing one's "luck" (or the baby's) and that prudence and unnecessary risk avoidance should be the order of the day. Inappropriate economy and "cost containment" in this important area is not worth a single baby's life!

CONCLUSION

Inguinal hernias in infancy and childhood long have sustained the operative skills and financial security of pediatric surgeons who would otherwise have both starved and rusted technically as competent and well-honed pediatric surgeons. Inguinal hernias in this age group also provide a most satisfying and technically challenging and interesting operative challenge which never dulls the attention nor diminishes the excitement of the technical challenge for the best, most competent and most experienced of pediatric surgeons.

REFERENCES

1. Shun A, Puri P. Inguinal hernia in the newborn: A 15-year review. Pediatr Surg Int 1990; 3:156-157.
2. Rajput A, Gauderer MWL, Hack M. Inguinal hernias in very low birth weight infants: Incidence and timing of repair. J Pediatr Surg 1992; 27:1322-1324.
3. Baguley PE, Fizgerald PG, Srinathan SK et al. Emergency room reduction of incarcerated inguinal hernia in infants: Is routine hospital admission necessary? Pediatr Surg Int 1992; 7:366-367.
4. Davies N, Najmaldin A, Burge DM. Irreducible inguinal hernia in children under two years of age. Br J Surg 1990; 77: 1291-1292.
5. Rothenberg RE, Barnett T. Bilateral herniotomy in infants and children. Surgery 1955; 37:947-950.
6. Clausen EG, Jake RJ, Binkley FM. Contralateral inguinal exploration of unilateral hernia in infants and children. Surgery 1958; 44:735-740.
7. Rowe MI, Clatworthy HW. The other side of the pediatric inguinal hernia. Surg Clin North Am 1971; 51:1371-1376.
8. McGregor DB, Halverson K, McVay CB. The unilateral pediatric inguinal hernia: Should a contralateral side be explored? J Pediatr Surg 1980; 15:313-317.
9. Shandling B, Janik JS. The vulnerability of the vas deferens. J Pediatr Surg 1981; 16:461-464.
10. Janik JS, Shandling B. The vulnerability of the vas deferens (II): The case against routine bilateral inguinal exploration. J Pediatr Surg 1982; 17:585-588.
11. Given JP, Rubin SZ. Occurrence of contralateral inguinal hernia following unilateral repair in a pediatric hospital. J Pediatr Surg 1989; 24:963-965.
12. Steward DJ. Preterm infants are more prone to complications following minor surgery than are term infants. Anesthesiology 1982; 56:304-306.
13. Liu LMP, Cote CJ, Goudsouzian NG et al. Life threatening apnea in infants recovering from anesthesia. Anesthesiology 1983; 59:506-510.

14. Rescorla FJ, Grosfeld JL. Inguinal hernia repair in the perinatal period and early infancy: Clinical considerations. J Pediatr Surg 1984; 19:832-837.

15. Kurth CD, Spitzer, Broennle AM et al. Postoperative apnea in preterm infants. Anesthesiology 1987; 66:483-488.

16. Mayhew JF, Bourke DL, Guinee WS. Evaluation of the premature infant at risk for postoperative complications. Can J Anesth 1987; 34:627-631.

17. Melone JH, Schwartz MZ, Tyson KRT et al. Outpatient inguinal hernioraphy in premature infants: Is it safe? J Pediatr Surg 1992; 27:203-208.

18. Caniano DA. Discussion of paper by Melone JH et al. J Pediatr Surg 1992; 27:207.

Appendix A

Publications by the author relating to clinical and experimental pediatric surgery

1. Gross RE, Moore TC. Duplication of the urethra. Arch Surg 1950; 60:749-761.
2. Shumacker HB Jr., Moore TC. Surgical management of traumatic chylothorax. Surg Gynec Obstet 1951; 93:46-50.
3. Moore TC. The management of intussusception in infants and children. Ann Surg 1952; 135: 184-192.
4. Moore TC, Shumacker HB Jr. Intussusception of ileum through persistent omphalomesenteric duct. Surgery 1952; 31:278-284.
5. Moore TC. Congenital cysts of the mesentery. Quart Bull Ind Univ Med Center 1952; 14:29-33.
6. Moore TC, Lawrence EA. Congenital malformations of the rectum and anus; I. Clinical features and surgical management in 120 cases. Surgery 1952; 32:352-366.
7. Moore TC, Lawrence EA. Congenital malformations of the rectum and anus; II. Associated anomalies encountered in a series of 120 cases. Surg Gynec Obstet 1952; 95:281-288.
8. Moore TC. Congenital obstruction of the gastrointestinal tract in infants and children. Bull Hoosier State M.A. 1952; 3:31-35.
9. Moore TC, Battersby JS. Congenital duplications of the small intestine; Report of 11 cases. Surg Gynec Obstet 1952; 95:557-567.
10. Moore TC, Stokes GE. Gastroschisis: Report of two cases treated by a modification of the Gross operation for omphalocele. Surgery 1953; 33:112-120.
11. Moore TC. Annular pancreas. Surgery 1953; 33:138-148.
12. Moore TC. Congenital atresia of the extrahepatic bile ducts: Report of 31 proved cases. Surg Gynec Obstet 1953; 96:215-225.
13. Moore TC, Shumacker HB Jr. Unsuitability of transventricular autogenous slings for diminishing valvular insufficiency. Surgery 1953; 33:173-182.
14. Moore TC, Shumacker HB Jr. Congenital and experimentally produced pericardial defects. Angiology 1953; 4:1-11.
15. Shumacker HB Jr., Moore TC. Surgical closure of atrial septal defects: A preliminary report. Quart Bull Ind Univ Med Center 1953; 15:3-6.
16. Moore TC, Shumacker HB Jr. Experimental creation of atrial septal defects, with some notes on the production of a right to left atrial shunt. Angiology 1953; 41:244-252.
17. Moore TC. Common duct exploration and drainage for obstructive neonatal jaundice. Ann Surg 1953; 138:111-114.
18. Shumacker HB Jr., Moore TC, King H. The experimental closure of atrial septal defects. J Thoracic Surg 1953; 26:551-570.
19. Moore TC, Stokes GE. Congenital stenosis and atresia of the small intestine. Surg Gynec Obstet 1953; 97:719-730.
20. Moore TC. Early operation for congenital atresia of the bile ducts: An editorial. American Surgeon 1953; 19:1012-1013.
21. Moore TC, Hurley AG. Congenital duplication of the gall bladder. Surgery 1954; 35:283-289.
22. Moore TC, Harris EJ. Congenital malformations which may produced gastrointestinal tract obstruction in infancy and childhood. J Indiana State M.A. 1954; 47: 1390-1398.
23. Moore TC, Siderys H. The use of pliable plastics in the repair of abdominal wall defects. Ann Surg 1955; 142:973-979.
24. Moore TC, Shumacker HB Jr. Adrenalin producing tumors in childhood. Ann Surg 1956; 143:256-265.
25. Moore TC, Silver RA. Kartagener's syndrome: Report of a case treated by middle lobectomy. American Surgeon 1956; 22:595-597.
26. Moore TC. Congenital intrinsic duodenal obstruction: Report of 32 cases. Ann Surg 1956; 144:159-164.
27. Moore TC. Omphalomesenteric duct anomalies. Surg Gynec Obstet 1956; 103:569-580.
28. Moore TC. Annular pancreas, common duct compression and cholelithiasis. A.M.A. Arch Surg 1956; 73:1050-1054.
29. Moore TC. Transmesenteric hernia in infancy; with a note on operative intestinal decompression in infancy. Surgery 1957; 41:438-443.
30. Moore TC. Congenital cysts of the mesentery: Report of four cases. Ann Surg 1957; 145:428-436.
31. Moore TC, Martinez H, Enerson DH. In-

trathoracic mixed neuroblastoma and ganglioneuroma in childhood. J Indiana State M.A. 1957; 50:564-567.

32. Moore TC, Battersby JS, Roggenkamp MW, Campbell JA. Congenital posterolateral diaphragmatic hernia in the newborn. Surg Gynec Obstet 1957; 104:675-689.

33. Moore TC. Lobectomy for post-pneumonic lung abscess in infancy and childhood. Surgery 1958; 44:741-757.

34. Moore TC, Bounous G. Experimental use of nylon mesh for esophageal support. J Thoracic Surg 1959; 37:224-230.

35. Moore TC, Goldstein J. Use of intact omentum for closure of full-thickness esophageal defects. Surgery 1959; 45:899.

36. Battersby JS, Moore TC. Esophageal replacement and by-pass with the ascending and right half of the transverse colon for the treatment of congenital atresia of the esophagus. Surg Gynec Obstet 1959; 109:207-215.

37. Moore TC. Esophageal obstruction due to anomalous right subclavian artery. J Indiana State M.A. 1959 52:1117-1120.

38. Moore TC, Bounous G. Experimental use of nylon mesh supported pericardial grafts for closure of full-thickness esophageal defects. J Thoracic Surg 1959; 38:108-114.

39. Moore TC, Battersby JS. Pulmonary abscess in infancy and childhood: Report of 18 cases. Ann Surg 1960; 151:496-500.

40. Moore TC, Goldstein J, Bounous G. Experimental closure of large full-thickness esophageal defects. Bull Soc Int de Chir 1961; 20:15-22.

41. Moore TC, Goldstein J, Teramoto S. Use of intact lung for closure of full-thickness esophageal defects. J Thoracic Cardiovasc Surg 1961; 41:336-341.

42. Moore TC, Heimberger I, Teramoto S. Experimental use of synthetic mesh for support of esophageal anastomoses. J Thoracic Cardiovasc Surg 1961; 42:219-224.

43. Armbruster EJ, Moore TC. Experimental use of crimped women teflon for esophageal replacement. Quart Bull Ind Univ Med Center 1962; 24:8-11.

44. Speck CR, Moore TC, Stout FE. Antenatal roentgen diagnosis of meconium peritonitis. Am J Roentgenol 1962; 88:566-570.

45. Moore TC. Intestinal obstruction in the newborn. J Indiana State M.A. 1962; 55:607-613.

46. Siderys H, Moore TC, Shumacker HB Jr. Left hepatic lobectomy for hemangioma of the liver in the newborn. Surgery 1962: 502-504.

47. Moore TC. Giant cystic meconium peritonitis. Ann Surg 1963; 15:566-572.

48. Moore TC. Chondroedtederma dysplasis (Ellis-van Creveld) with bronchial malformation and neonatal tension lobar emphysema. J Thoracic Cardiovasc Surg 1963; 46:1-10.

49. Moore TC. Gastroschisis with antenatal evisceration of intestines and urinary bladder. Ann Surg 1963; 158:263-269.

50. Hathaway WE, Moore TC. Hypoglycemia and perforated peptic ulcers in infancy. Clin Pediat 1963; 2:425-427.

51. Moore TC. Gastroschisis, Chapter 22 in Hernia, ed. by Nyhus LN, Harkins HN. J.B. Lippincott Co: Philadelphia, 1964: 334-337.

52. Moore TC. Gastrectomy in infancy and childhood; I. Report of two cases of gastrectomy in early infancy. Ann Surg 1964; 160:245-250.

53. Moore TC. Gastrectomy in infancy and childhood; II. Results of an international survey. Ann Surg 1965; 162:91-99.

54. Judd DR, Wince LL, Moore TC. Gastroschisis: Report of two cases with survival. Surgery 1965; 58:1033-1036.

55. Thompson DP, Moore TC. Acute thoracic distress in childhood due to spontaneous rupture of a large mediastinal teratoma. J Pediatr Surg 1969; 4:416-423.

56. Moore TC, Salzberg AM, Talman EA. Jejuno-ileo-colic intubation and plication for intestinal obstruction with massive adhesions in infancy. Surgery 1970; 67:364-368.

57. Patton JJ, Moore TC. Massive megacolon and mega-ileum in childhood due to tuberculosis of the ascending colon. Surgery 1970; 67:513-518.

58. White PH, Hirose FH, Moore TC. Rhabdomyosarcoma of the superior portion of the urinary bladder in childhood. J Pediatr Surg 1971; 6:178.

59. Orlando JC, Moore TC. Splenectomy for trauma in childhood: Report of 36 cases.

Surg Gynec Obstet 1972; 134:94-96.

60. Hollister DW, Rimoin DL, Reed W, Lachman RS, Moore TC, Weil M. Disappearing fingers and toes-Hereditary acroosteolysis with peripheral neuropathy and vasospasm. Clin Res 1972; 20:261-264.

61. Moore TC, Sinclair MC. Is conservative care of minor splenic injury feasible? Forum. Modern Medicine. Feb. 19, 1973;99.

62. Weber GA, Finklestein JZ, Lemmi CAE, Moore TC. Effect of repeated SRBC immunization on mouse splenic histidine decarboxylase response to Gross leukemia virus tumor transplantation. IRCS Medical Science, (73-6) 42-2-10, June 1973.

63. Ban JL, Hirose FH, Lachman RS, Moore TC. Pendunuculated cystic lymphagioma of the splenocolic ligament in childhood. Am J Surg 1972; 24:410-412.

64. Castagna JT, Moore TC. Use of the appendix as a colon substitute in vesico-intestinal extrophy. J Pediatr Surg 1973; 8:331.

65. Ban JL, Moore TC. Intrathoracic tension incarceration of stomach and of liver through right-sided congenital posterolateral diaphragmatic hernia. J Thoracic Cardiovasc Surg 1973; 66:969-971.

66. Moore TC. Internal hernia with high jejunal obstruction in infancy due to adhesions from antenatal meconium peritonitis. J Pediatr Surg 1973; 6:971-972.

67. Asch MJ, Lachman R, Lippmann M, Moore TC. Truck aerial impalement injury of the thorax: Report of a case in an 8 year-old boy. J Pediatr Surg 1974; 9:251-252.

68. Sinclair MC, Moore TC. Major surgery for abdominal and thoracic trauma in childhood and adolescence. J Pediatr Surg 1974; 9:155-162.

69. Johnson D, Moore TC. Large intra-thoracic superior sucus cystic mass arising from brachial plexus in childhood. J Pediatr Surg 1974; 9:403-404.

70. Moore TC, Fine RN, Asch MJ, Berne TV, English TS. Early post transplant function in childhood of 33 machine preserved human cadaveric kidneys. Pediatrics 1974; 54:773-778.

71. Sinclair MC, Moore TC, Asch MJ, Brosman SA. Injury of hollow abdominal viscera from blunt trauma in childhood and adolescence.

Am J Surg 1974; 128:693-698.

72. Asch MJ, Cohen AH, Moore TC. Hepatic and splenic lymphangiomatosis with skeletal involvement: Report of a case and review of the literature. Surgery 1974;76: 334-339.

73. Asch MJ, Liebman W, Lachman RS, Moore TC. Esophageal achalasia: Diagnosis and cardiomyotomy in a newborn infant. J Pediatr Surg 1974; 9:911-912.

74. Sinclair MC, Moore TC, Asch MJ. Penetrating abdominal injuries in childhood and adolescence. Am Surg 1975; 41:342-346.

75. Asch MJ, Sperling M, Fisher R, Leake R, Moore TC, Oh W. Metabolic and hormonal studies comparing three parenteral nutrition regimens in infants. Ann Surg 1975; 182:62-65.

76. Kwong M, Moore TC, Lemmi CAE, Oh W, Thibeault DW. Histidine decarboxylase in fetal intrauterine growth-retarded rats. Pediatric Research 1975; 9:278.

77. Moore TC. Massive bile peritonitis in infancy due to spontaneous bile duct perforation with portal vein occlusion. J Pediatr Surg 1975; 10:537-538.

78. Shabot MM, Asch MJ, State D, Moore TC. Benign obstructing papilloma of the ampula of Vater in infancy. Surgery 1975; 78: 560-563.

79. Moore TC, Finklestein JZ, Lachman R, Hirose F. Spntaneous perforation and closure of the small intestine in association with childhood leukemia. J Pediatr Surg 1975; 10:955-957.

80. Kwong MS, Moore TC, Lemmi CAE, Oh W, Thibeault DS. Histidine decarboxylase activity in fetal intrauterine growth-retarded rats. Pediatric Research 1976; 10:737.

81. Moore TC, Leake RD. Infra-umbilical entry into the peritoneal cavity through a small incision for the identification and cannulation of an umbilical artery. J Pediatr Surg 1977; 12:247-249.

82. Moore TC. Gastroschisis and omphalocele: Clinical differences. Surgery 1977; 82: 561-568.

83. Moore TC. Atresia of the colon at the splenic flexure with absence of the distal colon and ischemic destruction of the proximal colon. J Pediatr Surg 1978; 8:89-90.

84. Kobayashi RH, Moore TC. Ovarian teratomas in childhood. J Pediatr Surg 1978; 8:419-422.

85. Moore TC, Peter M. Thru-and-thru gunshot penetration of distal abdominal aorta in a 4 year-old child managed by aortic transection, debridement and reanastomosis with survival. J Trauma 1979; 19:537-539.

86. Moore TC, Landers DB, Lachman RS. Hirschsprung's disease discordant in monozygotic twins: A study of possible environmental factors in the production of colonic aganglionosis. J Pediatr Surg 1979; 14:158-161.

87. Shabot MM, Asch MJ, Moore TC. Cecal perforation due to blunt abdominal trauma in childhood. Zeitschr f Kinderchirurgie 1979; 28:272-277.

88. Moore TC, Lachman RS. Obstructing non-granulomatous transmural colitis in early infancy. Zeitschr f Kinderchirurgie 1980; 29:78-80.

89. Moore TC, Lachman RS. Distal mechanical small bowel obstruction as a sequelae of blunt trauma pancreatitis in childhood. Zeitschr f Kinderchirurgie 1981; 34: 296-298.

90. Moore TC, Cobo JC. Massive symptomatic cystic hygroma confined to the thorax in early childhood. J Thoracic Cardiovasc Surg 1985; 89:459-462.

91. Moore TC, Hyman PE. Extrahepatic biliary atresia in one human leukocyte identical twin. Pediatrics 1985; 76:604-606.

92. Moore TC, Nur K. An international survey of gastroschisis and omphalocele (490 cases): I. Nature and distribution of additional malformations. Pediatr Surg Int 1986; 1:46-50.

93. Moore TC, Nur K. An international survey of gastroschisis and omphalocele (490 cases) II. Relative incidence, frequency and environmental factors. Pediatr Surg Int 1986; 1:105-109.

94. Moore TC, Cameron RB. Spontaneous perforation of the extrahepatic biliary tract in infancy and childhood: Review of 77 operatively managed cases. Pediatr Surg Int 1986; 1:206-209.

95. Moore TC. Jejunal atresia with midgut deletion J Pediatr Surg 1986; 21:951-952.

96. Moore TC. Pathogenesis of biliary atresia. Pediatrics 1986: 78:182-183.

97. Moore TC, Nur K. An international survey of gastroschisis and omphalocele (490 cases): III. Factors influencing outcome of surgical management. Pediatr Surg Int 1987; 2:27-32.

98. Moore TC. Non-operative management of blunt abdominal trauma in childhood. Surgery 1987; 101:380-381.

99. Gamal R, Moore TC. Massive acquired omental cyst as a complication of ventriculo peritoneal shunting. J Pediatr Surg 1988; 23:1041-1042.

100. Moore TC. Elective pre-term seciton for improved primary repair of gastroschisis. Pediatr Surg Int 1988; 4:25-27.

101. Moore TC. Management of necrotizing enterocolitis by "patch, drain and wait". Pediatr Surg Int 1989; 4:110-113.

102. Dubrow TJ, Gorrin NR, Wacklym FA, Abdul-Rasool IH, Moore TC. Malignant hyperthermia: Experience in the prospective management of eight children. J Pediatr Surg 1989; 24:163-166.

103. Moore TC, Gamal R. Early and late (15-17 year) transplant functions of 33 machine preserved cadaveric kidneys from pediatric age donors 13 and under. Transplantation 1989; 47:720-722.

104. Lami JL, Moore TC. Colectomy for necrotizing amoebic colitis in early childhood with survival. J Pediatr Surg 1989; 24:1174-1176.

105. Moore TC. Advantages of performing the saggital anoplasty operation for imperforate anus at birth. J Pediatr Surg 1990; 25:276-277.

106. Gorrin NR, Moore TC, Asch MJ. Glass shrapnel injuries to children resulting from "dry ice bomb" explosions: Report of three cases. J Pediatr Surg 1990; 25:296.

107. Baumgartner F, Moore TC. Angiographic embolization of post-traumatic hematobilia in a six-year old boy. Digestive Diseases & Sciences 1990; 35:261-263.

108. Gamal R, Moore TC. Appendicitis in children 13 years and under: Report of 230 cases. Am J Surg 1990; 159:589-592.

109. Baumgartner F, Moore TC, Mitchner J. Recurrent ventriculoperitoneal shunt

pseudocyst in a nine-year old girl. Klin Wchnschr 1990; 68:485-487.

110. Moore TC. Management of midgut volvulus with extensive necrosis by "patch, drain and wait" in early infancy and childhood: Report of three cases. Pediatr Surg Int 1991; 6:313-317.

111. Baumgartner F, Moore TC. Atretic, obstructive duodenal mass associated with annular pancreas and malrotation in a newborn male. Eur J Pediatr Surg 1992; 2:42-44.

112. Suede M, Moore TC. Mid-gut non-rotation with a large dumb-bell shaped, abscessed and air-containing right paraduodenal hernia in early childhood. Pediatr Surg Int 1992; 7:149-151.

113. Moore TC. Role of labor in gastroschisis bowel thickening and its prevention by elective pre-term and pre-labor cesarian section. Pediatr Surg Int 1992; 7:256-259.

114. Lai E, Cunningham TJ, Moore TC. In utero intussusception producing meconium peritonitis with and without free air: Report of 2 cases and a review of the literature. Pediatr Surg Int (Submitted for publication). (Accepted pending revision).

AUTHOR INDEX

SUBJECT INDEX